Children and Exercise XXIV

W0230114

Children and Exercise XXIV presents the latest scientific research into paediatric exercise physiology, endocrinology, kinanthropometry, growth and maturation, and youth sport. Including contributions from a wide range of leading international experts, the book is arranged into six thematic sections addressing:

- children's health and well-being
- physical activity patterns
- exercise endocrinology
- élite young athletes
- aerobic and anaerobic fitness
- muscle physiology.

Offering critical reviews of current topics and reports of current and ongoing research in paediatric health and exercise science, this is a key text for all researchers, teachers, health professionals and students with an interest in paediatric sport and exercise science, sports medicine and physical education.

Toivo Jürimäe is Professor and Chair of Sport Pedagogy at the Institute of Sport Pedagogy, University of Tartu, Estonia.

Neil Armstrong is Professor of Paediatric Exercise Physiology and Director of the Children's Health and Exercise Research Centre at the University of Exeter. He is also Deputy Vice-Chancellor of the University of Exeter.

Jaak Jürimäe is Associate Professor in the Faculty of Exercise and Sport Sciences at the University of Tartu, Estonia.

The papers contained within this volume were first presented at the 24th Pediatric Work Physiology meeting, held in Tallinn, Estonia, in September 2007.

Children and Exercise XXIV

The proceedings of the 24th Pediatric Work Physiology Meeting

Edited by Toivo Jürimäe, Neil Armstrong and Jaak Jürimäe

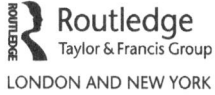

Routledge
Taylor & Francis Group

LONDON AND NEW YORK

First published 2009
by Routledge
2 Park Square, Milton Park, Abingdon, Oxon, OX14 4RN

Simultaneously published in the USA and Canada
by Routledge
711 Third Avenue, New York, NY 10017

*Routledge is an imprint of the Taylor & Francis Group,
an informa business*

First issued in paperback 2011

© 2009 Toivo Jürimäe, Neil Armstrong and Jaak Jürimäe editorial matter
and selection; individual chapters the contributors

Typeset in Goudy by Keyword Group Ltd

All rights reserved. No part of this book may be reprinted or reproduced or
utilised in any form or by any electronic, mechanical, or other means, now
known or hereafter invented, including photocopying and recording, or in
any information storage or retrieval system, without permission in writing
from the publishers.

British Library Cataloguing in Publication Data
A catalogue record for this book is available
from the British Library

Library of Congress Cataloging-in-Publication Data
Children and exercise XXIV: the proceedings of the 24th Pediatric
   Work Physiology Meeting / edited by Toivo Jürimäe, Neil Armstrong
   and Jaak Jürimäe.
     p. cm.
   Includes bibliographical references
   1. Exercise for children–Congresses. I. Jürimäe, T. II. Armstrong, Neil.
     III. Jürimäe, Jaak. IV. Title. V. Title: Children and exercise 24.
     VI. Title: Children and exercise twenty-four.
   [DNLM: 1. Exercise–physiology–Congresses. 2. Child. 3. Health
     Behavior–Congresses. 4. Physical Fitness–physiology–
     Congresses. QT 255 P3728c 2008]
   RJ133.P422 2008
   613.7'1083–dc22   2008012546

ISBN 10: 0-415-45147-7 (hbk)
ISBN 10: 0-415-66692-9 (pbk)
ISBN 10: 0-203-89085-X (ebk)

ISBN 13: 978-0-415-45147-5 (hbk)
ISBN 13: 978-0-415-66692-3 (pbk)
ISBN 13: 978-0-203-89085-1 (ebk)

Contents

Preface

Children and Exercise XXIV contains the Proceedings of the XXIVth International Symposium of the European Group of Pediatric Work Physiology (PWP) held in Tallinn, Estonia from 5–9 September 2007. The Symposium was hosted by the Centre of Behavioural and Health Sciences, University of Tartu and chaired by Professor Toivo Jürimäe.

The European Group of Pediatric Work Physiology has organised the following international symposia:

Symposium	Date	Place	Chair
I	1968	Dortmund, Germany	J. Rutenfranz
II	1969	Liblice, Czechoslovakia	V.S. Seliger
III	1970	Stockholm, Sweden	C. Thoren
IV	1972	Netanya, Israel	O. Bar-Or
V	1973	De Haan, Belgium	M. Hebblinck
VI	1974	Sec, Czechoslovakia	M. Macek
VII	1975	Trois Rivieres, Canada	R.J. Shephard
VIII	1976	Bisham Abbey, UK	C.T.M. Davies
IX	1978	Marstand, Sweden	B.O. Eriksson
X	1981	Jousta, Finland	J. Ilmarinen
XI	1983	Papendahl, Netherlands	R.A. Binkhorst
XII	1985	Hardenhausen, Germany	J. Rutenfranz
XIII	1987	Hurdal, Norway	S. Oseid
XIV	1989	Leuven, Belgium	G. Beunen
XV	1989	Seregelyes, Hungary	R. Frenkl
XVI	1991	St Sauves, France	J. Coudert/E. Van Praagh
XVII	1993	Hamilton, Canada	O. Bar-Or
XVIII	1995	Odense, Denmark	K. Froberg
XIX	1997	Exeter, UK	N. Armstrong
XX	1999	Rome, Italy	A. Calzolari
XXI	2001	Corsedonk, Belgium	D. Matthys
XXII	2003	Porto, Portugal	J. Maia
XXIII	2005	Gwatt, Switzerland	S. Kriemler/N. Farpour Lambert
XXIV	2007	Tallinn, Estonia	T. Jürimäe

The XXIV Symposium attracted delegates from 29 countries and followed PWP tradition with an emphasis on discussion of issues relating to children and exercise. This volume reflects the formal programme and contains a tribute to Professor Oded Bar-Or who inspired a generation of paediatric exercise physiologists, six of the keynote presentations and 49 of the free communications. The book offers invited expert reviews of key topics and reports current and on-going research in paediatric exercise science. If it stimulates further interest in the exciting study of the exercising child it will have served its purpose.

Acknowledgements

The editors would like to thank the following reviewers:

Adam Baxter-Jones (Canada)

Mark Tremblay (Canada)

Karsten Froberg (Denmark)

Han Kemper (The Netherlands)

Gaston Beunen (Belgium)

Jorge Mota (Portugal)

Albrecht Claessens (Belgium)

Willem van Mechelen (The Netherlands)

Part I
Keynote lectures

1 The 2007 Jozef Rutenfranz lecture

A behavioural and ecological perspective to energy-balance-related behaviours in children

W. van Mechelen

VU University Medical Center, Department of Public & Occupational Health, Body@Work–Research Center Physical Activity, Work and Health, TNO-VUmc, EMGO Institute, The Netherlands

Introduction

Professor Jozef Rutenfranz was one of the founders of the European Group of Pediatric Work Physiology. He passed away in 1989, having produced as an author or co-author 149 PubMed-listed publications. From this impressive list of work it can be learned that Professor Rutenfranz had a broad interest in many topics. Two of these topics seem to have been of his prime interest: i.e. occupational work physiology applied to the assessment of an acceptable physiological load at work and issues related to the paediatric exercise field in its broadest sense.

Related to the latter, Berndt *et al.* had already recommended, in their 1975 publication, participation in regular lessons of physical education in order to prevent childhood adiposity. Interestingly, the main trigger for this recommendation was their observation that obese children were perceived as being less popular by their classmates compared to normal weight children.

When looking at current overweight and obesity rates amongst children it can only be concluded that the situation has worsened tremendously since 1975. In a recent review by Katzmarzyk *et al.* (2007), the current overall worldwide overweight and obesity prevalence rates were estimated at 10 per cent and 2–3 per cent, respectively, with extreme overweight plus obesity rates in the US and Europe estimated at 30 per cent and 20 per cent, respectively.

From our own research in the Amsterdam Growth and Health Longitudinal Study we know that there is a large degree of tracking of overweight and obesity (Van Lenthe *et al.*, 1996). This indicates that overweight and obese children are bound to become overweight and obese adults, which in turn is associated with major health problems for both the individual and society. Problems for society not only lie in the direct medical costs, but also in the indirect costs associated with productivity loss and increased work disability rates.

Given this current state of affairs the question is not if we need to do something about this overweight and obesity epidemic, but how? Answering the 'how' question, however, requires insight into the mechanisms and concepts that determine this epidemic. Therefore, the purpose of this paper is to share some personal thoughts on the mechanisms and concepts behind the current childhood overweight and obesity epidemic and to speculate about potential options for change.

A behavioural and ecological perspective to energy-balance-related behaviours in children

Childhood overweight and obesity result from a chronic, subtle, imbalance between energy intake (food consumption) and energy expenditure (physical [in-]activity). Clearly, both energy intake and energy expenditure are energy-balance-related human behaviours.

However, not all food consumption and not all physical (in-)activity contribute in an equal manner to this balance. It is therefore necessary to indentify certain sub-behaviours correlated most with this imbalance, ultimately leading to overweight and obesity.

Not attempting to give an in-depth overview, a number of food consumption correlates (including succinct behaviours) have been identified to contribute to the problem, such as portion size, snacking in-between meals, consumption of sugar containing drinks, skipping breakfast, low frequency of family meals, presence of fast food options, marketing, pricing policy, etc. With regard to physical (in-) activity correlates (again including succinct behaviours) such as watching TV, reduced active commuting to and from school, family support, neighbourhood safety, urban sprawl, neighbourhood walkability, convenience of car use, crime rates, etc. have been identified to contribute to the problem (e.g. Singh *et al.*, 2006; Katzmarzyk *et al.*, 2007; van der Horst *et al.*, 2007).

In an attempt to group these correlates into distinct categories, individual, socio-cultural and environmental-political correlates have been distinguished, with individual correlates being proximal to food consumption and physical (in-)activity behaviour and environmental-political correlates being more distal. The proximal correlates include person-related variables such as attitude, self-efficacy, beliefs, age, educational level, ethnicity, etc.

To make things even more complex, it is clear that all these factors overlap and interact with each other at various levels.

The complexity of the multi-level, multi-factorial nature of food consumption and physical (in-)activity behaviour is exemplified for physical activity in Figure 1.1 by what is called a social-ecological model of health behaviour. When trying to change both food consumption and physical (in-)activity behaviour, such conceptual models should be used to drive the agenda forward.

However, when addressing the overweight and obesity problem by applying such a model a number of key issues can be raised.

First, it is often assumed that food consumption and physical (in-)activity behaviour is primarily the product of individual reasoning and is therefore under major control of constructs such as knowledge, attitudes, self-efficacy, perceived behavioural control and intention towards a certain (sub-)behaviour.

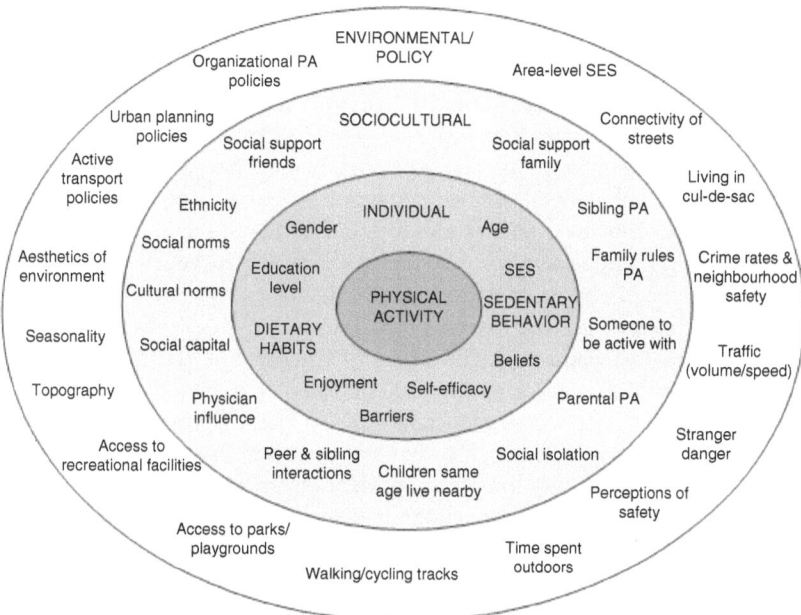

Figure 1.1 A social-ecological model for physical activity, taking into account individual, socio-cultural and environmental-political correlates (used with courtesy of Dr. Clare Hume, Deakin University, Melbourne, Australia).

This assumption is reflected in the names of theories explaining health behaviour from such a standpoint; e.g. the Theory of Reasoned Action, the Theory of Planned Behaviour (TBP), etc. However, analyses testing the internal validity of the TPB in a sample of 221 adolescents showed that current physical activity was most strongly associated with past physical activity and was neither associated with attitude, subjective norm nor perceived behavioural control, thus giving ground for the notion that current physical activity behaviour might be determined by habit strength, rather than by cognitive reasoning (de Bruijn *et al.*, 2006). So, perhaps theories like the Theory of Reasoned Action and the Theory of Planned Behaviour should be renamed the Theory of Unreasoned Action and the Theory of Unplanned Behaviour. At least analyses like the one conducted by de Bruin *et al.* must have implications for the design and content of interventions aimed at changing these behaviours, by taking the habitual nature of behaviour into account. Such a finding implies also that more testing of conceptual models regarding specified food consumption and physical (in-)activity sub-behaviours is needed before sound interventions can be set up.

Second is the question whether intervention emphasis should be placed on proximal (i.e. on individual) or on more distal (i.e. on social-cultural and/or environmental-political) correlates of food consumption and physical (in-)activity behaviour. Basically, the answer to this question depends on which of the two following statements one adheres to: i.e. 'nowadays food consumption and physical (in-)activity behaviour are abnormal reactions to a normal environment', or whether these behaviours 'are normal reactions to an abnormal environment'. If the first statement is true, interventions should primarily be aimed at the individual needing to change its abnormal behaviour. However, if the latter statement is true, behavioural change can only be induced by changing the abnormal environment, in whatever way. Of course the answer to this question is not a black and white issue, but there is good reason to believe that more emphasis should be placed on changing the obesogenic environment in order to solve childhood overweight and obesity problems.

The third and last point to mention in this context is the lack of high quality, experimental studies with a long(-er) duration of follow-up. High quality implies that trials are conducted along the lines of the CONSORT statement (www.consort-statement.org), but also that the intervention is developed in a planned way, according to the Intervention Mapping protocol (e.g. Singh et al., 2006). Longer duration of follow-up implies in my perspective at least a follow-up of two years.

Food for thought?

In 2007, two studies were published which exemplify the complex nature of the obesity epidemic and which are worth reporting in the context of this lecture.

The study of Christakis et al. (2007) describes the longitudinal spread of obesity over a 32-year period in the social network of the Framingham Heart Study cohort. This study showed the presence of discernible clusters of obese persons in this social network up to three degrees of social separation. The study also showed: a 57 per cent increased risk to become obese if a friend had become obese in a given time interval; a 40 per cent increased risk to become obese if one's sibling became obese and; a 37 per cent increased risk to become obese if one's spouse became obese. These effects were, however, not seen among neighbours in the immediate geographic location. It was also seen that persons of the same sex had a relatively greater influence on each other than those of the opposite sex. The findings of this study point to strong social influences on the spread of obesity.

Robinson et al. (2007) studied in an experimental study the effects of fast food branding on taste preferences of children aged 3.5–5.4 years. To do so they offered five pairs of identical foods and drinks in McDonald's packaging and in matched, unbranded ('plain') packaging. The children were asked to indicate whether the food substances offered tasted the same or if one tasted better. The results showed that the children preferred the tastes of the foods and drinks if they thought they were from McDonalds. Moderator analysis found significantly greater effects of branding among children with more TV sets in their homes and among children who ate food at McDonalds more often. These findings show that food branding plays an important role in taste preferences of young children for food and drinks often associated with the obesity epidemic. Therefore it should be considered to regulate branding of food and drinks aimed at young children, but perhaps also for the public in general.

'Solving' the childhood obesity problem: self-regulation and self-responsibility or 'the nanny state'?

It seems as if the obesity epidemic is getting out of hand. Data show that we are not dealing with a linear phenomenon, but with an exponentially increasing phenomenon (Katzmarzyk *et al.*, 2007, Noovens *et al.*, 2008).

In attempts to halt the childhood obesity epidemic we might, given the exponential increase of the problem, not be able to wait long enough before sound evidence is available regarding appropriate preventive action. Given this, it is important to discern on what kind of action to spend limited financial resources. So far most of the 'bets' have been on interventions mainly aimed at changing individual behaviour. These interventions aimed at individual behaviour have been conducted from the political perspective of self-regulation and self-responsibility. In other words, these interventions assume that individuals are by and large responsible for their own behaviour, are capable in a self-regulatory manner to change their behaviour and should thus change their behaviour by themselves. In countries where such a political standpoint is present most prominently (e.g. the USA, Australia) this approach has clearly not worked.

The opposite approach recognizes the prime dominance of the environmental-political and social-cultural environment on human health behaviour. This approach entails governmental influence through generic measures or legislation (i.e. 'Nanny knows best!'), thereby 'dictating' to people how to behave. There are a number of Public Health interventions along this approach that have shown success, with the classical example of John Snow as a starting point (Mackenbach, 2007). There are, to my knowledge, no experiments showing that this approach will work with regard to food consumption and physical (in-)activity. However, there is some evidence that the built environment can influence physical activity levels (Katzmarzyk *et al.*, 2007). Consequently, building codes can for instance be adjusted in such a way that builders and urban planners will be 'forced' to take the food consumption and physical (in-)activity aspects of their plans into consideration. The same approach holds true when structuring the school, work, community and family environment.

Of course modern society is not in need of a nanny state; but, by constructing a physical, social, political and cultural environment which favours healthy choices with regard to food consumption and physical activity, the goal of a normal weight society will in my opinion be reached much easier, compared to a current environment which systematically favours unhealthy food consumption and physical inactivity behaviour.

If such an approach needs more firm political action, so be it, because by the end of the day we are not dealing with a health care problem, but with a problem which is the end-product of continuous societal and political choice.

References

Berndt, I., Rehs, H.-J. and Rutenfranz, J., 1975, Sportpädagogische Gesichtspunkte zur Profylaxe der Adipositas im Kindesalter. *Öff. Gesundh.-Wesen*, **37**, pp. 1–9.

Christakis, N.A. and Fowler, J.H., 2007, The spread of obesity in a large social network over 32 years. *New England Journal of Medicine*, **357**, pp. 370–379.

de Bruijn, G.J., Kremers, S.P.J., Lensvelt-Mulders, G., de Vries, H., van Mechelen, W. and Brug, J., 2006, Modeling individual and physical environmental factors with adolescent physical activity. *American Journal of Preventive Medicine*, **30**, pp. 507–512.

Katzmarzyk, P.T., Bauer, L.A., Blair, S.N., Lambert, E.V., Oppert, J.M. and Riddoch, C., 2007, International Conference on Physical Activity and Obesity: Summary Statement and Recommendations. *International Journal of Pediatric Obesity*, pp. 1–19.

Mackenbach, J., 2007, Sanitation: pragmatism works. *British Medical Journal*, **334**, Suppl. 1, p. s17.

Noovens, A.C.J., Visscher, T.L.S., Verschuren W.M.N., Schuit, A.J., Boshuizen H.C., van Mechelen, W. and Seidell, J.C., 2008, Age, period and cohort effects on body weight and body mass index in adults: The Doetinchem Cohort study. In: *Epidemiological Studies on Weight Gain and its Determinants*, by Nooyens A.C.J. PhD thesis, VU University Amsterdam, The Netherlands (in press).

Robinson, T.N., Borzekowski, D.L.G., Matheson, D.M. and Kraemer, H.C., 2007, Effects of fast food branding on young children's taste preferences. *Archives of Pediatric and Adolescent Medicine*, **161**, pp. 792–797.

Singh, A.S., Chin, A., Paw, M.J.M., Kremers, S.P., Visscher, T.L., Brug, J. and van Mechelen, W., 2006, Design of the Dutch Obesity Intervention in Teenagers (NRG-DOiT): Systematic development, implementation and evaluation of a school-based intervention aimed at the prevention of excessive weight gain in adolescents. *BioMed Central Public Health*, **16**, p. 304.

van der Horst, K., Chin, A., Paw, M.J., Twisk, J.W. and van Mechelen, W., 2007, A brief review on correlates of physical activity and sedentariness in youth. *Medicine and Science in Sports and Exercise*, **39**, pp. 1241–1250.

van Lenthe, F.J., Kemper, H.C., van Mechelen, W. and Twisk, J.W., 1996, Development and tracking of central pattern of subcutaneous fat in adolescence and adulthood: The Amsterdam Growth and Health Study. *International Journal of Epidemiology*, **25**, pp. 1162–1171.

2 Oded Bar-Or

Science and beyond

B. Falk

Department of Physical Education and Kinesiology, Brock University, Canada

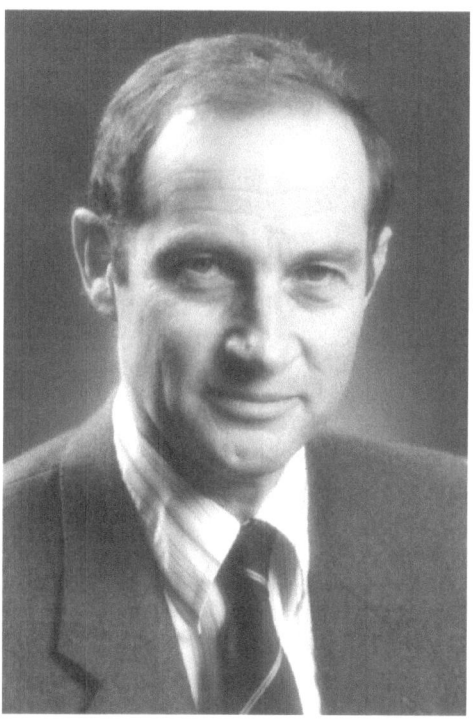

Oded Bar-Or was a superb physiologist, a brilliant scientist, a gifted teacher, a caring clinician and a dear friend to so many. It is a humbling experience for me to deliver this memorial paper to so many of his colleagues, his former students and his friends.

Oded was an incredible speaker. One of the best of his always excellent talks was in 1999, at the Paediatric Work Physiology (PWP) meeting in Sabadia, Italy, in honour of P.O. Astrand – a brilliant speaker himself. The title was: 'There is nothing new under the sun', a verse taken from the book of Ecclesiastes (Chapter 1:9, NIV). Oded eloquently demonstrated that so many of our so called 'new' findings in paediatric exercise physiology were actually demonstrated numerous years earlier by Astrand.

That incredible talk is the inspiration of the present paper. In the May 2006 issue of *Pediatric Exercise Science*, Tom Rowland wrote about Oded:

> The impact that this extraordinary man had on the well-being of children and the role he served as educator, motivator, and friend cannot be overstated.
>
> (Rowland *et al.*, 2006).

In the following pages I would like to pick out a few of Oded's works, accomplishments and, more importantly, his attributes, and demonstrate the *impact* he and his work had on the scientific community, professionals, children and families, colleagues, students, and friends.

In 1970, Oded founded the Department of Research and Sports Medicine at the Wingate Institute. He started out with a team of two which since then has grown over ten-fold. Much of the Wingate Institute's international reputation can be directly traced to Oded's work there.

In 1982, Oded founded the world's first paediatric medical clinic dedicated entirely to the application of exercise physiology to the diagnosis and treatment of children's diseases and pathologies. The 'Children's Exercise and Nutrition Centre' at Chedoke Hospital (McMaster University) has been a model of symbiotic relationships, academic research and clinical practice. Many around the world have attempted to duplicate this unique approach, but only a few succeeded to a similar extent.

A year after founding the Centre, Oded published his seminal book: *Pediatric Sports Medicine for the Practitioner* (Bar-Or, 1983). The first of its kind, the book was entirely dedicated to paediatric sports medicine and exercise physiology. For over 20 years it remained the only book of its kind. In it, Oded described the inactive child as a 'sick' child. He demonstrated that exercise could be used to prevent, diagnose or treat numerous diseases and conditions (e.g. obesity, exercise-induced asthma, cerebral palsy). An updated version, co-authored with Tom Rowland, was published in 2004 (Bar-Or and Rowland, 2004).

A pillar in Oded's work, taken for granted today by all of us PWP members, was the notion that 'children are not small adults'. Likely, it was Oded who eventually succeeded in instilling this idea in the highly conservative medical profession. This notion was the backbone of much of Oded's work. Maybe the best known example is in the area of thermoregulation.

For example, in a 1980 study (Bar-Or *et al.*, 1980), Oded and his team at the Wingate Institute's Research Centre demonstrated that children voluntarily dehydrate during exercise in the heat. In other words, even when children can consume as much water as they please, they do not drink sufficiently and progressively dehydrate. At the time, the phenomenon was termed 'involuntary dehydration'. In their recent book, Oded and Tom Rowland renamed the phenomenon 'voluntary dehydration'. The actual finding was similar to what had been observed in adults. The performance, health and safety implications, however, were quite different. It turned out that for a similar percentage of loss in body mass (dehydration), children's core temperature rose nearly twice as much compared with adults.

That same year (1980), Oded published a landmark review of paediatric thermoregulation during exercise in the heat (Bar-Or, 1980). That paper directly led to the publication of the American Academy of Pediatrics' Position Statement on Heat Stress and the Exercising Child in 1982 (American Academy of Pediatrics, 1982), which was later updated in 2000 (American Academy of Pediatrics, 2000). For the first time, the 1982 statement provided practical guidelines for children's participation in exercise in the heat and recommendations for their proper hydration before, during, and after such exertions.

From the mid-1990s on, Oded, with the help of Bogdan Wilk and dedicated students, extended the earlier dehydration studies with a series of investigations on fluid replacement during exercise in the heat. They examined flavour preferences and optimal fluid composition, as well as child-oriented hydration strategies. They were followed up by very practical recommendations regarding acclimatization/acclimation and hydration strategies for children exercising or competing in hot environments.

Some of Oded's most recent studies in thermoregulation have not yet been published. Those were conducted at the request of General Motors, North America's largest car manufacturer, following several heat fatalities of young children that were left in hot parked cars. The studies quantified the rate of rise of body temperature in infants and children trapped in closed parked cars under various climatic conditions. Consequently, car manufacturers are now developing automatic protective systems that would hopefully prevent such fatalities.

Exercise-induced asthma (EIA) was another area in which Oded had a considerable impact on the scientific and clinical community, and more importantly, on children and their families. In one of the early studies in Israel, Oded and his team investigated the effect of dry versus humid air on EIA sufferers (Bar-Or *et al.*, 1977), typically children. Contrary to prevailing notions the study elegantly demonstrated that ambient dry air was most deleterious, while in humid air pulmonary function was minimally affected. This was a major revelation. For years, asthmatic children were sent and their entire families often moved to dry desert or mountain regions. It turned out that the air in those regions was typically cleaner which was beneficial to allergenic-type asthma patients, some of which were EIA sufferers as well. These and subsequent findings were instrumental in turning recommendations 180° around and, rather than moving to the desert, children with EIA were recommended to take up swimming or other water-related sports. Up to that time, EIA patients were often afraid of or instructed to avoid all physical activity. Recommending exercise was revolutionary enough but Oded and his colleagues were also instrumental in showing that intermittent exercise, often as a preliminary warm-up, was highly effective in averting EIA attacks even in non-water sports. EIA patients were consequently made able to reap the benefits of exercise.

Cerebral palsy (CP) was another children's affliction that caught Oded's interest. The definitive study of physical training of CP children was published by Oded and his colleagues as early as 1976 (Bar-Or *et al.*, 1976). The 12-months, twice-per-week training programme they employed resulted in an 8 per cent increase in $\dot{V}O_2$ max. This study was revolutionary in that, until that time, like EIA patients, CP sufferers were told to avoid vigorous physical activity. It was probably very much due to this study that aerobic exercise training has been included in many rehabilitation programmes for CP children and adolescents.

Oded later went on to investigate the reasons behind children's high cost of locomotion in general, and CP children, in particular. In a series of studies, he and his students examined muscle EMG, metabolic response, and gait kinematics in children with and without CP. This was a perfect example of the multidisciplinary approach which Oded encouraged, preached for, and believed in. A consistent finding in those studies was the high cost of locomotion in children with CP, due at least, in part, to the much greater extent of agonist-antagonist co-contraction during walking. That is, they were activating their antagonist muscles to a much greater degree than healthy children at a price of a much higher energy cost of locomotion and associated effort.

In a recent work Oded and Desiree Maltais, his Ph.D. student, showed a negative correlation between physical activity levels and the oxygen cost of locomotion in children with CP (Maltais *et al.*, 2005). The lower their locomotive oxygen cost was, the higher was their physical activity level. The question became then: Would an intervention to reduce the oxygen cost of locomotion increase physical activity levels? Or, would increasing physical activity levels result in a decreased oxygen cost in these children? The answer likely lies in both approaches.

Cystic fibrosis (CF) is a genetic progressive disease that affects many organs, notably the lungs. Disease management has improved in leaps and bounds since Oded studied CF, but at that time, the fate of these patients was much bleaker than it is today. Oded always regarded CF as a tragic disease, but there was not much he could do for the patients who would come in every few months for functional capacity testing. This was one of the most difficult populations for him to deal with, because invariably, their condition deteriorated from visit to visit.

In a 1992 paper, published in *The Lancet* (Bar-Or *et al.*, 1992), Oded and his team showed that CF children can exercise in the heat, but while doing so they drink even less and, consequently, dehydrate more than healthy children, whom he had already shown to suffer from involuntary dehydration. Therefore, a potentially critical implication of these findings was that CF children are at a significantly greater thermoregulatory risk and should be vigorously encouraged to drink while exercising. Despite his more than 180 peer-reviewed publications, this was among those he was most proud of. He had not only helped CF sufferers by demonstrating the merits of exercise, but also showed them how to reap those benefits safely.

Almost a decade later, we embarked on an exercise intervention study of Israeli CF children. The study was conducted in cooperation with the Israeli

CF Foundation and Oded served as a consultant. From the initial planning stages, Oded stressed the importance of a proper hydration regimen in any kind of exercise intervention. The CF Foundation in Israel, a powerful and influential organization, does quite a bit for its members. Among other things, it publishes an extensive newsletter every few months. Following Oded's involvement, every summer issue of this official publication reiterates and stresses the importance of hydration and proactive beverage consuming during exercise.

Oded's first peer-reviewed publications dealt with obesity (Bar-Or *et al.*, 1968, 1969). At Elsworth Buskirk's lab at Penn State University, he investigated the thermoregulatory response to exercise in the heat of lean and obese men and women. In 1975 he was ahead of his time in advocating exercise for obese children (Bar-Or, 1975). A PubMed search ('obesity' OR 'overweight' AND 'children' AND 'exercise') shows only seven publications on this topic up to 1975. By contrast, in 2005 alone, more than 160 such manuscripts were published (Rowland *et al.*, 2006).

No talk about Oded would be complete without highlighting the Wingate Anaerobic Test (WAnT). It was introduced in 1974 (Ayalon *et al.*, 1974) and has since been employed in hundreds of studies and countless fitness tests in laboratories around the world. It is the most widely accepted test of anaerobic power. It has been shown highly reliable in very diverse populations; in healthy or disabled children, adults, and the elderly, as well as in athletes. It is an integral feature in almost every exercise physiology laboratory around the world and appears in almost every exercise physiology textbook.

As is the case with so many of Oded's concepts and ideas, the WAnT's greatest merit is its simplicity. In fact, Oded had an outstanding ability to simplify concepts and explanations of complex physiological phenomena, or at least make them seem simple. This fact, in addition to the now-obvious core merit of his ideas, has been instrumental in spurring much past and ongoing research as well as fruitful, constructive discussions in the field of paediatric exercise science.

Oded was self-assured yet a very humble and unpretentious man. The WAnT is a case in point. Its naming was not exploited for self-glorification (and was not named the Bar-Or test, after the man most responsible for its development), but rather, to acknowledge the Wingate Institute in which it had been conceived and developed.

Nevertheless, there *is* a 'Bar-Or Test'. Not many are aware of this fitness test outside Israel. However, anyone who has served in the Israeli Military since 1970, which means the majority of the population, knows exactly what the Bar-Or Test is and has likely performed it more than once (and despised whoever that 'Bar-Or' was ...). In fact, the military promotion of many has partly depended on passing the test. The development of that test, at the Military's request, was one of the very first projects Oded undertook at the newly founded Department of Research and Sports Medicine at the Wingate Institute. With some modifications the test is still administered today. Upon visiting Israel in 1998, Oded was rewarded with a special Israeli Defense Forces award, which he highly cherished, in recognition of this contribution.

The concept of 'globalization', if not the actual term, was probably 'invented' by Oded long before it became a household term. Oded had close colleagues and disciples all over the world, including Brazil, England, Finland, Germany, Guatemala, Holland, Israel, Japan, Korea, Poland, Switzerland, and the United States (a partial list). It is not surprising therefore that international visitors of one kind or another were a permanent feature at the Children's Exercise and Nutrition Centre, whether they came for a day, a week, several months, or even several years. Oded himself rarely stayed put and was truly a 'Frequent Flyer'. It was an inseparable part of his work and mission. He was invited to collaborate, lecture, or serve as a consultant in practically every continent (except Antarctica).

Oded's last scientific talk was at the PWP meeting in Switzerland, September 2005. It was titled 'Energy cost of locomotion in paediatric health and disease'. That talk was very important to Oded, and although he was in inconceivable pain, he managed to electrify everyone who was present. It was an experience never to be forgotten.

Approaching the end of this paper, I ask myself how Oded would have wanted to end this paper. Being the humble man he was, he would surely not have wanted this paper to end with a tribute to his accomplishments but rather with a message.

Indeed, in one of his last lectures (summer of 2005), at Brock University, Oded addressed the Ontario Chapter of the Diabetic Association of Native Americans. It was an audience of the native community members, families and children, most of whom were diabetic. Almost all of them, including children, were overweight or obese. Despite the highly heterogeneous background of his audience, Oded managed to clearly and effectively deliver his message to each and every individual. He spoke about physical activity and children's obesity and

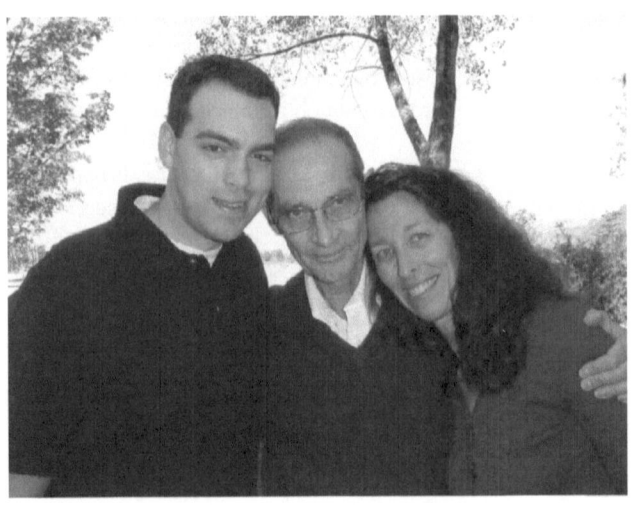

explained the importance for children to be active. He did not leave it at that and provided a clear and simple practical advice to parents: 'just send them outside and let them play!', he said. No need for structure or sophisticated equipment. Given the opportunity, children will invariably be active in their play.

Oded was an educator at heart. Upon his explicit request the photo on page 14 was taken at Oded's last conference – the 2005 PWP in Switzerland. I was Oded's first Ph.D. graduate in Canada, Brian Timmons his last. I believe this photo holds in it something Oded wanted of all of us: to pass along and build upon his legacy of insight and far-reaching vision.

I could have quoted many more of Oded's works and accomplishments and I am certain that there are many more notable impacts I could have enumerated today. Many of you, the readers of these pages, can probably come up with tales and anecdotes of your own acquaintance with Oded. I hope you do, and in doing so, allow his legacy to live on.

Note

At the conference Professors Han C.G. Kemper and Emmanuel Van Praagh also presented personal tributes to Oded Bar-Or's contribution to paediatric exercise physiology.

References

American Academy of Pediatrics Committee on Sports Medicine, 1982, Climatic heat stress and the exercising child. *Pediatrics*, **69**, pp. 808–809.

American Academy of Pediatrics Committee on Sports Medicine and Fitness, 2000, Climatic heat stress and the exercising child and adolescent. *Pediatrics*, **106(1 Pt 1)**, pp. 158–159.

Ayalon, A., Inbar, O. and Bar-Or, O., 1974, Relationships between measurements of explosive strength and anaerobic power. In: *International Series on Sports Sciences: Vol 1, Biomechanics IV*, edited by Nelson, R.C. and Morehouse, C.A. Baltimore: University Park Press, pp. 527–532.

Bar-Or, O., 1975, The obese child and physical exercise (in Hebrew). *Eitanim*, **28**, pp. 264–267.

Bar-Or, O., 1980, Invited Review – Climate and the exercising child. *International Journal of Sports Medicine*, **1**, pp. 53–65.

Bar-Or, O., 1983, *Pediatric Sports Medicine for the Practitioner. From Physiologic Principles to Clinical Applications*. New York: Springer Verlag.

Bar-Or, O., Lundegren, H.M., Magnusson, L.L. and Buskirk, E.R., 1968, Distribution of heat-activated sweat glands in obese and lean men and women. *Human Biology*, **40**, pp. 234–248.

Bar-Or, O., Lundegren, H.H. and Buskirk, E.R., 1969, Heat tolerance of exercising obese and lean women. *Journal of Applied Physiology*, **26**, pp. 403–409.

Bar-Or, O., Inbar, O. and Spira, R., 1976, Physiological effects of a sports rehabilitation program on cerebral palsied and post-poliomyelitic adolescents. *Medicine and Science in Sports*, **8**, pp. 157–161.

Bar-Or, O., Neuman, I. and Dotan, R., 1977, Effect of dry and humid climates on exercise-induced asthma in children and pre-adolescents. *Journal of Allergy and Clinical Immunology*, **69**, pp. 163–167.

Bar-Or, O., Dotan, R., Inbar, O., Rotshtein, A. and Zonder, H., 1980, Voluntary hypohydration in 10 to 12-year-old boys. *Journal of Applied Physiology*, **48**, pp. 104–108.

Bar-Or, O., Blimkie, C.J.R., Hay, J.A., MacDougall, J.D., Ward, D.S. and Wilson, W.M., 1992, Voluntary dehydration and heat intolerance in cystic fibrosis. *The Lancet*, **339**, pp. 696–699.

Bar-Or, O. and Rowland, T.W., 2004, *Pediatric Exercise Medicine. From Physiologic Principles to Health Care Application*. Champaign, IL: Human Kinetics.

Maltais, D., Pierrynowski, M., Galea, V.A. and Bar-Or, O., 2005, Physical activity level is associated with the O_2 cost of walking in cerebral palsy. *Medicine and Science in Sports and Exercise*, **37**, pp. 347–353.

Rowland, T.W., Falk, B., Van Praagh, E., Blimkie, C.J.R., Kemper, H.C.G., Unnithan, V.B., Riddell, M.C., Ward, D.S. and Morgan, D.W., 2006, Remembering a cherished friend and colleague. *Pediatric Exercise Science*, **18**, pp. 145–170.

3 Exercise metabolism during growth and maturation

N. Armstrong
Children's Health and Exercise Research Centre,
University of Exeter, UK

Introduction

In a longitudinal study, Armstrong and Welsman (2001) reported that, over the age range 12–17 years, peak power, as determined on the Wingate anaerobic test, increased by about 120 per cent in boys and 66 per cent in girls, whereas increases in peak $\dot{V}O_2$ were somewhat less, at about 70 per cent and 50 per cent for boys and girls respectively. These data indicate that there are age- and sex-related changes in anaerobic and aerobic power which are not synchronous and suggest that both sexes may experience a more marked increase in anaerobic metabolism than aerobic metabolism as they move from childhood, through adolescence and into young adulthood. However, metabolic profiles estimated from exercise tests are the sum of numerous factors and do not provide the quality and specificity of data required to tease out changes in exercise metabolism during growth and maturation.

Studies of substrate utilization (Boisseau and Delmarche, 2000), exercise blood lactates (Pfitzinger and Freedson, 1997), hormonal responses to exercise (Berg and Keul, 1998), and recovery from high intensity exercise (Ratel et al., 2003) have contributed to our understanding of the interplay of anaerobic and aerobic metabolism but ethical considerations have limited potentially more informative studies at muscle cell level. Data from a few muscle biopsy studies of energy stores and utilization (Eriksson, 1980), enzyme activity (Haralambie, 1982), and muscle fibre type (Jansson, 1996) are available but they are difficult to interpret and clouded by small sample sizes and methodological problems, such as having to be collected at rest or post-exercise rather than during exercise.

Current evidence suggests that during exercise children have relatively higher oxidative metabolic activity than adolescents or adults and that there is a progressive increase in glycolytic metabolic activity, with growth and maturation at least into adolescence and perhaps into young adulthood. However, understanding of exercise metabolism during growth and maturation is incomplete and noninvasive methods of interrogating muscle during exercise are required to promote further understanding of the mechanisms involved. In this paper, I will explore the current and potential contribution of two non-invasive techniques which have been recently introduced to paediatric physiology, namely breath-by-breath respiratory gas analysis ($\dot{V}O_2$ kinetics) and ^{31}P magnetic resonance spectroscopy ($^{31}PMRS$).

Oxygen uptake kinetics

The assessment and interpretation of $\dot{V}O_2$ kinetic responses to changes in exercise intensity is complex, but with the application of suitable methodology and appropriate modelling techniques the data have been shown to provide a non-invasive window into metabolic activity at the muscular level (Rossiter *et al.*, 1999). To provide a framework in which to explore paediatric data I will initially outline the characteristics of the $\dot{V}O_2$ kinetic response to exercise in different domains.

Oxygen uptake kinetics are studied in the laboratory by the use of a step transition where a period of low intensity exercise (e.g. unloaded pedalling on a cycle ergometer) is followed by a sudden increase in exercise intensity to a predetermined level. The $\dot{V}O_2$ kinetic response is then described in relation to four well-defined exercise domains which are termed moderate, heavy, very heavy and severe.

Moderate intensity exercise does not involve a sustained anaerobic contribution to adenosine triphosphate (ATP) resynthesis and the upper marker of this domain is therefore the anaerobic threshold or a suitable derivative such as the lactate threshold, or, more usually with children, the non-invasive ventilatory threshold (T_{vent}). During exercise above T_{vent} anaerobic glycolysis makes a larger contribution to energy needs than during moderate exercise but within the heavy exercise domain blood lactate accumulation stabilizes over time, reflecting a balance between the rate of appearance and rate of removal. The upper marker of the heavy exercise domain is therefore the maximal lactate steady state (MLSS). Determination of the MLSS requires multiple blood samples, so critical power (CP), which occurs at about 70–80 per cent of peak $\dot{V}O_2$, is the preferred variable for use with children. However, as the determination of children's CP is very demanding, in practice 40 per cent of the difference between T_{vent} and peak $\dot{V}O_2$ is normally used as the upper threshold of the heavy exercise domain. This easily determined threshold is appropriate as it falls below the CP of most children. Exercise above CP but below peak $\dot{V}O_2$ is regarded as falling within the very heavy domain where $\dot{V}O_2$ continues to rise almost linearly until a slow component of $\dot{V}O_2$ results in the achievement of peak $\dot{V}O_2$. In the severe exercise domain, where the projected $\dot{V}O_2$ is greater than peak $\dot{V}O_2$, the response is truncated with the rapid achievement of peak $\dot{V}O_2$. As rigorously determined paediatric data are only available for moderate and heavy exercise I will focus on these domains.

With a step transition in exercise there is an almost immediate increase in cardiac output which occurs prior to the arrival at the lungs of venous blood from the exercising muscles. Phase 1 (the cardiodynamic phase), which lasts about 15s, is therefore independent of $\dot{V}O_2$ at the mouth and is predominantly a reflection of the increase in pulmonary blood flow with exercise. Phase 2, the primary component, features a rapid exponential rise in $\dot{V}O_2$ that arises from hypoxic and hypercapnic blood from the exercising muscles arriving at the lung. The speed of the phase 2 $\dot{V}O_2$ kinetics is described by the time constant (τ) which is the time taken to reach 63 per cent of the change in $\dot{V}O_2$. Phase 2 $\dot{V}O_2$ has been shown to reflect muscle $\dot{V}O_2$ despite some disassociation due to muscle utilization of oxygen stores and differences in blood flow at the muscle and lung (Rossiter *et al.*, 1999).

During moderate exercise, $\dot{V}O_2$ reaches a steady state (phase 3) within about 2 min with an O_2 cost (or gain) of about 10 mL min^{-1} W^{-1} above that found during unloaded pedalling. In phases 1 and 2 ATP resynthesis cannot be met fully by the $\dot{V}O_2$ and the additional energy requirements are met primarily from the breakdown of phosphocreatine (PCr), with minor contributions from O_2 stores and glycolysis. The O_2 equivalent of these sources is termed the O_2 deficit and the faster the τ the smaller the O_2 deficit. During heavy exercise, the phase 2 gain is similar to that observed during moderate exercise but glycolysis makes a larger contribution to the O_2 deficit. Within 2–3 min of the onset of exercise a slow component of $\dot{V}O_2$ is superimposed upon the primary $\dot{V}O_2$ response, the O_2 cost of exercise becomes elevated over time and it might be 10–15 min before a steady state is achieved. The mechanisms underpinning the slow component are elusive but the most plausible theory proposes a combined influence of muscle fibre distribution, motor unit recruitment, and the matching of O_2 delivery to active muscles. Figure 3.1 describes the three phases of $\dot{V}O_2$ kinetics in the four exercise domains.

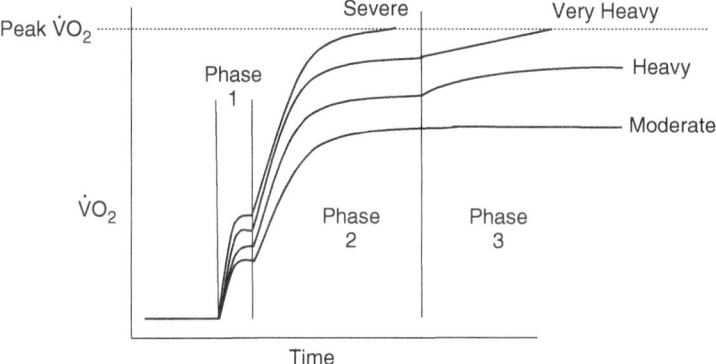

Figure 3.1 The three phases of the kinetic rise in pulmonary oxygen uptake in response to a step change in exercise in four different exercise intensity domains (reprinted with permission from Fawkner, S.G. and Armstrong, N., 2003. Oxygen uptake kinetic response to exercise in children. *Sports Medicine* 33, pp. 651–669.)

Oxygen uptake kinetics in children

Data from children are sparse and many paediatric studies lack methodological rigour. For example, during a step transition large breath-by-breath variations and small $\dot{V}O_2$ amplitudes characterize children's responses and, in order to improve the signal-to-noise ratio and maintain 95 per cent confidence intervals (CIs) within accepted limits, it is necessary to align and average several identical transitions. Few studies have averaged multiple identical transitions, used appropriate modelling techniques, exhibited strict adherence to exercise domains and reported the 95 per cent CIs of their data.

Moderate intensity exercise

Several studies have investigated the effect of age on the phase 2 $\dot{V}O_2$ response and data are equivocal, although the trend is towards a faster τ and an elevated O_2 cost per unit of work in children than in adults. In the only study to date to satisfy the above criteria, Fawkner *et al.* (2002) compared the $\dot{V}O_2$ kinetics of 11–12-year-old children with those of young adults during a step change to exercise below 80 per cent of T_{vent}. Up to 10 transitions were averaged for each participant and those in whom the CIs exceeded 5s were excluded from the study, leaving 12 boys, 11 girls, 13 men and 12 women. The phase 2 τ was significantly faster in boys than men (19.0s vs 27.9s) and in girls than women (21.0s vs 26.0s) with no sex differences observed in either children or adults. $\dot{V}O_2$ amplitude, O_2 deficit, and O_2 deficit relative to $\dot{V}O_2$ amplitude, were all significantly higher in adults than in children.

Children's faster τ and therefore lower anaerobic contribution to ATP resynthesis might be due to a more efficient O_2 delivery system, a greater relative capacity for O_2 utilization at the muscle, or both. There is no evidence to suggest that O_2 delivery to the mitochondria is enhanced in children compared with adults or that increased availability of O_2 speeds $\dot{V}O_2$ kinetics during moderate exercise.

Children's faster τ and lower relative O_2 deficit are therefore likely to reflect an enhanced capacity for oxidative phosphorylation.

Heavy intensity exercise

Although they do not meet fully the above criteria, the published studies which have compared the responses of children (>90 per cent boys) to adults have observed significantly faster τ and indicated greater O_2 gains during the primary component in children (Barstow and Scheuermann, 2006).

In two studies using appropriate modelling techniques in which the 95 per cent CIs of the τ were within 5s, Fawkner and Armstrong (2004 a,b) investigated prepubertal children's responses to a step change to exercise at 40 per cent of the difference between T_{vent} and peak $\dot{V}O_2$. In the first study they monitored changes in 22 children's $\dot{V}O_2$ responses over a 2-year period. On the first test occasion, a greater O_2 gain during phase 2 and a significantly faster τ were observed in both the girls (21.1s vs 26.4s) and the boys (16.8s vs 21.7s) than on a subsequent test 2 years later. A slow component of $\dot{V}O_2$ was observed in both tests. In the first test the slow component contribution was about 10 per cent of the final $\dot{V}O_2$ after 9 min exercise, and in the second test it increased to about 15 per cent. The O_2 cost by the end of the exercise period was equal on both test occasions, which suggests that the phosphate turnover required to maintain heavy exercise was independent of age but in the second test a lesser proportion of the required O_2 was achieved in the primary phase. In the second study, they observed the responses of 25 boys and 23 girls and reported that the τ was significantly faster in boys than in girls (17.6s vs 21.9s) and that the slow component contribution to the change in $\dot{V}O_2$ amplitude was significantly greater in girls than in boys (11.8 per cent vs 8.9 per cent).

Explanations for age-related changes in the speed of τ, the size of the slow component and the O_2 cost of the primary component are difficult to substantiate with confidence but several hypotheses exist. There is no strong evidence to suggest that O_2 delivery during exercise is either impaired in healthy subjects or that it decreases with age. A more plausible proposal indicates the presence of a developmental influence on the mitochondrial O_2 utilization potential that supports an enhanced oxidative function during childhood. These responses are also characteristic of subjects with a high ratio of type 1 to type 2 muscle fibres and, although the data are equivocal, a critical review of the literature concluded that the percentage of type 1 fibres in the vastus lateralis decrease, at least in males between the age of 10 and 35 years (Jansson, 1996).

Why there are sex differences in $\dot{V}O_2$ responses to a step change to exercise above T_{vent} but not below T_{vent} is not readily apparent. In adults, the proportion of type 1 fibres has been shown to be negatively correlated with τ and the slow component during heavy but not moderate exercise (Jones *et al.*, 2006). So, if has been reported in at least one study, girls have a lower percentage of type 1 fibres than boys (Jansson, 1996) this would be consistent with the sex differences observed by Fawkner and Armstrong (2004b).

^{31}P Magnetic resonance spectroscopy

^{31}PMRS spectra obtained during rest, exercise and recovery allow the monitoring of ATP, phosphocreatine (PCr) and inorganic phosphate (Pi) in real time and provide a non-invasive window into muscle metabolism. The decline in PCr and the corresponding rise in Pi with exercise can be monitored and the ratio Pi/PCr is used in the interpretation of ^{31}PMRS spectra. Intracellular pH can be calculated from the shift in the Pi spectral peak relative to the PCr peak and this reflects the acidification of the muscle and provides an indirect measure of glycolysis. During a progressive, incremental exercise test to exhaustion, initial shallow slopes in Pi/PCr and pH plotted against power output are followed by steeper slopes with increasing exercise intensity and the transition point is known as the intracellular threshold (IT). Armstrong *et al.* (2006) demonstrated that, with 9–11-year-olds,

ITs occur at a similar relative exercise intensity as the T_{vent} during cycle ergometry (59 per cent of peak power vs 58 per cent of peak $\dot{V}O_2$, respectively).

^{31}PMRS studies in children

Published paediatric ^{31}PMRS studies have required the child to participate in single leg calf or quadriceps exercise on a non-magnetic ergometer while lying supine or prone in an MR scanner. The small size of children's calf muscles leads to a low signal-to-noise ratio and potential difficulties in curve fitting the spectra. Furthermore, the gastrocnemius is composed mainly of type 2 fibres and the soleus mainly of type 1 fibres, so if there are varying amounts of these muscles in the volume of calf muscle being interrogated, this might bias the interpretation, particularly when comparing muscles of different sizes. A challenge with young subjects is that ^{31}PMRS studies require exercise within a small bore tube and the further requirement that the acquisition of data be synchronized with the rate of muscle contraction. This can be problematic with young children and published studies to date, which are outlined in the following paragraph, have seldom addressed habituation to the prescribed exercise.

Zanconato et al. (1993) reported data from eight boys and two girls and five men and three women who carried out supine, progressive calf exercise to voluntary exhaustion. A slow phase and a fast phase of Pi/PCr increase and pH decrease were detected in 75 per cent of the adults and 50 per cent of the children. Below the ITs the Pi/PCr and pH slopes were similar in children and adults but above the ITs the incline in Pi/PCr and decline in pH were both steeper in adults than in children who achieved an end-exercise Pi/PCr only 27 per cent of adult values. Although it is not readily apparent why so few ITs were detected, these data indicate age-related differences in energy metabolism during high intensity exercise. Zanconato et al.'s findings were subsequently supported by Kuno et al. (1995), who collected ^{31}PMRS data from 14 trained and 23 untrained boys and six adults during quadriceps exercise to exhaustion. Lower values of pH and the ratio PCr/(PCr+Pi) were reported in the adults at exhaustion with no significant differences between the trained and untrained boys. Kuno et al. also reported no differences between adults and boys in the recovery τ of PCr, a finding in conflict with that of Taylor et al. (1997), who reported a faster PCr recovery half-time in 6–12-year-olds than in adults following maximal calf exercise and suggested that this indicated an enhanced oxidative capacity during childhood. Physiological (cellular acidosis), anatomical (comparing calf with quadriceps) and methodical (only 1 transition) limitations preclude firm conclusions to be drawn from these recovery studies. Peterson et al. (1999) compared the responses of nine prepubertal and nine pubertal trained girl swimmers to 2 min of plantar flexion exercise at light (40 per cent maximal work capacity, MWC) and severe (140 per cent MWC) intensities. No significant differences were observed, implying that, in conflict with previous ^{31}PMRS studies, glycolytic metabolism during high intensity exercise is not maturity-dependent. However, the magnitude of the pubertal/prepubertal difference

(66 per cent) in the Pi/PCr ratio, the high variability and the small sample sizes suggests that the observed difference between the groups might have biological meaning.

The few published ^{31}PMRS paediatric studies have provided valuable insights into muscle metabolism during exercise but need to be interpreted with respect to the muscles interrogated, the use of small, mixed age and/or sex samples and the rigour of habituation, data collection, data analysis and interpretation. The potential of the technique remains relatively unexplored in paediatric exercise physiology and in the next section I will briefly outline some of our recent research, which has, to date, mainly been published in abstract form (Armstrong *et al.*, 2006; Barker *et al.*, in press, 2007).

For this series of studies we constructed a to-scale replica scanner which enables children to overcome fears of exercising in a prone position within a tube and to practise until they can follow the up-down movement of the leg via a metronomic cursor projected onto a visual display, without using expensive magnet time. The knee extensions are practised at a cadence in unison with the magnetic pulse sequence to be used in the MR scanner. It is only when the children are fully habituated to exercising in the replica scanner and capable of maintaining the required knee extension cadence that they transfer to the MR scanner, where, to prevent displacement of the muscle volume of interest relative to the ^{31}PMRS coil and to minimize adjacent muscle contribution to the exercise, they are secured with Velcro straps over the lower back, legs and hips. Following this methodology, Barker *et al.* (2006) demonstrated a Pi/PCr IT detection rate of 93 per cent with 11–12-year-olds and it is worthy of note that they observed mean end Pi/PCr ratios >2.0 compared with the children's mean end Pi/PCr ratios of 0.54 reported by Zanconato *et al.* (1993). Good reliability of Pi/PCr ITs were reported with a typical error, expressed as percentage coefficient of variation, across 3 trials a week apart of about 10 per cent.

Barker *et al.* (in press) examined the influence of age and sex on the muscle metabolic responses of 15 boys, 15 girls, eight men and eight women who completed a single-leg quadriceps incremental exercise test to exhaustion. Muscle mass was quantified using MR imaging scans scaled to power output measures using log-linear allometric procedures. No significant age- or sex-related changes in Pi/PCr were noted at the IT or in peak power output scaled for muscle mass. The rest to end-exercise change in Pi/PCr was significantly lower in children compared to adults and sex differences were observed in children but not in adults. These data generally support those from earlier ^{31}PMRS studies and indicate comparable oxidative metabolism during moderate exercise but a greater contribution from glycolysis during heavy exercise in adults than in children and in girls than in boys. They are in agreement with reported age- and sex-related $\dot{V}O_2$ kinetic responses to heavy exercise but not moderate exercise.

To explore further age- and sex-related responses to moderate exercise, Barker *et al.* (2007) determined the PCr kinetic responses to the onset of moderate exercise of eight boys, ten girls, eight men and eight women. The subjects completed repeat constant exercise transitions (children, range 3–9; adults 2–5) corresponding to 80 per cent of their Pi/PCr IT. The 95 per cent CIs of PCr τ were, on average, 6s. No significant age- or sex-related differences in τ were detected, suggesting, in conflict with the extant $\dot{V}O_2$ kinetic data, comparable capacity for mitochondrial oxidative phosphorylation in child and adult muscle.

To investigate the relationship between $\dot{V}O_2$ and PCr kinetics in children, Armstrong et al. (2006) used the techniques described above to determine the $\dot{V}O_2$ kinetic τ, during moderate cycling exercise, and the PCr kinetic τ, during moderate knee extension exercise in an MR scanner, of 12 children. There was no significant difference in the PCr and $\dot{V}O_2$ τs; despite the relative homogeneity the τs were significantly correlated; and the PCr and $\dot{V}O_2$ τs 95 per cent CIs overlapped in 92 per cent of the kinetic responses. Taken together these findings suggest that, as previously shown in adults (Rossiter et al., 1999), the kinetic responses of PCr and $\dot{V}O_2$ to the onset of exercise are mechanistically linked.

Current data from ^{31}PMRS and $\dot{V}O_2$ kinetic studies are in agreement and suggest that there are age- and sex-related differences in responses to heavy exercise but data from moderate exercise are equivocal and demand further study. The kinetic responses of PCr and $\dot{V}O_2$ at the onset of moderate exercise appear to be mechanistically linked.

Conclusion

The weight of evidence indicates that during exercise of different intensities there is an interplay of aerobic and anaerobic metabolism in which children exhibit a relatively higher oxidative capacity than adults with an age-related increase in glycolytic metabolism. Our understanding of paediatric exercise metabolism is, however, limited by ethical and methodological constraints. Few studies have rigorously assessed and interpreted PCr and $\dot{V}O_2$ kinetics during exercise and innovative analysis of breath-by-breath respiratory gas responses and ^{31}PMRS spectra provides a relatively unexplored potential to provide further insights into paediatric exercise metabolism. Further research using ^{31}PMRS is required but the close relationship between PCr and $\dot{V}O_2$ kinetics encourages the use of more child-friendly and less expensive $\dot{V}O_2$ kinetics as a non-invasive window into exercise metabolism during growth and maturation.

References

Armstrong, N. and Welsman, J.R., 2001, Peak oxygen uptake in relation to growth and maturation in 11–17 year old humans. European Journal of Applied Physiology, **85**, pp. 546–551.

Armstrong, N., Barker, A.R., Fulford, J., Welford, D., Welsman, J.R. and Williams, C.A., 2006, Kinetics of muscle phosphocreatine and pulmonary oxygen uptake during moderate intensity exercise in children. In: Proceedings of the 11th Annual Congress of the European College of Sport Sciences, edited by Hoppeler, H., Reilly, T., Tsolakidis, E., Gfeller, L., Klossner, S. Cologne: Sportverlag Strauss, p. 443.

Barker, A., Welsman, J., Welford, D., Fulford J., Williams, C.A. and Armstrong, N., 2006, Reliability of ^{31}P magnetic spectroscopy during an exhaustive incremental exercise test in children. *European Journal of Applied Physiology*, **98**, pp. 556–565.

Barker, A.R., Welsman, J.R., Fulford, J., Welford, D. and Armstrong, N., 2007, Muscle phosphocreatine kinetics during moderate intensity exercise in children and adults. *Acta Kinesiologiae Universitatis Tartuensis*, **12(Suppl)**, p. 47.

Barker, A.R., Welsman, J.R., Fulford, J., Welford, D. and Armstrong, N., in press. Quadriceps muscle energetics during an exercise test to exhaustion in children and adults. In: *Proceedings of the Annual Conference of the British Association of Sport and Exercise Sciences*. Bath, UK.

Barstow, T.J. and Scheuermann, B.W., 2006, Effects of maturation and aging on $\dot{V}O_2$ kinetics. In: *Oxygen Uptake Kinetics in Sport, Exercise and Medicine*, edited by Jones, A.M. and Poole, D.C. London: Routledge, pp. 332–352.

Berg, A. and Keul, J., 1998, Biochemical changes during exercise in children. In: *Young Athletes*, edited by Malina, R.M. Champaign, IL: Human Kinetics, pp. 61–78.

Boisseau, N. and Delmarche, P., 2000, Metabolic and hormonal responses to exercise in children and adolescents. *Sports Medicine*, **30**, pp. 405–422.

Eriksson, B.O., 1980, Muscle metabolism in children – a review. *Acta Physiologica Scandinavica*, **283**, pp. 20–28.

Fawkner, S.G. and Armstrong, N., 2003, Oxygen uptake kinetic response to exercise in children. *Sports Medicine*, **33**, pp. 651–669.

Fawkner, S.G. and Armstrong, N., 2004a. Longitudinal changes in the kinetic response to heavy intensity exercise. *Journal of Applied Physiology*, **97**, pp. 460–466.

Fawkner, S.G. and Armstrong, N., 2004b, Sex differences in the oxygen uptake kinetic response to heavy intensity exercise in prepubertal children. *European Journal of Applied Physiology*, **93**, pp. 210–216.

Fawkner, S., Armstrong, N., Potter, C. R. and Welsman, J.R., 2002, Oxygen uptake kinetics in children and adults after the onset of moderate-intensity exercise. *Journal of Sports Sciences*, **20**, pp. 319–326.

Haralambie, G., 1982, Enzyme activities in skeletal muscle of 13–15 year old adolescents. Bulletin Européen Physiopathologie Respiratoire, **18**, 16–74.

Jansson, E., 1996, Age-related fiber type changes in human skeletal muscle. In: *Biochemistry of Exercise IX*, edited by Maughan, R.J. and Shirreffs, S.M. Champaign, IL: Human Kinetics, pp. 297–307.

Jones, A.M., Pringle, J.S.M. and Carter, H., 2006, Influence of muscle fibre type and motor unit recruitment on $\dot{V}O_2$ kinetics. In: *Oxygen Uptake Kinetics in Sport, Exercise and Medicine*, edited by Jones, A.M. and Poole, D.C. London: Routledge, pp. 261–293.

Kuno, S., Takahashi, H., Fujimoto, K., Akima, H., Miyamaru, M., Nemoto, I., Itai, Y. and Katsuta, S., 1995, Muscle metabolism during exercise using phosphorus-31 nuclear magnetic resonance spectroscopy in adolescents. *European Journal of Applied Physiology*, **70**, pp. 301–304.

Peterson, S.R., Gaul, C.A., Stanton, M.M. and Hanstock, C.C., 1998, Skeletal muscle metabolism during short-term high intensity exercise in prepubertal and pubertal girls. *Journal of Applied Physiology*, **87**, pp. 2151–2156.

Pfitzinger, P. and Freedson, P., 1997, Blood lactate responses to exercise in children. Part 2. Lactate threshold. *Pediatric Exercise Science*, **9**, pp. 299–307.

Ratel, S., Lazaar, N., Williams, C.A., Bedu M. and Duche, P., 2003, Age differences in human skeletal muscle fatigue during high intensity intermittent exercise. *Acta Paediatrica*, **92**, pp. 1248–1254.

Rossiter, H.B., Ward, S.A., Doyle, V.L., Howe, F.A., Griffiths, J.R. and Whipp, B.J., 1999, Inferences from pulmonary oxygen uptake with respect to intramuscular (phosphocreatine) kinetics during moderate exercise in humans. *Journal of Physiology*, **518**, pp. 921–932.

Taylor, D.J., Kemp, G.J., Thompson, C.H. and Raddar, G.K., 1997, Ageing: Effects on oxidative function of skeltal muscle in vivo. *Molecular and Cellular Biochemistry*, **174**, pp. 321–324.

Zanconato, S., Buchthal, S., Barstow, T. J. and Cooper, D. M., 1993, ^{31}P-magnetic resonance spectroscopy of leg muscle metabolism during exercise in children and adults. *Journal of Applied Physiology*, **74**, pp. 2214–2218.

4 The overtraining syndrome

Are there clear markers?

R. Meeusen

Vrije Universiteit Brussel Department of Human Physiology and Sports Medicine, Brussels, Belgium

Introduction

The goal of training competitive athletes is to provide training loads that are effective in improving performance. During this process, athletes may go through several stages within a competitive season of periodised training. These phases of training range from undertraining, during the period between competitive seasons or during active rest and taper, to 'overreaching' and 'overtraining' which includes maladaptations and diminished competitive performance (Meeusen *et al.*, 2006). When prolonged and excessive training happens concurrent with other stressors and insufficient recovery, performance decrements can result in chronic maladaptations that can lead to the overtraining syndrome (OTS). Literature on 'overtraining' has increased enormously; however, the major difficulties are the lack of common and consistent terminology as well as a gold standard for the diagnosis of overtraining.

Definition

Intensified training can result in a decline in performance; however, when appropriate periods of recovery are provided, a 'supercompensation' effect may occur, with the athlete exhibiting an enhanced performance when compared to baseline levels. Recently, the European College of Sports Science published a 'consensus statement' which defined the several stages of the training and overtraining states of the athletes (Meeusen *et al.*, 2006).

Most papers document athletes going on a short training camp in order to create a 'functional overreaching' (FOR). They typically follow athletes not only during the increased training (volume and/or intensity), but also register recovery from this training status.

When this 'intensified training' continues, the athletes can evolve into a state of extreme overreaching or 'non-functional overreaching' (NFOR), which will lead to a stagnation or decrease in performance that will not resume for several weeks or months.

Both 'functional' and 'non-functional' overreached athletes will be able to fully recover after sufficient rest. As it is possible to recover from short-term or FOR within a period of two weeks, the recovery from the NFOR state is less clear. This is probably because not many studies tried to define the subtle difference that exists between extreme overreaching, which needs several weeks or even months to recover (Meeusen et al., 2006), and the OTS. Athletes who suffer from the OTS may need months or even years to completely recover, leading frequently to cessation of a (top) sports career.

The difficulty lies in the subtle difference that might exist between extreme overreached athletes and those having OTS. In using the expression 'syndrome', we emphasise the multifactorial aetiology, and acknowledge that exercise (training) is not necessarily the sole causative factor of the syndrome.

Mechanisms

Probably because of the difficulty in detecting straightforward mechanisms responsible for OTS, many speculations have been made as to the 'real' reason for the genesis of OTS. This has led to many papers that present a possible hypothesis for the origin of OTS (Meeusen et al., 2006).

Although these theories have potential, these theories remain speculative until more prospective studies are carried out where a longitudinal follow-up of athletes (who may develop OTS) is performed, or specific diagnostic tools are developed.

There have been several proposals of which physiological and biochemical measures might be indicative of OR or OTS. Reduced maximal heart rates after increased training may be the result of reduced sympathetic nervous system activity, decreased tissue responsiveness to catecholamines, changes in adrenergic receptor activity, or simply the result of a reduced power output achieved with maximal effort. Several other reductions in maximal physiological measures (oxygen uptake, heart rate, etc.) might be a consequence of a reduction in exercise time and not related to abnormalities per se, and it should be noted that changes of resting heart rate are not consistently found in athletes suffering from OTS (Meeusen et al., 2006).

There are many reports of upper respiratory track infections (URTI) due to increased training, and also in OR and OTS athletes. The amount of scientific information to substantiate these arguments is, however, limited. It is unknown if immune function is seriously impaired in athletes suffering from OTS, as there is insufficient scientific data available. However, anecdotal reports from athletes and coaches of an increased infection rate with OTS (Smith, 2000) have been supported by a few empirical studies (Kingsbury et al., 1998; Reid et al., 2004).

The current information regarding the immune system and OR confirms that periods of intensified training result in depressed immune cell functions, with little or no alteration in circulating cell numbers. However, although immune parameters change in response to increased training load, these changes do not vary between those athletes who successfully adapt to OR and those who maladapt and develop symptoms of OTS.

For several years, it has been hypothesised that a hormonal-mediated central disregulation occurs during the pathogenesis of OTS, and that measurements of blood hormones could help detect OTS (Kuipers and Keizer, 1988; Fry and Kraemer, 1991; Urhausen et al., 1995, 1998a; Fry et al., 1997; Keizer, 1998; Fry et al., 2006). Meeusen et al. (2004) recently published a test protocol with two consecutive maximal exercise tests separated by 4 hours. With this protocol, they found that in order to detect signs of OTS and distinguish them from normal training responses or FOR, this method may be a good indicator not only of the recovery capacity of the athlete but also of the ability to normally perform the second bout of exercise. The use of two bouts of maximal exercise to study neuroendocrine variations showed an adapted exercise-induced increase of adrenocorticotrope hormone, prolactin, and growth hormone to a two-exercise bout (Meeusen et al., 2004). The test could therefore be used as an indirect measure of hypothalamic-pituitary capacity. In a FOR stage, a less pronounced neuroendocrine response to a second bout of exercise on the same day is found, while in an NFOR stage, the hormonal response to a two-bout exercise protocol shows an extreme increased release after the second exercise trigger (Meeusen et al., 2004). With the same protocol, it has been shown that athletes suffering from OTS have an extremely large increase in hormonal release in the first exercise bout, followed by a complete suppression in the second exercise bout (Meeusen et al., 2004). This could indicate hypersensitivity of the pituitary, followed by insensitivity or exhaustion afterwards. Previous reports that used a single exercise protocol found similar effects (Meeusen et al., 2004). It appears that the use of two exercise bouts is more useful in detecting overreaching for preventing overtraining. Early detection of overreaching may be very important in the prevention of overtraining.

Diagnosis

Although the knowledge of the pathomechanisms of OTS has significantly increased in recent years, there is still a strong demand for relevant tools for the early diagnosis of OTS. OTS is characterised by a 'sports-specific' decrease in performance, together with persistent fatigue and disturbances in mood-state (Armstrong and Van Heest, 2002; Urhausen and Kindermann, 2002; Halson and Jeukendrup, 2004; Meeusen et al., 2006). Importantly, as there is no diagnostic tool to identify an athlete as suffering from OTS, diagnosis can only be made by excluding all other possible influences on changes in performance and mood-state. Therefore, if no explanation for the observed changes can be found, OTS is diagnosed. Early and unequivocal recognition of OTS is virtually impossible because the only certain sign of this condition is a decrease in performance during competition or training. The definitive diagnosis of OTS always requires the exclusion of an organic disease, e.g. endocrinological disorders (thyroid or adrenal gland, diabetes), iron deficiency with anaemia, or infectious diseases

(Meeusen *et al.*, 2006). Other major disorders or eating disorders, such as anorexia nervosa and bulimia, should also be excluded. However, it should be emphasised that many endocrinological and clinical findings due to NFOR and OTS can mimic other diseases. The borderline between under- and overdiagnosis is very difficult to judge (Meeusen *et al.*, 2006).

Conclusion

A difficulty in recognising and conducting research into athletes with OTS is defining the point at which OTS develops. The majority of studies aimed at identifying markers of ensuing OTS are actually reporting markers of excessive exercise stress, resulting in the acute condition of OR and not the chronic condition of OTS. Until there is a definite diagnostic tool, it is of utmost importance to standardise measures that are now thought to provide a good inventory of the training status of the athlete. It is very important to emphasise the need to distinguish OTS from OR and other potential causes of temporary under-performance, such as anaemia, acute infection, muscle damage, and insufficient carbohydrate intake.

The physical demands of intensified training are not the only elements in the development of OTS. It seems that a complex set of psychological factors are important in the development of OTS, including excessive expectations from coach or family members, competitive stress, personality structure, social environment, relationships with family and friends, monotony in training, personal or emotional problems, and school- or work-related demands. While no single marker can be taken as an indicator of impending OTS, the regular monitoring of a combination of performance and physiological, biochemical, immunological, and psychological variables would seem to be the best strategy to identify athletes who are failing to cope with the stress of training.

Much more research is necessary to get a clear-cut answer to the origin and detection of OTS. Therefore, we encourage researchers and clinicians to report as much as possible on individual cases of athletes who are underperforming and, by following the exclusion diagnosis, find if they are suffering from OTS.

References

Armstrong, L. and VanHeest, J., 2002, The unknown mechanisms of the overtraining syndrome. Clues from depression and psychoneuroimmunology. *Sports Medicine*, **32**, pp. 185–209.

Fry, A. and Kraemer, W., 1997, Resistance exercise overtraining and overreaching. *Sports Medicine*, **23**, pp. 106–129.

Fry, A., Steinacker, J. and Meeusen, R., 2006, Endocrinology of overtraining. In: Kraemer, W. and Rogol, A. (eds), 'The Endocrine System in Sports and Exercise', Volume XI of the *Encyclopaedia of Sports Medicine*. Blackwell Publishing USA.

Fry, R., Morton, A. and Keast, D., 1991, Overtraining in athletes, *Sports Medicine*, **12**, pp. 32–65.

Halson, S. and Jeukendrup, A., 2004, Does overtraining exist? An analysis of overreaching and overtraining research. *Sports Medicine*, **34**, pp. 967–981.

Keizer, H., 1998, Neuroendicrine aspects of overtraining. In: Kreider, R., Fry, A.C., O'Toole, M. (eds), *Overtraining in Sport*. Champaign IL: Human Kinetics, pp. 145–168.

Kingsbury, K.J., Kay, L. and Hjelm, M., 1998, Contrasting plasma amino acid patterns in elite athletes: Association with fatigue and infection. *British Journal of Sports Medicine*, **32**, pp. 25–33.

Kuipers, H. and Keizer, H., 1988, Overtraining in elite athletes. *Sports Medicine*, **6**, pp. 79–92.

Meeusen, R., Piacentini, M.F., Busschaert, B., Buyse, L., De Schutter, G. and Stray-Gundersen, J., 2004, Hormonal responses in athletes: The use of a two-bout exercise protocol to detect subtle differences in (over)training status. *European Journal of Applied Physiology*, **91**, pp. 140–146.

Meeusen, R., Duclos, M., Gleeson, M., Rietjens, G., Steinacker, J. and Urhausen, A., 2006, Prevention, diagnosis and the treatment of the Overtraining Syndrome. *European Journal of Sport Science*, **6**, pp. 1–14.

Reid, V.L., Gleeson, M, Williams, N. and Clancy, R.L., 2004, Clinical investigation of athletes with persistent fatigue and/or recurrent infections. *British Journal of Sports Medicine*, **38**, pp. 42–45.

Smith, L., 2000, Cytokine hypothesis of overtraining: A physiological adaptation to excessive stress? *Medicine and Science in Sports and Exercise*, **32**, pp. 317–331.

Urhausen, A., Gabriel, H. and Kindermann, W., 1995, Blood hormones as markers of training stress and overtraining. *Sports Medicine*, **20**, pp. 251–276.

Urhausen, A., Gabriel, H. and Kindermann, W., 1998, Impaired pituitary hormonal response to exhaustive exercise in overtrained endurance athletes. *Medicine and Science in Sports and Exercise*, **30**, pp. 407–414.

Urhausen, A., Kindermann, W., 2002, Diagnosis of overtraining, what tools do we have? *Sports Medicine*, **32**, pp. 95–102.

5 The evolution of paediatric fitness test performance

G.R. Tomkinson

School of Health Sciences, University of South Australia, Australia

Introduction

There has been considerable interest in both the lay and scientific literature regarding whether today's children and adolescents are fitter than yesterday's children and adolescents. On the back of considerable anecdotal and lay speculation, it is now widely believed that the fitness of children and adolescents has declined in recent decades (Savage and Scott, 1998). Sedentary technologies, the easy availability of energy-rich food, and declines in community-based physical activity have been implicated (French et al., 2001). While there is certainly some scientific evidence which argues that paediatric fitness has declined (DiNubile, 1993), not all available evidence is supportive, with others arguing that it has not changed at all (Armstrong et al., 1991) or that we can not be confident either way (Rowland, 2002).

The fact that most of the available scientific evidence has made only informal secular comparisons, with occasional rigorous statistical treatment, means that very little is known about secular changes in paediatric fitness. Furthermore, only a few studies have actually reported on secular changes in criterion measures of fitness. Nonetheless, some clues can be gleaned by examining secular changes in paediatric fitness test performance. While various factors (e.g. practice, environmental conditions, motivation, pacing, etc.) influence field test performances, there is good reason to believe that field tests are reliable and reasonably valid estimators of underlying fitness components (Docherty, 1996). The aim of this study therefore, is to quantify the global evolution of children's aerobic and anaerobic fitness test performance over the last part of the twentieth century.

Methods

Hitherto, the reviews of Tomkinson (2007) and Tomkinson and Olds (2007) provide the most complete commentary on secular changes in paediatric aerobic and anaerobic fitness test performance. Using a meta-analytical strategy, Tomkinson (2007) and Tomkinson and Olds (2007) reviewed 42 studies which examined the secular changes in power (single jump tests), speed (sprint and sprint-agility running tests) and aerobic (distance, timed and endurance shuttle running tests) test performances requiring maximal effort. The reviews included only studies which explicitly commented on secular changes in fitness test performances across at least two time points, spanning a minimum range of three years, on comparable populations. Secular changes were calculated at the country × age × sex × test level using least squares linear regression weighted by the square root of sample size, and were expressed as a percentage of the weighted mean value for all data points in the regression. Negative values were used to indicate secular declines, and positive values secular improvements.

Results

Secular changes in power ($n = 20,802,929$), speed ($n = 28,320,308$) and aerobic ($n = 25,455,527$) performance were calculated for 6–19-year-olds from 32 countries (representing five geographical regions) between 1958 and 2003. Over the 45-year period, power and speed test performances improved at +0.03 per cent and +0.04 per cent per annum (p.a.), respectively, while aerobic performances declined at –0.36 per cent p.a.

Secular differences in boys and girls, and children and adolescents

Over the period 1958–2003, weighted mean changes for boys and girls were strikingly similar for power (+0.03 per cent vs +0.04 per cent p.a.) and speed (+0.05 per cent vs +0.05 per cent p.a.), with boys declining at a greater rate than girls for aerobic performance (–0.40 per cent vs –0.31 per cent p.a.). A similar pattern emerged for children and adolescents, with similarities for power (0.00 per cent vs +0.06 per cent p.a.) and speed (0.00 per cent vs +0.08 per cent p.a.), and greater declines in children than in adolescents for aerobic performance (–0.47 per cent vs –0.27 per cent p.a.).

Secular differences among geographical regions

Secular changes were reasonably similar for different geographical regions. Since 1970, there has been little overall change in power test performance, with improvements in Africa and the Middle East (+0.34 per cent p.a.), Australasia (+0.08 per cent p.a.), and North America (+0.26 per cent p.a.), and declines in Asia (–0.03 per cent p.a.) and Europe (–0.09 per cent p.a.). There has also been little overall change in speed test performance, with improvements in Europe (+0.03 per cent p.a.) and North America (+0.03 per cent p.a.), and declines in Africa and the Middle East (–0.09 per cent p.a.), Asia (–0.03 per cent p.a.) and Australasia (–0.06 per cent p.a.). On the other hand, aerobic test performances have declined globally at –0.46 per cent p.a. over this time, with only the performances of Asian (–0.44 per cent p.a.) and European (–0.31 per cent p.a.) children and adolescents declining at rates less than the global decline.

The time-related patterns of change and performance

The secular changes however, have not always been consistent over time (Figure 5.1; panel a). Changes for both power and speed were initially positive (i.e. improvements); however, in about 1985 there was a crossover from positive to negative (i.e. declines) for power, and a drop from positive to zero (i.e. no change) for speed. Aerobic changes were also initially positive, from the late

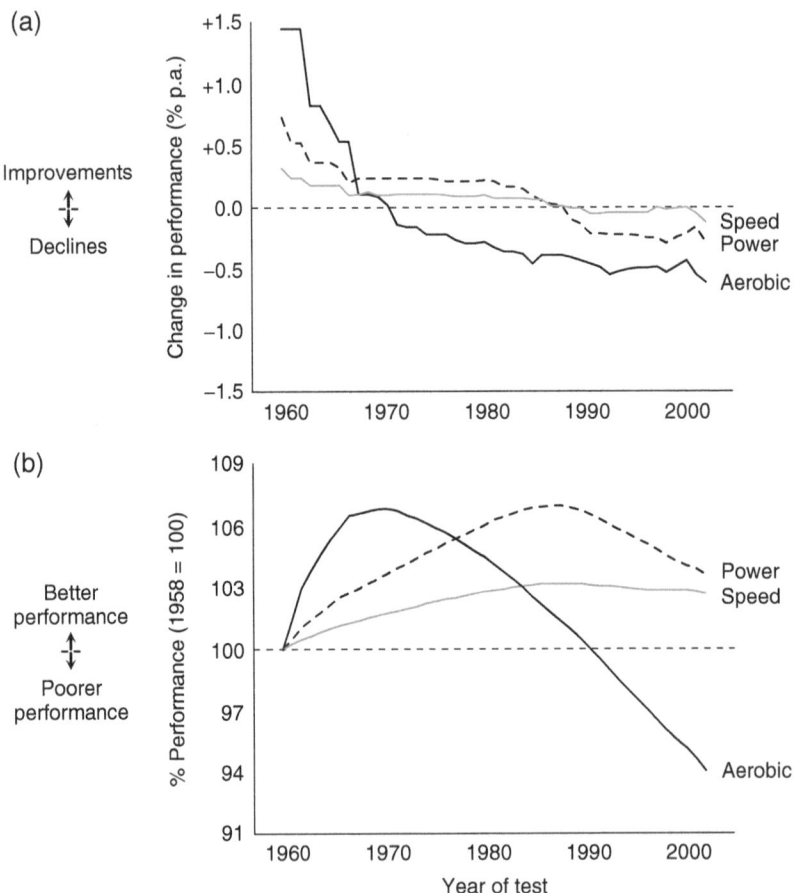

Figure 5.1 Global time-related patterns of (a) change and (b) performance for aerobic fitness tests (black lines) and anaerobic fitness tests of power (dotted lines) and speed (grey lines) for the period 1958–2002. The anaerobic test data are from Tomkinson (2007) and the aerobic test data from Tomkinson and Olds (2007). In (a), higher values (i.e. those greater than zero) indicate improvements in performance; in (b) higher values (i.e. those greater than 100) indicate better performance. Adapted by permission from Tomkinson (2007) and Tomkinson and Olds (2007).

1950s through to about 1970, where changes crossed from positive to negative, increasing in magnitude every decade thereafter.

Figure 5.1 (panel b) describes the time-related patterns of performance, standardised to 1958 = 100. Power test performances consistently improved from the late 1950s until the early 1980s, stabilising until the late 1980s, followed by a 15-year decline. Speed test performances, on the other hand, steadily increased over the period 1958–1985, and plateaued thereafter. Aerobic performances improved sharply from the late 1950s until the mid-1960s, where there was a performance shoulder until the mid-1970s, followed by a 25–30 year decline.

Discussion

Using data on over 74 million children and adolescents from 32 countries tested between 1958 and 2003, these data show that, over the past three decades, there has been a sharp decline in aerobic performance and relative stability in anaerobic performance. Secular changes were remarkably similar for boys and girls, for children and adolescents, and reasonably similar for different geographical regions. This section offers an interpretation of the secular declines in aerobic performance, and speculates on why aerobic performances have declined and anaerobic performances have remained relatively stable.

Causes of the secular declines in aerobic performance

What is causing this recent decline in aerobic performance? It has been argued that secular declines in aerobic performances requiring maximal effort are caused by a network of social, behavioural, physical, psychosocial and physiological factors (Tomkinson and Olds, 2007). Proximate causes of declines in running performance requiring maximal effort are essentially changes in maximal oxygen uptake, mechanical efficiency and the sustainable fraction of maximal oxygen uptake (Sjödin and Svedenhag, 1985). Furthermore, a reduction in psychosocial aspects of maximal performance, both affective (e.g. motivation) and cognitive (e.g. pacing), may also be important. These changes are in turn affected by physical changes, such as increased fat mass and reduced cardiovascular function (Westerstahl *et al.*, 2003). So what has caused these physical changes? Ultimately, they are the result of behavioural changes such as excessive energy intake relative to expenditure, reduced energy expenditure, and reduced vigorous physical activity (Tomkinson *et al.*, 2003). Finally, these behavioural changes, in turn, are likely mediated by a changing social and built environment (e.g. a changing family profile, a breakdown of local communities, the increased use of sedentary technologies, and a shift towards suburbanisation), which is becoming 'toxic for exercise' (Tomkinson *et al.*, 2003).

Though this model describes plausible underlying causal mechanisms, it is the changes in fitness test performance which are of primary interest, rather than the underlying mechanisms. It is the ability to run fast, play harder and keep moving longer which is important for children's physical activity levels, irrespective of the mechanistic factors responsible for the changes.

Secular differences in aerobic and anaerobic performances

Why have aerobic performances declined over recent decades, and anaerobic performances remained relatively stable? While the answer is not obvious, these secular differences may be due to the differential effects of fat mass and fat-free mass on aerobic and anaerobic performances (Tomkinson, 2007). Advances in the rate of maturation (and therefore differences in the age-related changes in performance) may also play a role (Tomkinson *et al.*, 2006). It is also possible that skill contributes more to paediatric anaerobic performance, and without evidence of secular changes in paediatric motor skills, anaerobic performances could be less susceptible to secular change (Tomkinson and Olds, 2007). Though not complete, these are at least three reasons for the secular differences in aerobic and anaerobic performances.

Conclusion

These data provide overwhelming evidence of secular declines in paediatric aerobic performance in recent decades, and relative stability in anaerobic performance. The aetiology of the secular change in aerobic performance is difficult to pinpoint, although it is likely caused by a network of social, behavioural, physical, psychosocial and physiological factors.

References

Armstrong, N., Williams, J., Balding, J., Gentle, P. and Kirby, B., 1991, The peak oxygen uptake of British children with reference to age, sex, and sexual maturity. *European Journal of Applied Physiology*, **62**, pp. 369–375.

DiNubile, N.A., 1993, Youth fitness – problems and solutions. *Preventive Medicine*, **22**, pp. 589–594.

Docherty, D., 1996, Field tests and test batteries. In: *Measurement in Pediatric Exercise Science*, edited by Docherty, D. Champaign, IL: Human Kinetics, pp. 285–334.

French, S.A., Story, M. and Jeffery, R.W., 2001, Environmental influences on eating and physical activity. *Annual Review of Public Health*, **22**, pp. 309–335.

Rowland, T., 2002, Declining cardiorespiratory fitness in youth: Fact or supposition? *Pediatric Exercise Science*, **14**, pp. 1–8.

Savage, M.P. and Scott, L.B., 1998, Physical activity and rural middle school adolescents. *Journal of Youth and Adolescence*, **27**, pp. 245–253.

Sjödin, B. and Svedenhag, J., 1985, Applied physiology of marathon running. *Sports Medicine*, **2**, pp. 83–99.

Tomkinson, G.R., 2007, Global changes in anaerobic fitness test performance of children and adolescents (1958–2003). *Scandinavian Journal of Medicine and Science in Sports*, **17**, pp. 497–507.

Tomkinson, G.R. and Olds, T.S., 2007, Secular changes in pediatric aerobic fitness test performance: The global picture. In: *Pediatric Fitness: Secular Trends and Geographic Variability*, Vol. 50 (Medicine and Sport Science Series), edited by Tomkinson, G.R. and Olds, T.S. Basel: Karger, pp. 46–66.

Tomkinson, G.R., Léger, L.A., Olds, T.S. and Cazorla, G., 2003, Secular trends in the performance of children and adolescents (1980–2000): An analysis of 55 studies of the 20 m shuttle run in 11 countries. *Sports Medicine*, **33**, pp. 285–300.

Tomkinson, G.R., Hamlin, M.J. and Olds, T.S., 2006, Secular trends in anaerobic test performance in Australasian children and adolescents. *Pediatric Exercise Science*, **18**, pp. 314–328.

Westerstahl, M., Barnekow-Bergkvist, M., Hedberg, G. and Jansson, E., 2003, Secular trends in body dimensions and physical fitness among adolescents in Sweden from 1974 to 1995. *Scandinavian Journal of Medicine and Science in Sports*, **13**, pp. 128–137.

6 Cytokines and exercise in children

A. Eliakim and D. Nemet

Child Health and Sports Center, Pediatric Department, Meir Medical Center, Sackler School of Medicine, Tel-Aviv University, Israel

Introduction

Physical activity or inactivity may have profound effects on children's health. These effects are mediated, at least partially, by the relationship between physical activity, anabolic and/or catabolic hormones and circulating inflammatory mediators/cytokines. These relationships are not limited to individuals participating in competitive sports, but also exist for the healthy child and adolescent, and even for the chronically ill child. When studying the complex relations between exercise and these mediators, one should differentiate between the acute effects of a brief, single exercise bout and the adaptations that occur in physically active people or in response to long-term programmes of endurance training.

This paper demonstrates some of the effects of a single exercise bout as well as exercise training on these anabolic/catabolic hormones and inflammatory mediators in each of these conditions.

The young athlete

The efficiency of exercise training depends on the intensity, volume, duration and frequency of training, as well as on the athlete's ability to tolerate it. Thus, many efforts are made to quantify the balance between training load and the athlete's tolerance by objective parameters.

Recent reports suggest, rather surprisingly, that a brief single exercise leads to a simultaneous increase in antagonistic mediators. On the one hand, exercise stimulates anabolic components of the Growth Hormone (GH) → Insulin-like Growth Factor-I (IGF-I) axis, a family of hormones, growth factors, binding proteins and receptors that play a major role in the physiological adaptation to exercise and exercise training (Eliakim *et al.*, 1999; Schwarz *et al.*, 1996). On the other hand, exercise elevates catabolic pro-inflammatory cytokines such as Interlukin-6 (IL-6), IL-1 and tumor necrosis factor-α (TNF-α) (Nemet *et al.*, 2002). These inflammatory mediators are secreted from the muscles, immune cells (e.g. white blood cells) and adipocytes. The net anabolic effect of exercise (e.g. muscle hypertrophy, and as a consequence improved fitness) is determined by the exercise-induced balance between these growth factors and inflammatory mediators. Therefore, it is suggested that assessment of the changes in these circulating mediators following different types of exercise (anaerobic and aerobic-type) may help to quantify the training loads. It is believed that the changes in the GH-IGF-I axis following brief exercise suggest exercise-related anabolic adaptations, and increases of inflammatory cytokines like IL-6 may indicate their important role in muscle tissue repair following exercise.

In contrast, the response of these mediators to prolonged exercise training is more complicated and often bi-phasic (Eliakim *et al.*, 2005). An imposition of a training programme which is associated with substantial increase in energy expenditure leads initially to a marked increase in pro-inflammatory cytokines, and as a consequence, to decreases in anabolic components of the GH-IGF-I axis. Further, if and when the training adaptation is successful, the pro-inflammatory cytokines fall, and with that decrease, the suppression of the GH-IGF-I diminishes, an anabolic 'rebound' in the GH-IGF-I axis may occur, and IGF-I level exceed the pre-training level (Nemet *et al.*, 2004, Figure 6.1).

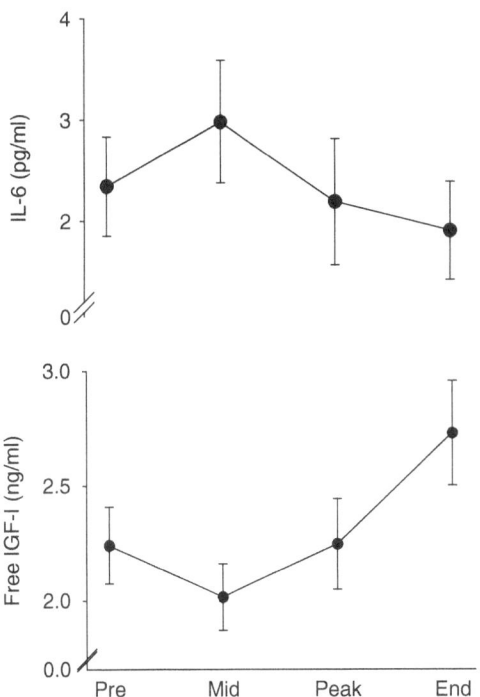

Figure 6.1 Circulating levels of free IGF-I (bottom panel) and IL-6 (top panel) during a training season. During periods of heavy training levels of IL-6 increase, and IGF-I decrease. Tapering down prior to the competition period results in a marked decrease in IL-6 and a sharp anabolic rebound of IGF-I.

Exactly how and when this change occurs, and whether the initial catabolic-type stage is necessary for the ultimate anabolic adaptation remains unknown.

The chronically ill child

In the last two decades childhood obesity has gained epidemic proportions in westernized countries. The mechanisms responsible for the increasing prevalence of childhood obesity are not completely understood, but life-style changes associated with increased caloric intake and decreased energy expenditure probably play an important role. Childhood obesity is associated with increased risk of hypertension, hyperlipidaemia, insulin resistance and the development of type-2 diabetes, increased coagulopathy, and endothelial dysfunction (Dietz, 1998).

Recent studies have shown that circulating levels of inflammatory adipocytokines (mainly IL-6) are elevated in obese children and adolescents. These results suggest that low grade chronic inflammation may play a possible important role in the pathogenesis of *childhood* obesity and the development of its related cardio-vascular complications later in life.

Consistent with the effect of exercise in the young elite athlete, a single exercise leads to a simultaneous transient increase in circulating cytokines and anabolic components of the GH-IGF-I axis. However, the exercise associated increase in GH is significantly attenuated in obese children and adolescents compared to normal weight, age and maturity-matched controls (Eliakim *et al.*, 2006; McMurray *et al.*, 2007). The mechanisms for the blunted exercise-associated increase in GH levels are not completely understood. However, it was suggested that the attenuated GH response to exercise is related to an obesity-associated generalized impairment of the adrenergic and, in particularly, the dopaminergic response to exercise. It is possible that the coupled blunted GH and catecholamine response to exercise leads to reduced carbohydrate and fat utilization during exercise and as a result to a greater protein utilization. This may lead to a lower effect of training in obese children, and may explain the limited success of weight-reduction interventions in changing body composition and improving physical fitness in obese children and adolescents.

Interestingly, very few studies examined the effect of exercise training or weight reduction programmes on inflammatory cytokines in obese children and adolescents. Gallistl *et al.* (2001) examined the effect of a three-week school-based, summer vacation, combined dietary and physical activity intervention on body weight and inflammatory mediators in 49 overweight (BMI > 85 per cent) children and adolescents. Diet consisted of daily caloric intake of 3.5–5 MJ, and physical activity was performed three times each day. However, the type, duration and intensity of exercise were not characterized, fitness was not evaluated and there was no control group. The programme resulted in a significant decrease in body weight, BMI and fat mass, and there was a significant decrease in resting heart rate. The programme was also associated with a significant decrease in IL-6 (by ~100 per cent). In addition, the decrease in IL-6 correlated, although not strongly, with the decrease in BMI. The long-term effects of the programme were not studied.

Consistent with that, Balagopal *et al.* (2005) studied the effect of a combined three-month dietary-behavioural-physical activity intervention on body weight and inflammatory markers in a small group (eight intervention, seven controls) of obese adolescents (BMI > 30 kgm^{-2}). Participants performed 45 minutes of aerobic-type activities (three per week), and were followed by a nutritionist once a week. Nutritional consultations were aimed to reduce consumption of high-caloric beverages and snacks, as well as meal size and reduce sedentary activities such as screen time. The programme led to a significant decrease in body fat, improvement of insulin resistance (determined by HOMA-IR), and to a remarkable decrease in C-reactive protein, fibrinogen and IL-6 (Figure 6.2). Fitness level was not assessed.

These studies indicate that weight reduction programmes which include aerobic-type exercise training in obese children and adolescents result in a decrease in circulating cytokines, and suggest that the exercise preventive role in obesity is mediated, at least partially, by attenuation of the inflammatory response. However, the relative contribution of weight and adiposity loss, or improvement of physical fitness, could not be estimated. Moreover, due to the paucity of studies, further research in larger and specific populations is needed to clarify the mechanisms that link physical activity, fitness and inflammation in childhood obesity.

The healthy child

The health consequences of being overweight during childhood and adolescence are now very well recognized, and the preponderance of evidence suggests that physical inactivity plays a role in the development of obesity (typically determined

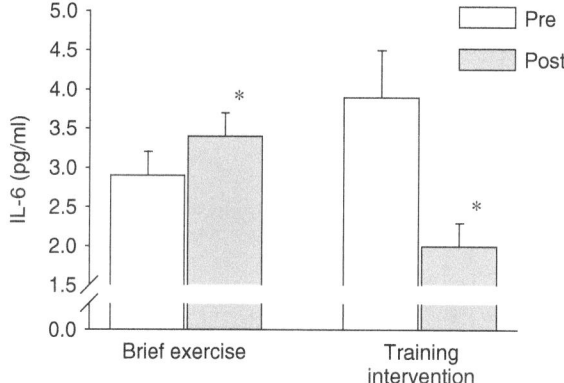

Figure 6.2 The effect of a brief exercise (left panel) and exercise training (right panel) on circulating IL-6 levels in obese children. While a brief exercise leads to an increase in IL-6 levels, training is associated with a decreased inflammatory state.

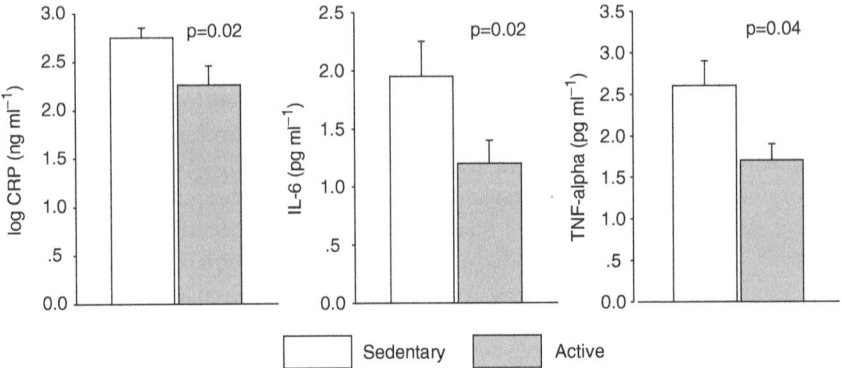

Figure 6.3 Levels of inflammatory mediators in active and sedentary normal weight healthy adolescent girls. Increased physical activity was associated with reduced circulating levels of inflammatory mediators.

by body mass index [BMI]). However, what remains enigmatic are the specific roles of body fat and physical activity per se. The question – how would an active and inactive adolescent, each with the same BMI, compare in terms of health risk assessment – has been difficult to approach and answer.

In order to begin to gauge independent effects of physical activity on health risk, we matched by BMI two groups of *normal-weight* adolescent females (BMI percentile ~ 58). One group was physically active – all participated in high school sports; and one was sedentary (Ischander *et al.*, 2007). Active girls had significantly greater muscle mass and were fitter, had lower inflammatory cytokines levels (i.e. CRP, IL-6, and TNF-α; Figure 6.3) and leptin. In addition, the active girls had higher levels of adiponectin, a recently discovered adipocytokine which is unique in that its circulating levels are inversely related to fat mass in both children and adults, and was found to protect against adverse consequences of obesity such as insulin resistance.

In adolescent girls, the choice of a lifestyle involving high-school sports is characterized by circulating mediators and a body composition pattern that, if sustained, is associated with generally lower long-term risk of cardiovascular disease later in life. Therefore, efforts should be made to promote physical activity in this unique population, since levels of physical activity decline dramatically in girls during puberty.

Summary

The exercise-associated adaptations of anabolic/catabolic hormone and inflammatory cytokines indicate that these markers may be used to gauge the training intensity of aerobic and anaerobic-type exercise and exercise training.

The effect of exercise training on pro-inflammatory cytokines is potentially beneficial for healthy children, for children with chronic diseases and for children involved in competitive sports.

References

Balagopal, P., George, D., Patton, N., Yarandi, H., Roberts W.L., Bayne, E. and Gidding, S., 2005, Lifestyle-only intervention attenuates the inflammatory state associated with obesity: A randomized controlled study in adolescents. *Journal of Pediatrics*, **146**, pp. 342–348.

Dietz, W.H., 1998, Health consequences of obesity in youth: Childhood predictors of adult disease. *Pediatrics*, **101**, pp. 518–525.

Eliakim, A., Brasel, J.A. and Cooper, D.M., 1999, GH response to exercise: Assessment of the pituitary refractory period, and relationship with circulating components of the GH-IGF-I axis in adolescent females. *Journal of Pediatric Endocrinology and Metabolism*, **12**, pp. 47–55.

Eliakim, A., Nemet, D. and Cooper D.M., 2005, Exercise, training and the GH-IGF-I axis. In: *The Endocrine System in Sports and Exercise*. Oxford: Blackwell Publishing, pp. 165–179.

Eliakim, A., Nemet, D., Zaldivar, F., McMurray, R.G., Culler, F.L., Galassetti, P. and Cooper D.M., 2006, Reduced exercise-associated response of the GH-IGF-I axis and catecholamines in obese children and adolescents. *Journal of Applied Physiology*, **100**, pp. 1630–1637.

Gallistl, S., Sudi, K.M., Aigner, R. and Borkenstein, M., 2001, Changes in serum interleukin-6 concentrations in obese children and adolescents during a weight reduction program. *International Journal of Obesity and Related Metabolic Disorders*, **25**, pp. 1640–1643.

Ischander, M., Zaldivar, F. Jr., Eliakim, A., Nussbaum, E., Dunton, G., Leu, S.Y., Cooper, D.M. and Schneider, M., 2007, Physical activity, growth, and inflammatory mediators in BMI-matched female adolescents. *Medicine and Science in Sports and Exercise*, **39,** pp. 1131–1138.

McMurray, R.G., Zaldivar, F., Galassetti, P., Larson, J., Eliakim, A., Nemet, D. and Cooper, D.M., 2007, Cellular immunity and inflammatory mediator responses to intense exercise in overweight children and adolescents. *Journal of Investigative Medicine*, **55**, pp. 120–129.

Nemet, D., Oh, Y., Kim, H.S., Hill, M. and Cooper, D.M., 2002, Effect of intense exercise on inflammatory cytokines and growth mediators in adolescent boys. *Pediatrics*, **110**, pp. 681–689.

Nemet, D., Pontello, A.M, Rose-Gottron, C. and Cooper, D.M., 2004, Cytokines and growth factors during and after a wrestling season in adolescent boys. *Medicine and Science in Sports and Exercise*, **36**, pp. 794–800.

Schwarz, A.J., Brasel, J.A., Hintz, R.L., Mohan, S. and Cooper, D.M., 1996, Acute effect of brief low and high intensity exercise on circulating IGF-I, II, and IGF-I binding protein-3 and its proteolysis in young healthy men. *Journal of Clinical Endocrinology and Metabolism*, **81**, pp. 3492–3497.

Part II
Health and well-being

7 Does the positive effect of physical activity during childhood and adolescence on bone mass accrual persist into early adult life?

A.D.G. Baxter-Jones,[1] *R.L. Mirwald,*[1]
R.A. Faulkner,[1] *K.C. Kowalski*[1] *and D.A. Bailey*[1,2]
[1]College of Kinesiology, University of Saskatchewan, Saskatoon, Saskatchewan, Canada and [2]School of Human Movement Studies, University of Queensland, Brisbane, Australia

Introduction

It is thought that bone accrual and mineralization should be maximized as a primary means of preventing osteoporosis. Bone may be most receptive to the influence of physical activity during childhood and adolescence. Numerous studies have provided evidence of increased bone mineral content (BMC), not only in child and adolescent athletes involved in high impact activities, but also children and adolescents who simply had a more physically active lifestyle (Janz *et al.*, 2001; Cooper *et al.*, 2005). It remains inconclusive, however, if these affects of physical activity on BMC during the growing years persist into early adulthood.

We previously showed that physical activity significantly affected bone mineral accrual in growing children over a 6-year period (Bailey *et al.*, 1999). We now have continuous longitudinal data on this same group of subjects into their young adult years. We hypothesize that those adults who were classified as active as children will have greater BMC than adults who were classified as inactive in childhood.

Methods

Participants were from the Saskatchewan Pediatric Bone Mineral Accrual Study (PBMAS), which used a mixed longitudinal cohort design. Individuals were repeatedly measured for up to seven consecutive years from 1991 through to 1997 and then again from 2002 through to 2007. In 1991 the parents of 228 students (113 boys and 115 girls) provided written consent. After seven years of data collection 109 males and 121 females had been measured on two or more occasions (median six years). Between 2002 and 2007, 169 subjects were measured on at least one more occasion (age range 18.2 to 29.5 years). The present analysis uses longitudinal data from 66 females and 61 males.

Anthropometric measurements, including stature and body weight, were taken at six-month intervals following standard protocols. Maturity status was measured by establishing the age at peak height velocity (PHV) using a cubic spline procedure fitted to whole-year height velocities.

Bone mineral content (BMC, g) of the total body (TB), lumbar spine (LS, L1–L4), total hip (TH) and the femoral neck (FN) was measured annually by dual-energy X-ray absorptiometry using the Hologic QDR 2000 (Hologic, Inc., Waltham, MA, USA).

Physical activity was assessed using the Physical Activity Questionnaire for Children (PAQ-C) or Adolescents (PAQ-A) (Crocker et al., 1997). During adulthood, the Physical Activity Questionnaire for Adults (PAQ-AD) was developed and used (Copeland et al., 2005). For each individual an age and gender specific Z score was determined for each test administration. An average childhood and adolescent Z score was then calculated, as was an adult average. Quartiles of the Z scores were then formed. Individuals whose activity Z score fell in the highest quartile were classified as active, those in the lowest quartile were classified as inactive.

All data were analyzed using SPSS for Windows, version 15.0 (SPSS, Inc., Chicago, IL, USA). Analysis of variance (ANOVA) was used to examine adult within gender differences between the three childhood physical activity groupings for all anthropometric characteristics, physical activity and bone variables (TB, TH, FN and LS BMC). Two (gender) by three (physical activity groups) analysis of covariance (ANCOVA) analysis were performed to evaluate the effects of childhood activity on each BMC site in adulthood. Significance level was set at $p < 0.05$.

Results

At follow-up the average age was 22.9 years (range 18.2 to 29.5 years). Somatic maturity (attainment of peak height velocity (PHV)) had occurred, on average, 10.3 years previously (range 5.5 to 14.7 years).

Within genders, no significant differences were found between physical activity groups for chronological age, maturity age, height or weight ($p > 0.05$). However, adult and childhood normalized mean physical activity scores were significantly different, with the active childhood group having the highest normalized values (Z-scores); $p < 0.05$. There was a significant correlation between the average childhood physical activity z-score and adult physical activity Z score; $r = 0.43$, $p < 0.05$.

In the factorial ANCOVA (covariates maturity age, chronological age, height, weight and adult physical activity) it was found that neither chronological age, maturity age nor adult physical activity were significant covariates for adult BMC values at any site; $p > 0.05$. In the factorial 2 (male, female) × 3 (inactive, average, active) ANCOVA (covariates mean adult height and weight) models no interaction effects were found for any of the dependent variables; $p > 0.05$. There were however significant main effects (gender and childhood activity groups) at each BMC site; $p < 0.05$. Males had significantly greater values of adjusted BMC, when physical activity group was ignored, compared to females at all sites (TB – 2731 ± 40.7 vs 2392 ± 38.8, TH – 43.8 ± 0.9 vs 33.7 ± 0.9, FN – 5.15 ± 0.10 vs 4.52 ± 0.09, LS – 69.9 ± 1.8 vs 61.5 ± 1.7; $p < 0.05$).

When the genders were combined the active childhood group had significantly greater adjusted mean adult BMC values at the TB, TH and FN than the inactive childhood group; $p < 0.05$. There were no significant differences between childhood activity groups at the LS; $p > 0.05$ (Figure 7.1).

Discussion

This study suggests that the positive effects of childhood physical activity during the time of peak bone mineral accrual persist into young adulthood.

There is increasing evidence that physical activity during the growing years affects bone mineral acquisition (Janz *et al.*, 2001; MacKelvie *et al.*, 2004), and we have reported previously in the present sample that regular every-day physical activity during the growing years affected bone mineral accrual (Bailey *et al.*, 1999). However, even if exercise during the growing years affects bone accrual, the importance of these effects from a clinical perspective depends on their permanence.

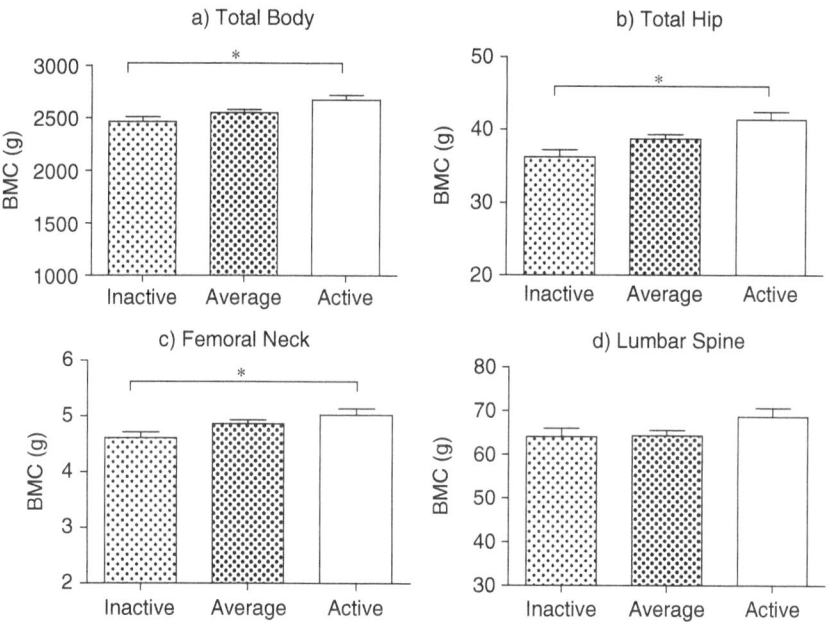

Figure 7.1 Comparison of adjusted mean (± SE) adult BMC values (covariates height and weight) between childhood activity groups (males and females combined) for (a) TB, (b) TH, (c) FN and (d) LS.
*Significantly different between groups; $p < 0.05$.

The results of the present study showed that subjects classified as active during childhood and adolescence maintained their advantage in BMC (at the TB, TH and FN sites) over those classified as inactive. Using the combined sample of males and females, the active group compared to the inactive group had 8 per cent greater BMC at the TB, 14 per cent greater at the TH and 9 per cent greater at the FN. Although not significant, the actives also had a 7 per cent advantage at the LS site. In our original study, one year after the attainment of peak bone mineral content, at the TB, the differences were 9 per cent in boys and 16 per cent in girls. Active boys had 7 per cent more BMC at the FN than inactive boys, and in girls the difference was 11 per cent (Bailey *et al.*, 1999). Thus, the current data provide strong support for the conjecture that physical activity related benefits of greater bone accrual during the growing years persists into young adult life.

In summary, there is increasing evidence that physical activity during the growing years affects components of bone strength such as bone mineral accrual; however, the importance of this observation for long-term skeletal health is not yet clear. The present study supports the conjecture that the effects of physical activity on bone mass persist into (at least) young adulthood. It has been speculated that a lower peak bone mass obtained during the growing years is related to increased fracture risk in later life (Seeman, 1994); thus the present study has implications for strategies to reduce lifetime risk of osteoporosis.

References

Bailey, D.A., McKay, H.A., Mirwald, R.L., Crocker, P.R., Faulkner, R.A., 1999, A six-year longitudinal study of the relationship of physical activity to bone mineral accrual in growing children. *Journal of Bone and Mineral Research*, **14**, pp. 1672–1679.

Cooper, C., Cawley, M., Bhalla, A., Egger, P., Ring, F., Morton, L., Barker, D., 1995, Childhood growth, physical-activity, and peak bone mass in women. *Journal of Bone and Mineral Research*, **10**, pp. 940–947.

Copeland, J.L., Kowalski, K.C., Donen, R.M., Tremblay, M.S., 2005, Convergent validity of the Physical Activity Questionnaire for Adults: The new member of the PAQ family. *Journal of Physical Activity and Health*, **2**, pp. 216–229.

Crocker, P.R.E., Bailey, D.A., Faulkner, R.A., Kowalski, K.C., McGrath, R., 1997, Measuring general levels of physical activity: Preliminary evidence for the physical activity questionnaire for older children. *Medicine and Science in Sports and Exercise*, **29**, pp. 1344–1349.

Janz, K.F., Burns, T.L., Torner, J.C., Levy, S.M., Paulos, R., Willing, M.C., Warren, J.J., 2001, Physical activity and bone measures in young children: The Iowa Bone Development Study. *Pediatrics*, **107**, pp. 1387–1393.

MacKelvie, K.J., Petit, M.A., Khan, K.M., Beck, T.J., McKay, H.A., 2004, Bone mass and structure are enhanced following a 2-year randomized controlled trial of exercise in prepubertal boys. *Bone*, **34**, pp. 755–764.

Seeman, E., 1994, Reduced bone density in women with fractures: Contribution of low peak bone density and rapid bone loss. *Osteoporosis International*, **4**(Suppl.1), pp. 15–25.

8 RER variability analysis by sample entropy

A preliminary comparison of obese and lean children

G.R. Biltz,[1] J.H. Harmon,[1] D.R. Dengel,[1] V.B. Unnithan[2] and G. Witten[3]

[1]School of Kinesiology, University of Minnesota, Minneapolis, MN, USA; [2]Sport Department, Liverpool Hope University, Liverpool, UK; [3]Department of Mathematics and Applied Mathematics, University of Cape Town, Cape Town, SA

Introduction

Research by Kelley *et al.* (2000) has shown an altered metabolic pattern in obese individuals that they call 'metabolic inflexibility'. In metabolic inflexibility (MI) fatty acid metabolism is not suppressed by rising insulin levels and it is not increased as expected in the basal or fasting state. Thus, the relative substrate flows appear 'inflexible' to changing metabolic conditions. This same observation was made by Caprio (1999) on obese adolescent females. An increased accumulation of intramuscular triglyceride appears to disrupt normal insulin signaling and results in insulin resistance for affected myocytes (Kelley *et al.*, 2000). The normal capacity to switch between carbohydrate and free fatty acid fuels based on availability and metabolic context is diminished – metabolic inflexibility.

The purpose of this study was to investigate breath-by-breath respiratory exchange ratio (RER) for features of metabolic inflexibility in obesity. We chose a form of variability analysis called sample entropy (SampEn), developed by Richman and Moorman (2000), that can be used to measure the regularity of any data sequence with or without time dependence. We hypothesize that obese children with metabolic inflexibility will have increased regularity within serial RER values compared to lean children. Also, we hypothesize that the SampEn scores for the RER series from the obese child will be less (greater regularity) than the scores from lean children during steady state activity.

Methods

Thirteen overweight ($\geq 85\%$ BMI for age and gender) plus obese ($\geq 95\%$ BMI for age and gender) children (4F, 9M: age $= 11.5 \pm 1.7$ y.) and nine lean ($\leq 85\%$ BMI

Table 8.1 Physical characteristics of subjects

	Lean	Obese	p-value
Number	9	13	–
Tanner stage	2.9 ± 0.3	2.8 ± 0.2	0.91
Age (y)	12.3 ± 0.7	11.5 ± 0.5	0.29
Weight (kg)	43.4 ± 4.0	70.1 ± 6.5	0.005
Height (m)	1.56 ± 0.04	1.60 ± 0.03	0.49
BMI (kg·m^{-2})	17.4 ± 0.7	26.9 ± 1.8	0.003

for age and gender) children (6F, 3M: age = 12.3 ± 2.2 y.) voluntarily participated in the study. See Table 8.1 for physical characteristics of the two groups.

Known medical problems that would have constrained the cycle ergometry testing were considered exclusion criteria for participating. None of the subjects were participating in systematic sport or exercise training. Verbal assent from the children and written informed consent from parents or guardians were obtained before participation. The study was approved by the local institutional review board.

All subjects underwent two continuous submaximal exercise stages at constant work rate on an electromagnetically-braked cycle ergometer (Excaliber, Lode, The Netherlands). The first stage was three minutes of unloaded cycling at 50 rpm cadence and the second stage was at 50W workload at 50 rpm cadence for all subjects. This 50W stage was sustained for five minutes. Following the two submaximal stages, the workload was increased by 25W every two minutes until volitional exhaustion. Criteria for achievement of peak exercise were a heart rate within 10 beats of 200 and an RER of ≥ 1.1. Expired oxygen and carbon dioxide concentrations and volumes were collected and analyzed using a Cosmed Quark metabolic cart (Rome, Italy). Prior to all tests, oxygen and carbon dioxide sensors were calibrated with standard gases of known oxygen (16 per cent) and carbon dioxide (5 per cent) concentrations. Resting and exercise data were calculated on a breath-by-breath basis. The determination of submaximal steady state and peak values was based on averaging 20-second epochs of the breath-by-breath data.

Breath-by-breath VCO_2, $\dot{V}O_2$, and RER data files were imported into a software program (Matlab, The Math Works, Inc., Natik, MA) for computation of RER variability using sample entropy analysis (SampEn) according to the recommendations of Richman and Moorman (2000). SampEn score is effectively a conditional probability: SampEn = − log A/B. Where B is the total number of matches of length **m** in the data series and A is the total number of matches at length **m+1** within the set of matches B. Data points within **m** and **m+1** are said to match if they agree within a pre-selected tolerance **r**. We chose **m** = 4 and **r** = 0.2 (std. dev.) for our SampEn analysis. Recommendations for selecting **m** and **r** and the determination of confidence intervals for SampEn can be found in Lake *et al.* (2002). All reported RER SampEn scores are for the single, five-minute, 50W cycling interval.

Table 8.2 Cycling oxygen uptake at 50W and peak workloads

	Lean	Obese	p-value
Peak $\dot{V}O_2$ (L·min^{-1})	1.50 ± 0.17	2.00 ± 0.13	0.027
Peak $\dot{V}O_2$ (mL·kg^{-1}·min^{-1})	34.8 ± 1.1	29.8 ± 1.6	0.019
Peak $\dot{V}O_2$ (mL·kgFFM^{-1}·min^{-1})	41.7 ± 1.7	45.4 ± 1.0	0.049
$\dot{V}O_2$ (L·min^{-1}) @ 50W	0.85 ± 0.03	1.02 ± 0.05	0.006
$\dot{V}O_2$ (mL·kg^{-1}·min^{-1}) @ 50W	20.5 ± 1.4	16.2 ± 0.7	0.006
$\dot{V}O_2$ (mL·kgFFM^{-1}·min^{-1}) @ 50W	24.5 ± 1.7	23.8 ± 1.6	0.781

Standard statistical analysis of RER data sequences and comparisons between obese and lean subjects were performed using Statview (Abacus Concepts, Inc., Berkeley, CA). An alpha level of 0.05 was accepted for statistical significance.

Results

A comparison of oxygen consumption characteristics for lean and obese subjects is found in Table 8.2. At 50W cycling there was not a significant difference between lean and obese in oxygen consumption relative to fat-free mass.

During 50W cycling the average RER values for the obese subjects were significantly lower than the lean group (0.86 ± 0.01 vs 0.92 ± 0.01, $p = 0.002$). The SampEn of the RER serial data was lower for the obese subjects as hypothesized (1.49 ± 0.08 vs 1.72 ± 0.13, $p = 0.06$). This is clearly suggestive of a trend toward increased regularity in the RER patterns of the obese subjects but not statistically significant.

Since body mass was significantly different between groups and all subjects pedaled at 50W for the RER sampling interval, we compared their relative oxygen consumption at 50W cycling. When O_2 consumption was adjusted relative to fat-free mass, the fractional utilization (50W $\dot{V}O_2$/Peak $\dot{V}O_2$) showed no significant difference between obese and lean ($52.2\% \pm 4.7$ vs $59.5\% \pm 2.7$, $p = 0.16$).

We also assessed whether SampEn scores across both groups correlated with other descriptors for obesity. There was a moderate correlation between SampEn score and per cent body fat ($r = -0.42$, $p = 0.049$).

Discussion

Serial RER data collected during steady state metabolic demand is a potential source of information about altered metabolism, metabolic inflexibility, as described by Kelley *et al.* (2000).

Variation in physiologic signals is more than just error around predetermined homeostatic mean values for the parameters (West, 2006). In fact, the loss of fine scale variation or the increased regularity of a physiologic signal is frequently a sign of altered or abnormal physiology (Goldberger *et al.*, 2002). The information in the patterns of data variability is beyond the usual statistics of central tendency – mean and standard deviation. This information can only be extracted with non-linear analysis of the data series (West, 2006; Goldberger *et al.*, 2002).

Variability analysis is a developing science for measuring the nature and degree of patterns of variation within a sequential data series in order to assess the underlying complex system that generates the physiologic signal being evaluated (Seely and Macklem, 2004). Heart rate variability (HRV) analysis has become an established investigative tool for evaluating cardiac parasympathetic-sympathetic balance. HRV analysis using time and frequency domain parameters has shown a difference between obese and non-obese children (Nagai *et al.*, 2003). This difference in pattern of HRV can distinguish active obese children from inactive obese children (Nagai and Moritani, 2004). RER variability also appears to differ for obese children.

In conclusion, this preliminary study suggests that RER variability patterns contain potential information about the underlying metabolic state – relative flexibility of substrate flows. Sample entropy provides a method to assess the regularity of sequential data and detect patterns in serial RER collected under appropriate data generating circumstances. A larger subject sample size with longer data series will be needed to further test our hypothesis that RER SampEn serves as a marker for metabolic inflexibility or, alternatively, metabolic fitness.

References

Caprio, S., 1999, Relationship between abdominal visceral fat and metabolic risk factors in obese adolescents. *American Journal of Human Biology*, **11**, pp. 259–266.

Goldberger, A.L., Amaral, L.A.N., Hausdorf, J.M., Ivanov, P.C., Peng, C.-K. and Stanley, H.E., 2002, Fractal dynamics in physiology: alterations with disease and aging. *Proceedings of the National Academy of Sciences*, **99**, pp. 2466–2472.

Kelley, D.E. and Mandarino, L.J., 2000, Fuel selection in human skeletal muscle in insulin resistance – a reexamination. *Diabetes*, **49**, pp. 677–683.

Lake, D.E., Richman, J.S, Griffin, M.P. and Moorman, J.R., 2002, Sample entropy analysis of neonatal heart rate variability. *American Journal of Physiology Regulatory, Integrative and Comparative Physiology*, **283**, pp. R789–R797.

Nagai, N. and Moritani, T., 2004, Effect of physical activity on autonomic nervous system function in lean and obese children. *International Journal of Obesity*, **28**, pp. 27–33.

Nagai, N., Matsumoto, T., Kita, H. and Moritani, T., 2003, Autonomic nervous system activity and the state and development of obesity in Japanese school children. *Obesity Research*, **11**, pp. 25–32.

Richman, J.S. and Moorman, J.R., 2000, *American Journal of Physiology, Heart and Circulatory Physiology*, **278**, pp. H2039–H2049.

Seely, A.J.E. and Macklem, P.T., 2004, *Critical Care*, **8**, pp. R367–R384.

West, B.J. 2006, Where medicine went wrong: Rediscovering the path to complexity. In: *Studies of Nonlinear Phenomena in Life Science – Vol. 11*, edited by West, B.J. Singapore: World Scientific, pp. 274–281.

9   Physical self-perceptions in non-overweight and overweight boys and girls

L. Foweather
Liverpool John Moores University, Liverpool, UK

Introduction

Previous research with children and adolescents has found that physical self-perceptions (PSP) are related to physical activity (Crocker *et al.*, 2000; Welk and Eklund, 2005). Overweight and obese children participate in less physical activity than normal-weight children (Trost *et al.*, 2001). This study investigated whether differences in PSP might be a contributing factor.

Methods

Participants and settings

231 children (Age mean 9.5 ± 0.5 years) were recruited from 11 local primary schools following ethical approval from the University Ethics Committee. Schools selected were matched according to enrolment size (large), and socioeconomic status of the area (low) to ensure a homogeneous sample. Informed consent was obtained from the Head Teacher, parents and children prior to the study.

Measures

Anthropometric measures

Children were individually measured for stature and body mass at the University laboratories. Body mass was measured using digital scales (Seca Ltd, Birmingham, UK) to the nearest 0.1 kg. Stature (m) was assessed on a fixed stadiometer (Leicester, UK) using the stretch stature method. Measurements were taken in light clothing and with footwear removed. Anthropometric measurements were then used to calculate body mass index (BMI).

Physical self-perceptions

PSP were measured using the Children and Youth Physical Self-Perception Profile (CY-PSPP, Whitehead, 1995), which has acceptable reliability and validity for use in children (Welk and Eklund, 2005). This 36-item inventory measures PSP in six constructs, including global self-esteem, general physical self-worth, and the scales of sports competence, body attractiveness, physical condition and physical strength.

Questionnaires were administered to children in small groups at the University laboratories by a member of the research team using standardised instructions. A researcher was available to provide assistance throughout the assessment, which was usually completed in 30–40 minutes.

Analyses

Participants were classified as non-overweight, overweight or obese according to UK referenced cut-off points (Chinn and Rona, 2004). Overweight and obese children were then combined into a single group termed 'overweight'. For PSP, summary scores were created for each of the CY-PSPP constructs, as well as a total score for the complete inventory.

Independent sample t-tests were used to assess differences between non-overweight and overweight children on all CY-PSPP scales, with separate analyses for boys and girls to allow for gender differences in PSP (Fox, 1990). All analyses were conducted using SPSS v.14, with statistical significance defined at $p < 0.05$.

Results

Descriptive statistics for non-overweight and overweight boys are presented in Table 9.1, whilst the findings for girls are shown in Table 9.2. For both boys and girls, the overweight group's BMI was significantly greater than the healthy weight group.

Overweight boys had significantly lower perceptions of sports competence, physical condition and body attractiveness than their non-overweight counterparts, and scored significantly lower on the CY-PSPP total score. For girls, no significant differences were found between groups on any of the CY-PSPP scales, nor on the total score.

Table 9.1 Descriptive statistics for non-overweight and overweight boys (M ± SD)

	Non-overweight (n = 52)	Overweight (n = 45)	Difference (P)
Age (years)	9.49 ± 0.5	9.55 ± 0.5	0.543
BMI (kg·m^{-2})	16.14 ± 1.3	21.4 ± 3.0	0.001
Sports competence	19.92 ± 3.0	18.16 ± 4.3	0.024
Physical condition	19.79 ± 3.4	17.73 ± 3.8	0.006
Body attractiveness	18.96 ± 4.1	16.67 ± 4.6	0.010
Physical strength	18.02 ± 3.9	17.47 ± 4.3	0.511
Physical self-worth	19.13 ± 3.9	17.91 ± 4.1	0.134
Self-esteem	20.29 ± 3.8	18.82 ± 4.2	0.074
CY-PSPP total	116.12 ± 17.6	106.76 ± 22	0.022

Table 9.2 Descriptive statistics for non-overweight and overweight girls (M ± SD)

	Non-overweight (n = 83)	Overweight (n = 51)	Difference (P)
Age (years)	9.48 ± 0.5	9.45 ± 0.4	0.745
BMI (kg·m^{-2})	16.44 ± 1.4	21.67 ± 2.5	0.001
Sports competence	17.69 ± 3.7	17.69 ± 2.6	0.999
Physical condition	17.67 ± 3.4	17.86 ± 3.1	0.751
Body attractiveness	17.10 ± 3.5	16.10 ± 3.6	0.119
Physical strength	15.88 ± 3.1	16.82 ± 3.3	0.100
Physical self-worth	17.71 ± 3.4	17.31 ± 2.6	0.450
Self-esteem	19.11 ± 3.4	18.65 ± 3.1	0.433
CY-PSPP total	105.16 ± 16.7	104.43 ± 12	0.771

Discussion

This study examined differences in PSP between non-overweight and overweight children. The results indicate that overweight boys have significantly lower perceptions of competence than their non-overweight counterparts for several facets of the physical-self; namely sports competence, physical condition and body attractiveness. However, for girls, no differences were observed between non-overweight and overweight groups.

The finding that overweight boys had lower perceptions of physical competence than non-overweight boys is consistent with recent research conducted in children (Southall *et al.*, 2004; Franklin *et al.*, 2006). Yet the finding that girls' PSP did not differ by weight status contradicts these studies and others (Phillips and Hill, 1998). Compared to boys, girls have lower perceptions of physical competence (Fox, 1990). This may explain the conflicting results of this study as a less differentiated profile may have mediated the differences between non-overweight and overweight girls.

Competence motivation theory (Harter, 1985) posits that individuals are more likely to be motivated to participate in behaviour if they perceive themselves as having the skills and abilities necessary to demonstrate competence. The results suggest that overweight boys had lower PSP than non-overweight boys in three of the six CY-PSPP constructs. This may be one reason why overweight boys engage in less physical activity than non-overweight boys (Trost *et al.*, 2001). Overweight boys who perceive themselves to be low in sports competence or physical fitness may be less likely to exert effort and continue participation in physical activity behaviours than non-overweight boys with higher perceptions of competence.

Perceptions of competence can be enhanced by increasing actual competence and through social support mechanisms (Harter, 1985). Interventions should seek to develop motor skills and improve physical fitness to increase actual competence. Socio-psychological mechanisms will best influence perceptions of competence (Fox, 2000). Therefore practitioners should seek to establish a fun, positive environment for physical activity participation with support, feedback and encouragement offered from peers, coaches, teachers and parents (Weiss, 2000).

In summary, this research indicates that low PSP might be an important factor in childhood obesity in boys, though other issues may contribute to difficulties in maintaining a healthy weight status in girls. Physical activity interventions seeking to combat obesity should include strategies to improve perceptions of competence.

References

Chinn, S. and Rona, R.J., 2004, Re: International definitions of overweight and obesity for children: A lasting solution? *Annals of Human Biology*, **31**, pp. 695–696.

Crocker, P.R.E., Eklund, R.C. and Kowalski, K.C., 2000, Children's physical activity and physical self-perceptions. *Journal of Sport Sciences*, **18**, pp. 383–394.

Fox, K.R., 1990, *The Physical Self-perception Profile Manual*, Dekalb, IL: Office for Health Promotion, Northern Illinois University.

Fox, K.R., 2000, Self-esteem, self-perceptions, and exercise. *International Journal of Sport and Exercise Psychology*, **31**, pp. 228–240.

Franklin, J., Denyer, G., Steinbeck, K.S., Caterson, I.D. and Hill, A.J., 2006, Obesity and risk of low self-esteem: A statewide survey of Australian children. *Pediatrics*, **118**, pp. 2482–2487.

Harter, S., 1985, Competence as a dimension of self-evaluation: Toward a comprehensive model of self-worth. In: *The Development of the Self*, edited by Leathy, R. New York: Academic Press, pp. 55–121.

Phillips, R.G. and Hill, A.J., 1998, Fat, plain, but not friendless: Self-esteem and peer acceptance of obese pre-adolescent girls. *International Journal of Obesity Related Metabolic Disorders*, **22**, pp. 287–293.

Southall, J.E., Okely, A.D. and Steele, J.R., 2004, Actual and perceived competence in overweight and nonoverweight children. *Pediatric Exercise Science*, **16**, pp. 15–24.

Trost, S.G., Kerr, L.M., Ward, D.S. and Pate, R.R., 2001, Physical activity and determinants of physical activity in obese and non-obese children. *International Journal of Obesity*, **25**, pp. 822–829.

Weiss, M.R., 2000, Motivating kids in physical activity. *Presidents Council on Physical Fitness and Sports Research Digest*, **3**, pp. 1–8.

Welk, G.J. and Eklund, B., 2005, Validation of the children and youth physical self perceptions profile for young children. *Psychology of Sport and Exercise*, **6**, pp. 51–65.

Whitehead, J.R., 1995, A study of children's physical self-perceptions using an adapted physical self-perception profile questionnaire. *Pediatric Exercise Science*, **7**, pp. 132–151.

10 Bone mineral density, anthropometry and body composition in 13–15-year-old physically active girls

R. Gruodyte,[1,2] M. Saar,[1] J. Jürimäe,[1] K. Maasalu[1] and T. Jürimäe[1]

[1]University of Tartu, Tartu, Estonia; [2]Lihuanian Academy of Physical Education, Kaunas, Lithuania

Introduction

Bone mineral density (BMD) increases during childhood and adolescence, until peak bone mass is reached. Peak bone mass is an important determinant of osteoporosis (Specker, 2001). Several studies have identified a positive association between the level of physical activity and BMD in children (Bass et al., 1998; MacKelvie et al., 2003). It is well documented that moderate exercise increases BMD in the prepubertal and early pubertal period but not in the postpubertal period (Morris et al., 1997; MacKelvie et al., 2002). One strategy to increase peak bone mass is a regular weight-bearing exercise. Weight-bearing exercise includes aerobics, jogging, jumping, volleyball and other sports that generate impact to the skeleton (Burrows, 2007). Sports participation during growth has been shown to increase BMD in the weight-loaded limbs by 10–20 per cent (Bass et al., 1998), which is greater if the exercise precedes pubertal growth (Bradney et al., 1998). Skeletal benefits of exercise have been shown to be greater when regular training is started prior to menarche (Heinonen et al., 2000). During puberty anthropometrical and body composition parameters change rapidly in adolescents. However, there are only very few studies available on the influence of anthropometry and body composition on the bone parameters in lean physically active girls. Only MacKelvie et al. (2002) concluded that body mass index (BMI) was significantly related to bone mineral accrual and may have played a role in dampening the effect of the jumping intervention. This study aimed to investigate the relationship between BMD, anthropometry and body composition in physically active pubertal girls.

Methods

This cross-sectional study involved 131 13–15-year-old physically active girls. They exercised three to six times per week and participated mostly in weight-bearing sport events such as sprinting, sport games, gymnastics, etc. The study was approved by the Medical Ethics Committee of the University of Tartu (Estonia).

Height (Martin metal anthropometer) and body mass (A&D Instrument, UK) of the participants were measured to the nearest 0.1 cm and 0.05 kg, respectively. Body mass index was calculated (BMI; $kg.m^{-2}$). According to the Tanner classification (Tanner, 1962), participants were at the pubertal stages 2–5. Body composition was assessed by dual-energy X-ray absorptiometry using DPX-IQ densitometer (Lunar Corporation, Madison, WI, USA) and analysed for body fat (FM) and fat-free (FFM) mass. At the same measurement, BMD at the spine (L2–L4) and femoral neck were measured.

Statistical analysis was performed with SPSS 11.0 for Windows (USA). Means and standard deviations (±SD) were determined. Pearson product moment correlation analysis was used to examine relationships between measured parameters. Stepwise multiple regression analysis was performed to determine the independent effect of the different anthropometric and body composition parameters to the spine and femoral neck BMD. The level of significance was set at $p < 0.05$.

Results

The mean anthropometrical, body composition and bone parameters are presented in Table 10.1.

In girls, both lumbar spine and femoral neck BMD correlated with body height ($r = 0.51-0.58$), body mass ($r = 0.60-0.62$), BMI ($r = 0.39-0.40$), FFM ($r = 0.61-0.63$) and body fat per cent ($r = 0.22-0.28$). The results of the stepwise multiple regression analysis are presented in Table 10.2.

Our results indicated that both basic anthropometric and body composition parameters highly and equally influenced BMD at the skeletal sites of lumbar spine and femoral neck in physically active pubertal girls. Analysing together anthropometrical and body composition parameters in the regression analysis, the influence of these parameters on lumbar spine and femoral neck BMD increased to 50.4 per cent ($R^2 \times 100$) and 46.8 per cent ($R^2 \times 100$), respectively.

Table 10.1 Mean (±SD) characteristics of the study subjects ($n = 131$)

Variable	Mean ± SD
Age (y)	13.6 ± 1.0
Height (cm)	165.9 ± 7.5
Body mass (kg)	54.7 ± 8.8
BMI ($kg \cdot m^{-2}$)	20.6 ± 2.5
Body fat (%)	24.1 ± 6.7
Fat free mass (kg)	41.2 ± 5.4
Lumbar spine BMD ($g \cdot cm^{-2}$)	1.098 ± 0.134
Femoral neck BMD ($g \cdot cm^{-2}$)	1.033 ± 0.118

Table 10.2 Stepwise multiple regression analysis results were dependent variables and spine and femoral neck BMD were independent variables of anthropometrical and body composition parameters

	BMD (lumbar spine)			BMD (femoral neck)		
	R^2	F	p	R^2	F	p
Height & weight	0.443	52.7	< 0.000	0.384	41.5	< 0.000
LBM & BF %	0.426	49.2	< 0.000	0.415	47.1	< 0.000

Discussion

The main finding of the present investigation was that there are close relationships between BMD variables, anthropometry and body composition in physically active pubertal girls.

All girls in our study were lean with relatively low body fat percentage values and relatively high physical activity levels. Accordingly, their BMD values were high compared to the results of other studies (Rautava *et al.*, 2007). In our study, we used physically active girls, who mostly used weight-bearing exercises in their everyday activities. However, it has to be considered that we do not know the possible effect of genetics (Krall *et al.*, 1993) and muscle gain effect to the development of specific BMD values.

Stepwise multiple regression analysis indicated that from the anthropometric parameters body height and body mass were selected. Surprisingly, BMI was not selected to characterise measured BMD values. On the other side, body mass also consists of bone mass. Low body mass has been declared to be a significant risk factor for the development of osteoporosis. However, obesity has been mentioned as a significant confounder of BMD (Holbrook and Barrett-Connors, 1993).

Body composition highly influences BMD values by at least three possible mechanisms: mechanical stress due to body mass, muscular forces and finally hormonal mechanisms (Lanyon, 1992). Lean body mass is a predictor of mechanical stress. In our study, both FFM and body fat percentage were selected to characterize measured BMD values (see Table 10.2). Probably the influence of fat tissue is relatively small, because studied girls were relatively lean. To date, previous results have been conflicting. For example, the study by Nichols *et al.* (1995) indicated that arm and leg FFM values were found to be significantly and positively correlated to the corresponding regional BMD in college females, while Reid *et al.* (1992) emphasised that body FM was an important determinant of whole body BMD in premenopausal women.

It was concluded that most of the measured anthropometrical (body height and body mass) and body composition (FFM and body fat percentage) are significant parameters to influence measured BMD values in physically active pubertal girls.

References

Bass, S., Pearce, G., Bradney, M., Hendrich, E., Delmas, P.D., Harding, A. and Seeman, E., 1998, Exercise before puberty may confer residual benefits in bone density in adulthood: Studies in active prepubertal and retired female gymnasts. *Journal of Bone and Mineral Research*, **13**, pp. 500–507.

Bradney, M., Pearce, G., Naughton, G., Sullivan, C., Bass, S., Beck, T., Carlson, J. and Seeman, E., 1998, Moderate exercise during growth in prepubertal boys: Changes in bone mass, volumetric density and bone strength: A controlled prospective study. *Journal of Bone and Mineral Research*, **13**, pp. 1818–1821.

Burrows, M., 2007, Exercise and bone mineral accrual in children and adolescents. *Journal of Sports Science and Medicine*, **6**, pp. 305–312.

Heinonen, A., Sievinen, H., Kannus, P., Oja, P., Pasanen, M. and Vuori, I., 2000, High impact exercise and bones of growing girls: A 9-month controlled trial. *Osteoporosis International*, **11**, pp. 1010–1017.

Holbrook, T.L. and Barrett-Connor, E., 1993, The association of lifetime weight and weight control patterns with bone mineral density in an adult community. *Bone and Mineral*, **20**, pp. 141–142.

Krall, E.A. and Pawson-Huges, B., 1993, Heritable and life-style determinants of bone mineral density. *Journal of Bone Mineral Density*, **8**, pp. 1–9.

Lanyon, L.E., 1992, Control of bone architecture by functional load bearing. *Journal of Bone and Mineral Research*, **7** (suppl.), pp. 5369–5375.

MacKelvie, K.J., Khan, K.M. and McKay, H.A., 2002, Is there a critical period for bone response to weight-bearing exercise in children and adolescence. A systematic review. *British Journal of Sports Medicine*, **36**, pp. 250–257.

MacKelvie, K.J., Khan, K.M., Petit, M.A., Janssen, P.A. and McKay, H.A., 2003, A school-based exercise intervention elicits substantial bone health benefits: A 2-year randomized controlled trail in girls. *Pediatrics*, **112**, pp. e447–e452.

Morris, F.L., Naughton, G.A., Gibbs, J.L., Carlson, J.S. and Wark, J.D., 1997, Prospective ten-month exercise intervention in premenarcheal girls: Positive effects on bone and lean mass. *Journal of Bone and Mineral Research*, **12**, pp. 1453–1462.

Nichols, D.L., Sanborn, C.F., Bonnick, S.L., Gengh, B. and Dimarco, N., 1995, Relationship of regional body composition to bone mineral density in college females. *Medicine and Science in Sport and Exercise*, **27**, pp. 178–182.

Rautava, E., Lehtonen-Veromaa, M., Kautiainen, H., Kajander, S., Heinonen, O.J., Viikari, J. and Möttönen, T., 2007, The reduction of physical activity reflects on the bone mass among young females: A follow-up study of 142 adolescent girls. *Osteoporosis International*, **18**, pp. 915–922.

Reid, I.R., Plank, L.D. and Evans, M.C., 1992, Fat mass is an important determinant of whole body bone density in premenopausal women, but not in men. *Journal of Clinical Endocrinology and Metabolism*, **75**, pp. 779–782.

Specker, B.L., 2001, The significance of high bone density in children. *Journal of Pediatrics*, **139**, pp. 473–475.

Tanner, J., 1962, *Growth at Adolescence*, 2nd edn. Oxford: Blackwell.

11 A process evaluation of a lifestyle intervention for 8–10-year-old children
The A-CLASS project

J. Hepples and G. Stratton
Liverpool John Moores University, Liverpool, UK

Introduction

This paper evaluates the development of the PASS (Physical Activity Signposting Scheme). PASS is a lifestyle intervention for children aimed at increasing physical activity levels. Qualitative methods are used to investigate the impact PASS has on children's physical activity behaviours.

Background

Whilst the benefits of physical activity for children have been well documented, about 50 per cent of children are not achieving recommended levels that would benefit their health (Biddle *et al.*, 2004).

Few lifestyle interventions have successfully reduced sedentary behaviour and increased physical activity levels in children (Campbell *et al.*, 2001). Robinson (1999) carried out a curriculum-based intervention, which included strategies such as self-monitoring and budgeting of TV use. This study resulted in reductions in TV use and body weight, although there was no increase in physical activity.

The Switch-Play programme (Salmon *et al.*, 2006) aimed to reduce sedentary behaviour, as well as increase physical activity. This study provided evidence to support programmes that combined physical activity and decreasing sedentary behaviours in a lifestyle intervention.

In Liverpool we have built on previous physical activity promotion work and design and implemented a lifestyle intervention programme alongside other more structured approaches. This programme focuses on the children's interaction with the environment as well as predisposing factors such as self-efficacy and enjoyment. In addition, reinforcing factors are acknowledged, by encouraging family and friend involvement through a lifestyle intervention.

The physical activity signposting scheme

PASS represents one of three physical activity interventions included in the A-CLASS project (see Ridgers *et al.*, 2006). PASS is a lifestyle intervention, designed to increase children's physical activity levels and decrease sedentary behaviour, whereas the other groups use structured exercise (incorporating both Fundamental Movement Skills (FMS) and high intensity exercise). The fourth group is a control.

Aims

The principal aim of the A-CLASS intervention is to increase children's activity levels and challenge sedentary behaviours. Subsequently the aims of PASS, are to:

- Assess children's physical activity levels during a lifestyle intervention;
- Assess how self-efficacy influences physical activity levels;
- Assess if the environment has an impact upon the physical activity levels; and,
- Process evaluation about how children interact with the missions (tasks).

Methods

Forty-five 8–10-year-old children from two primary schools in Liverpool took part in the study. The programme was delivered to a group of children at school in four six-weekly blocks (half an hour per week) with a six-week break between each block. Each weekly session consisted of a discussion of the previous week's task followed by the delivery of the subsequent week's physical activity task.

The design of the study is based upon action-research principles. When blocks of tasks are completed, the next set is designed as a result of feedback from interviews and focus groups. These focus groups and interviews take place with the children, parents and teachers.

At the time of writing the first three blocks of PASS have been completed. The focus group data from parents and teachers is being collected after block three and the next block of missions are being designed.

Behaviour change strategies in the current investigation are based upon prior successful approaches reported by Ory *et al.* (2002). These include: education, self-monitoring (pedometers, time spent in sedentary behaviours and physical activity) decision-making (intelligent TV viewing). Feedback and reinforcement were implemented (the children are rewarded at the end of each six weeks for completing all the missions).

Findings

All the children were unanimous in having enjoyed attending PASS, however some of the tasks were more popular than others.

Focus groups and interviews provided an insight into how effective tasks were at changing behaviour and also provided key information about the underlying factors, which influence physical activity participation. The following vignettes provide an overview of these findings. The qualitative data gathered from participants after the first block of tasks suggests that children's physical activity increased. 'We got to do more activity than we used to do and it helped us instead of being lazy we got to be active'.

One of the factors which may have affected the children's perception of an increase in physical activity is enjoyment. The children enjoyed attending PASS. In addition the children enjoyed being more active. 'It was fun doing something active everyday instead of watching TV'.

However, this was in contrast to a reluctance to carry out some of the tasks. The main task where some reluctance was evident was reducing television: 'I don't really like it when I can't watch the tele that much'.

Although the reducing television tasks were completed, it was rare if this behaviour change continued. To help sustain the behaviour change after the week of the task the next block of tasks were designed to be fun, motivating and enjoyable. In addition, a camera was issued for the second group of tasks. These were kept for the whole six weeks and the children took a number of pictures of the different activities they did each week.

A major underlying factor that influences children to participate in the tasks is an increase in self-efficacy. The children now believe that they are capable of being more active: 'before I thought I was fat now I don't cos I'm more active'.

The children also feel better about themselves as they feel that they are more active. For example: 'I'm so happy that I'm getting more fit'.

Although some children found some of the tasks difficult, they still appear to have achieved them. 'I found it hard to stop watching TV, but I stopped it in the end' (watching no more than two hours a day).

Achieving a task, which the children initially found difficult, may increase their self-efficacy of the task and suggests that self-esteem could be improved as a result of the PASS programme. In return activity levels may be increased, as the children believe that they can be more active. Therefore, tasks in the second block of work enabled children to be appropriately challenged.

The family also appears to have an impact on the child's participation in physical activity. However they may help their children, it appears that parents can sometimes be a hindrance. A lot of the children stated that a member of their family helped them with tasks and they appreciated this help. However some children found that their parents' help was off-putting: 'My mum kept prodding me with the chart, this made me not want to do it'.

In addition to parents nagging their children to do the tasks, others were seen as a hindrance as they would not always let their children do what they wanted to do; one child said: 'I had to nag mum to let me go outside because it was raining, she still wouldn't let me'.

Parents admitted that there were a number of reasons that they did not want their children going outside, these included safety and the weather. Parents also mentioned that at the end of the day at work it was too easy to say: 'just go on the computer or watch television, anything for peace and quiet'.

As the family has a great impact upon a child's physical activity levels, the second block of tasks aimed to encourage the family to be more involved. This is something most of the children were really enthusiastic about.

Conclusion

PASS aims to develop a sustainable lifestyle intervention to increase physical activity levels in 8–10-year-old children. The feedback from qualitative data suggests that the PASS scheme is having a positive influence on children's activity levels and self-esteem. The children enjoy the challenges set each week and it is relatively simple and cheap to deliver.

References

Biddle, S.J.H., Gorely, T. and Strensel, D.J., 2004, Health-enhancing physical activity and sedentary behaviour in children and adolescents. *Journal of Sports Sciences*, **22**, pp. 679–701.

Campbell, K., Waters, E., O'Meara, S. and Summerbell, C., 2001, Interventions for preventing obesity in children (Cochrane Review) In: *The Cochrane Library*, Issue 1. Oxford: Update Software.

Ory, M.G., Jordan, P.J. and Bazarre, T., 2002, The behaviour change consortium: Setting the stage for a new century of health behaviour change research. *Health Education Research*, **17**, pp. 500–511.

Ridgers, N., Stratton, G., Foweather, L., Henaghan, J., McWhannell, N. and Stone, M.R., 2006, The Active City of Liverpool, Active Schools and Sportslinx (A-CLASS) Project. *Education and Health*, **24**, pp. 26–29.

Robinson, T., 1999, Reducing children's television viewing to prevent obesity. *Journal of the American Medical Association*, **282**, pp. 1561–1566.

Salmon, J., Hume, C., Ball, K., Booth, M. and Crawford, D., 2006, Individual, social and home environment determinants of change in children's television viewing: The Switch-play intervention. *Journal of Science and Medicine in Sport*, **9**, pp. 378–387.

12 Time spent practicing fundamental motor skills during an eight-month preschool PE programme

Observational case study

S. Iivonen, A. Sääkslahti and J. Liukkonen

University of Jyväskylä, Department of Sport Sciences, Finland

Introduction

The developmental period during preschool years is critical if children are to master the Fundamental Motor Skills (FMS). FMS are needed to adopt a physically active lifestyle (Sääkslahti et al., 2004; Raudsepp and Päll, 2006). Time spent on physical activity alone is not enough to cause expected positive changes in preschool children's FMS (Fisher et al., 2005; Deli et al., 2006). Skill specific learning experiences are needed. According to Gallahue and Donnelly (2003) a developmentally appropriate curricular model of young children's PE is based on the phases of motor development and the stages of movement skill learning.

The present study examined the joint effects of five-year-old children's motor developmental status and the time spent practicing locomotor, manipulative, and body rolling skills as well as sedentary behaviour during the eight-month preschool Physical Education Curriculum (PEC). The PEC was designed to help children to understand the importance of a healthy lifestyle and to foster the development of social skills through the acquisition and development of motor skills (Zachopoulou et al., 2007). In the absence of earlier observational studies, investigating how much opportunity children actually get to practice motor skills during organized movement programs, the current study takes a new viewpoint on young children's PE activity.

Methods

The motor behaviours of four children (mean age 5.2 ± 0.4 y) were analyzed in this study. The APM-Inventory developed by Numminen (1995) was used to assess FMS in order to identify one skilful and one less skilful child from two PEC-participating preschools. The seven FMS measured were static balance, dynamic balance, running speed (10 m), standing broad-jump, throwing and catching a ball, throwing at a target, and kicking a ball at a target.

To analyze seven PEC-lessons out of the total 48 (see Table 12.1), the systematic video-observation based on actual continuous duration coding was used because

Table 12.1 Contents and end goals of the seven observed lessons of the PEC

Lesson No.	Preschoolers will develop in:
3	Moving in different ways by adjusting direction, level and speed
4	Balancing and body controlling skills
5	Balancing and body controlling skills Horizontal jumping and leaping skills
17	Understanding the function of perspiration Identifying the function of body temperature
23	Understanding the meaning of rest and contrasts between relaxation and tension Recognizing body functions while exercising and relaxing
27	Sending and receiving an object skills Being able to observe and give feedback
36	Moving quietly and carefully Understanding different kinds of feelings while moving Responding to stimuli

it gives a realistic measurement of the behaviour (McKenzie and Carlson, 1989). Computer software was constructed in the Department of Sport Sciences (2006) to provide precise measurement of total time (s) spent in seven motor skill observation categories and one category of sedentary behaviour. Because the appropriate observation times varied between children, the percentage of total time was used to describe children's engagement in skill specific practicing of FMS. In order to analyze the validity and reliability of the coding category system, two independent and trained observers' agreements were obtained: inter-observer percentage agreement scores varied between 83 and 100 per cent in observation categories of the present observation system.

Results

Practicing percentages and total observation times (seconds) of the seven motor skill categories and one category of sedentary behaviour are reported in Table 12.2. All the children spent more than 40 per cent of the total time of the seven PE lessons on sedentary behaviour. The skill specific practicing consisted mostly of walking and running activities (21–25 per cent) and secondly of different kinds of whole body manipulative activities (9–18 per cent). Connections between children's motor developmental status and the time spent practicing FMS were: (1) The practicing percents of locomotor skills were highest with the skilful child A; (2) The less skilful child C spent most of the time in sedentary behaviour. In addition, the practicing percentages of different kinds of jumping skills, upper and lower limb manipulative skills, whole body manipulative skills and body rolling skills were lowest with the less skilful child C; (3) The practicing per cent of upper limb manipulative skills was highest with the less skilful child D;

Table 12.2 Percentages of practice times (%) and total observation times (seconds) spent in seven skill practicing categories and sedentary behaviour during seven PE lessons

Skill observation categories	Skilful children				Less skilful children			
	Child A		Child B		Child C		Child D	
	%	(s)	%	(s)	%	(s)	%	(s)
Locomotor								
Walk, run	25	(1358)	21	(744)	25	(1338)	22	(788)
Crawl, creep, walking on fours	7	(356)	3	(117)	5	(266)	2	(76)
Leap, jump, hop, skip, slide, gallop	8	(443)	6	(224)	3	(165)	7	(257)
Manipulative								
Throw, catch, bounce, roll, strike, volley	4	(216)	6	(200)	1	(42)	9	(328)
Kick, trap, collect	1	(35)	1	(30)	1	(28)	1	(44)
Whole body manipulative	11	(607)	18	(639)	9	(490)	13	(467)
Body rolling	1	(38)	1	(46)	1	(29)	2	(56)
Sedentary	43	(2302)	43	(1522)	56	(3053)	43	(1513)

(4) The skilful child B got the highest practicing per cent in whole body manipulative skills.

Discussion

During this physical education curriculum all the observed children demonstrated the most engagement in not skill specific motor behaviour; that was lying, sitting or standing still by listening to instructions, waiting one's own turn or showing no interest in ongoing activities. The practice mostly consisted of walking and running skills, which usually begin to enter into mature developmental stage in five-year-old children (Gallahue and Donnelly, 2003). Practicing of upper and lower limb manipulative skills was remote. Lots of repetitions and learning experiences should take place to foster children's progression in throwing, catching, kicking and stopping skills, etc. because they are in the developmental level of a rapid change in five-year-old children (Sääkslahti *et al.*, 2004). Derri *et al.* (2007) found out that 7–8-year-old children's proficiency in motor tasks was related to the time devoted to skill specific practicing but not to the activities that were not skill specific. Also the findings of the current study highlight the importance of careful implementation of movement programs to include lots of developmentally appropriate skill practicing experiences, and to be carried out by professional physical educators with appropriate organizational skills (Sääkslahti *et al.*, 2004).

The present study showed that children's motor developmental status was not systematically connected to skill practice; rather the proportions of motor skill practice times were divided quite unsystematically between skilful and less skilful children. In terms of further studies, by observing live PE situations along with assessing children's motor proficiency, it will be possible to find out how children in PE situations actually behave and how movement programs and interventions designed to foster children's motor skills actually work. It is also important to find out whether such education induces more prominent and permanent changes in FMS later in life.

References

Deli, E., Bakle, I. and Zachopoulou, E., 2006, Implementing intervention movement programs for kindergarten children. *Journal of Early Childhood Research*, **4**, pp. 5–18.

Derri, V., Emmanoulidou, K., Vassiliadou, O., Kioumoirtzoglou, E. and Olave, E.L., 2007, Academic learning time in physical education (ALT-PE): is it related to fundamental movement skill acquisition and learning? *International Journal of Sport Science*, **3**, pp. 12–23.

Fisher, A., Reilly, J.J., Kelly, L.A., Montgomery, C., Williamson, A., Paton, J.Y. and Grant, S., 2005, Fundamental movement skills and habitual physical activity in young children. *Medicine and Science in Sports and Exercise*, **37**, pp. 684–688.

Gallahue, D. and Donnelly, F., 2003, *Developmental Physical Education for All Children.* Champaign, IL: Human Kinetics.

General Observation Software, 2006, University of Jyväskylä: Department of Sport Sciences.

McKenzie, T.L. and Carlson, B.R., 1989, Systematic observation and computer technology. In: *Analyzing Physical education and Sort Instruction*, edited by Darst, P.W., Zakrajsek, B. and Mancini, V.H.: Champaign, IL: Human Kinetics, pp. 81–89.

Numminen, P., 1995, *APM Inventory. Manual and Test Booklet for Assessing Preschool Children's Perceptual and Fundamental Motor Skills.* Jyväskylä: LIKES.

Raudsepp, L. and Päll, P., 2006, The relationship between fundamental motor skills and outside-school physical activity of elementary school children. *Pediatric Exercise Science*, **18**, pp. 426–435.

Sääkslahti, A., Numminen, P., Salo, P., Tuominen, J., Helenius, H. and Välimäki, I., 2004, Effects of a three-year intervention on children's physical activity from age 4 to 7. *Pediatric Exercise Science*, **16**, pp. 167–180.

Zachopoulou, E., Tzangaridou, N., Picup, I., Liukkonen, J. and Grammatikopoulos, P., 2007, *Early Steps 2007, Promoting Healthy Lifestyle and Social Interaction Through Physical Education Activities during Preschool Years.* Edition supported by EU Socrates Program, Comenius 2.1 Action. Thessasloniki: Xristodoulidi Publications.

13 Perceived teaching behaviours and motivation in physical education

Effect of age

A. *Koka*

Institute of Sport Pedagogy and Coaching Sciences, Centre of Behavioural and Health Sciences, University of Tartu, Estonia

Introduction

To date, physical education (PE) has been cited as a strategically useful network through which health-related physical activity messages can be conveyed virtually to all children (Hagger *et al.*, 2005). However, researchers have constantly shown that interest in PE and physical activity level declines with age (e.g. Biddle, 1995). It is crucial, therefore, to examine factors that influence students' motivation in PE with different age levels.

The teacher's behaviour has been considered as an important factor that can have an impact on students motivation in PE. Ntoumanis (2005), for example, in line with Deci and Ryan's (1985) self-determination theory, have shown that students who perceived their teacher's behaviour to support their psychological needs for competence, autonomy and relatedness in PE classes displayed enhanced motivation. There is limited evidence, however, regarding the role of teachers' behaviour on students' motivation in PE among different age groups. Therefore, this study was aimed to assess the relationships between different types of perceived teaching behaviours and students' psychological needs for competence, autonomy, and relatedness as well as motivation in PE among seventh- and twelfth-graders.

Methods

Participants and procedures

Participants were 98 students from one school in Estonia. From this sample, 45 students were in the seventh grade (M age = 13.1, SD = 0.66) and 53 were in the twelfth grade (M age = 17.9, SD = 0.24). Permission to carry out the study was obtained from the headmaster or from a class teacher. Also, parental consent was obtained for all children. Questionnaires were administered in quiet classroom conditions and these took approximately 15–20 min to complete. Students were assured that their answers would remain confidential.

Measures

The Revised Leadership Scale for Sport (RLSS, Zhang *et al.*, 1997), modified to PE context, was used to assess students' perceptions of different types of teaching behaviours on dimensions of democratic behaviour, autocratic behaviour, teaching and instruction, social support and situation consideration.

The Perceptions of the Teacher's Feedback questionnaire (PTF, Koka and Hein, 2005) was used to assess students' perceptions of different types of teachers' feedback in PE on dimensions of positive general feedback, informational feedback, positive non-verbal feedback and negative non-verbal feedback.

A five-item subscale of the perceived competence from the Intrinsic Motivation Inventory (IMI, McAuley *et al.*, 1989) was used to measure students' perceptions of competence in PE.

Students' sense of autonomy in PE was measured using three items derived from previous research assessing perceptions of autonomy in sport setting (Hollembeak and Amorose, 2005). Students were asked to reflect how they felt about the amount of choice or control they had when participating in PE.

Students' sense of relatedness in PE was assessed using five items derived from previous research assessing perceptions of relatedness in a sport setting (Hollembeak and Amorose, 2005). Items were modified by changing the relational context to PE.

Students' motivation toward PE was assessed by an adapted version of Mullan *et al.*'s (1997) Behavioural Regulations in Exercise Questionnaire (BREQ) with four different motivational types of intrinsic motivation, identified regulation, introjected regulation and external regulation. To reduce the number of variables without losing vital information, the method advocated by other researchers (e.g. Hagger *et al.*, 2005) was used to integrate four types of motivation into single relative autonomy index (RAI). Each subscale average score was weighted as follows: intrinsic motivation ($+2$), identified regulation ($+1$), interjected regulation (-1), and extrinsic regulation (-2), and an RAI was calculated based on the weighted composite of these scores.

Independent samples t-test was used to investigate age differences on all variables. Pearson product correlations coefficients were used to investigate relationships between the perceived teaching behaviours variables, psychological needs for competence, autonomy and relatedness and RAI. Correlational analyses were performed separately for seventh and twelfth-graders.

Results and discussion

Results indicated that twelfth-graders scored significantly higher than seventh graders on several perceived teaching behaviours such as teaching/instruction, social support, situation consideration and informational feedback, but lower on autocratic behaviour and negative non-verbal feedback (Table 13.1). Interestingly, twelfth-graders scored significantly higher on RAI, indicating that they had higher levels of autonomous forms of motivation in PE (i.e. intrinsic motivation

Table 13.1 Age differences for all study variables

Variable	M	SD	M	SD
	Seventh-graders		Twelfth-graders	
Democratic behaviour	3.10	0.91	3.14	0.90
Autocratic behaviour	2.46	0.82	1.81	0.69***
Teaching/instruction	3.36	0.66	3.98	0.59***
Social support	3.56	0.78	4.14	0.77***
Situation consideration	3.58	0.83	3.97	0.75**
Positive general feedback	3.25	1.13	3.46	0.91
Informational feedback	3.36	0.89	3.86	0.73**
Positive non-verbal feedback	2.58	0.94	2.94	0.93
Negative non-verbal feedback	2.19	1.05	1.67	0.71**
Perceived competence	3.53	0.98	3.53	0.83
Perceived autonomy	2.83	1.08	2.79	0.87
Perceived relatedness	4.84	1.47	4.69	1.34
RAI	2.65	3.87	4.13	3.36*

* $p < 0.05$, ** $p < 0.01$, *** $p < 0.001$.

Table 13.2 Correlations between perceived teaching behaviours, psychological needs for competence, autonomy and relatedness, and relative autonomy index (RAI) for both seventh- and twelfth-graders samples

Variable	Perceived competence	Perceived autonomy	Perceived relatedness	RAI
Seventh-graders				
Democratic behaviour	0.42**	0.64**	−0.09	0.34*
Autocratic behaviour	−0.21	−0.27	−0.02	−0.53**
Teaching/instruction	0.47**	0.47**	0.12	0.21
Social support	0.47**	0.58**	0.12	0.35*
Situation consideration	0.63**	0.48**	0.04	0.53**
Positive general feedback	0.54**	0.65**	0.14	0.36*
Informational feedback	0.26	0.51**	0.03	0.12
Positive non-verbal feedback	0.34*	0.34**	0.12	0.07
Negative non-verbal feedback	−0.20	−0.04	0.06	−0.41**
Twelfth-graders				
Democratic behaviour	0.20	0.57**	0.26	0.20
Autocratic behaviour	−0.27	−0.60**	−0.16	−0.13
Teaching/instruction	0.30*	0.22	0.21	0.20
Social support	0.30	0.48**	0.24	0.29*
Situation consideration	0.20	0.41**	0.28*	0.16
Positive general feedback	0.32*	0.69**	0.06	0.32*
Informational feedback	0.38**	0.37**	0.23	0.42**
Positive non-verbal feedback	0.23	0.57**	0.07	0.24
Negative non-verbal feedback	−0.15	−0.09	−0.01	0.08

* $p < 0.05$, ** $p < 0.01$.

and identified regulation). This is not consistent with previous research (Biddle, 1995).

Results of this study supported the tenet of self-determination theory (Decy and Ryan, 1985) and previous studies in the field (e.g. Ntoumanis, 2005), indicated that perceived teachers' behaviours that were positively related to student's psychological needs were, in general, positively related to motivation (Table 13.2). It is worth noting that different types of perceived teachers' behaviours were related to seventh- and twelfth-graders' motivation. As for seventh graders, students who perceived their teachers as situation considerate and not autocratic displayed enhanced motivation in PE. For twelfth graders, on the other hand, informational feedback from the teacher seemed to be most important for motivation to be enhanced (Table 13.2). In summary, PE teachers should consider the fact that different types of behaviours may be important to increase students' motivation at different ages.

Acknowledgement

This study was financially supported by the Estonian Science Foundation (grant no 7100). I thank Ülle Ernits for her assistance with collecting the data.

References

Biddle, S.J.H., 1995, Exercise motivation across life span. In: *European Perspectives on Exercise and Sport Psychology*, edited by Biddle, S.J.H. Human Kinetics Publishers, Inc., pp. 3–25.

Deci, E.L. and Ryan, R.M., 1985, *Intrinsic Motivation and Self-determination in Human Behaviour*. New York: Plenum Press.

Hagger, M.S., Chatzisarantis, N.L.D., Barkoukis, V., Wang, C.K.J. and Baranowski, J., 2005, Perceived autonomy support in physical education and leisure-time physical activity: A cross-cultural evaluation of the trans-contextual model. *Journal of Educational Psychology*, 97, pp. 287–301.

Hollembeak, J. and Amorose, A.J., 2005, Perceived coaching behaviors and college athletes' intrinsic motivation: A test of self-determination theory. *Journal of Applied Sport Psychology*, 17, pp. 1–17.

Koka, A. and Hein, V., 2005, The effect of perceived teacher feedback on intrinsic motivation in physical education. *International Journal of Sport Psychology*, 36, pp. 91–106.

McAuley, E., Duncan, T. and Tammen, V.V., 1989, Psychometric properties of the Intrinsic Motivation Inventory in a competitive sport setting: A confirmatory factor analysis. *Research Quarterly for Exercise and Sport*, 60, pp. 48–58.

Mullan, E., Markland, D. and Ingledew, D.K., 1997, A graded conceptualisation of self-determination in the regulation of exercise behaviour: Development of a measure using confirmatory factor analysis. *Personality and Individual Differences*, 23, pp. 745–752.

Ntoumanis, N., 2005, A prospective study of participation in optional school physical education using a self-determination theory framework. *Journal of Educational Psychology*, 3, pp. 444–453.

Zhang, J., Jensen, B.E. and Mann, B.L., 1997, Modification and revision of the leadership scale for sport. *Journal of Sport Behavior*, 20, pp. 105–122.

14 A profile of paediatric sports injuries at three types of medical practice

G. Naughton,[1] *C. Broderick,*[2,3] *N. Van Doorn,*[2]
G. Browne[3] *and L. Lam*[3]

[1]Australian Catholic University; [2]University of New South Wales, Australia; [3]Children's Hospital at Westmead, Sydney, Australia

Introduction

Childhood sporting experiences provide a milieu of benefits, but can also carry injury risks. While the vulnerability of the developing skeleton can increase injury risk, it is unreasonable to believe that injuries in sport are all growth-related. Paediatric sports injury surveillance helps to identify future directions for injury prevention in children's sport.

Injury profiles vary according to the setting. For example, strains and sprains are frequently reported when sports trainers provide data, but acute injuries are best profiled by hospital emergency departments. However, if injury reports occur in single settings such as hospitals or community sporting venues, the spectrum of injuries can be incomplete for adults (Baquie and Brukner, 1997; Finch *et al.*, 1999) and children (McMahon *et al.*, 1993). Profiles of injuries from multiple settings are considered to be more representative of the range and severity of all paediatric sports-related injuries.

Inherent in research on injuries is the frustration with the plethora of definitions used for 'injury and injury severity'. Reporting of injuries can also occur relative to seasons, years or hours of exposure. Exact comparisons are often improbable, but trends in the data often provide useful information for future research.

Within the limitations of injury research, existing trends include: boys incurring more injuries than girls (Skokan *et al.*, 2003), more severe injuries occurring in older than younger children (Browne and Lam, 2006) and games being more injurious than training (Radelet *et al.*, 2002). When team sports in young people are assessed, moderate to high impact sports such as football codes for boys and basketball for girls are described as the most injurious (Powell and Barber-Foss, 1999). Inclusion of a broader range of sports in injury surveillance results in 'high risk' individual sports (e.g. snowboarding, BMX cycling) being more injurious than team sports (Michaud *et al.*, 2001). Also, most reports of paediatric sporting injury surveillance have been generated from nations other than Australia.

Therefore, we conducted the Paediatric Sporting Injuries Study in Sydney, Australia. The study involved a 12-month surveillance study of 235 sporting injuries in young people (60 per cent male) aged five to 16 years. The objective was to profile and compare injuries presenting at three types of medical practice. We aimed to broaden the understanding of paediatric sports injuries and support development of appropriate recommendations for future injury prevention education.

Methods

Injury data were collected from patients on presentation for sports-related injuries at three types of medical practice: Sydney's largest paediatric emergency department (The Children's Hospital at Westmead) ($n =1$ site and 95 patients), sports physician practices ($n = 5$ sites and 88 patients) and general practices with a paediatric focus ($n = 5$ sites and 52 patients). Following hospital and university ethics approval, parents or guardians of young people with sports injuries were invited to participate in the study upon presentation with sports-related injuries at a site of one of three types of medical practice. A project coordinator managed data entry to clarify reports where necessary and eliminate the possibility of duplicating data. The instrument developed for the sports medicine injury surveillance project (Finch *et al.*, 1999; Finch and Mitchell, 2002) provided a standardized method for sports physicians to report injuries. The standardized survey formed the basis for the surveys completed for the present study and had a section for patients or parent and one for the physician. The patient forms had questions on the socio-demographics, sports history and description of incidents. Physician forms required information on diagnosis, injury and treatment as well as the likely severity in 'days of lost participation'.

Data were analyzed using the Stata statistical software programme. Since the study was of an exploratory nature, data were analyzed descriptively. Univariate statistics are presented in frequencies and percentages of survey responses. Bivariate analyses were conducted to examine unadjusted relationships between all characteristics variables and different types of medical practices. As all variables were categorized, Chi-squared tests were applied to examine the bivariate associations. Due to the multiple tests of hypotheses, the significant level for rejecting the null hypothesis in each test conducted was adjusted to the level 1 per cent instead of the conventional 5 per cent for two-tailed tests.

Results

Initial results showed specialist practices (40 per cent) and the children's hospital's emergency department (38 per cent) were most frequently visited by children with sporting injuries, but general practices (22 per cent) did not appear to see as many young patients with sporting injuries. Over two-thirds of the patients were aged between 12 and 16 years and only 25 per cent of injuries occurred in individual rather than team sports. Most injuries occurred in games.

Chi-squared analysis provided unadjusted associations of injury characteristics and the three different types of medical settings (Table 14.1). Associations were found in the higher percentage (63 per cent) of children with impact-related

Table 14.1 Profile of injuries at three types of medical practices

Characteristics of injuries		Type of medical practice frequency (%)		Results	
		Specialists	General practices	Hospitals	
Type of sports	Team sports	52 (63)	43 (84)	72 (82)	$\chi^2_2 = 11.36$,
	Individual sports	31 (37)	8 (16)	16 (18)	$p = 0.003$
Hours of training (per week)	≤ 5 hours	33 (44)	21 (43)	50 (76)	$\chi^2_2 = 18.05$,
	6 hours or more	42 (56)	28 (57)	16 (24)	$p < 0.001$
Mechanism of injury	Impact-related**	19 (24)	18 (35)	54 (63)	$\chi^2_2 = 26.97$,
	Non-impact-related	59 (76)	33 (65)	31 (36)	$p < 0.001$
Growth condition#	Yes	16 (17)	4 (8)	3 (3)	$\chi^2_2 = 9.67$,
	No	79 (83)	48 (92)	85 (97)	$p = 0.008$
Return to activity advice given	Able to return	46 (53)	12 (25)	11 (14)	$\chi^2_2 = 30.99$,
	Unable to return	40 (46)	36 (75)	68 (86)	$p < 0.001$
Imaging conducted	Yes	53 (56)	31 (60)	81 (92)	$\chi^2_2 = 32.31$,
	No	42 (44)	21 (40)	7 (8)	$p < 0.001$

**Impacted-related mechanism included: collision with fixed object; collision with player/tackle; struck by ball/or other sports equipment. Non-impact-related mechanism included: sudden stopping; jumping and falling; swerving and pivoting.
Growth-related conditions included: Osgood Schlatter, Sannsen Larsen Syndrome, Hypermobility and Severs Disease.

injuries and presentations at the emergency department, compared with 35 per cent at general practices and 24 per cent at specialist practices ($\chi^2_2 = 26.97$, $p < 0.001$). In contrast, presentations from individual sports (37 per cent) ($\chi^2_2 = 11.36$, $p = 0.003$) and young people with growth-related injuries (17 per cent) ($\chi^2_2 = 9.67$, $p = 0.008$) were higher at specialist practices than generalist practices and the emergency department. Approximately 76 per cent of children presenting with sports injuries at the hospital's emergency department participated in five hours or less of organised physical activity ($\chi^2_2 = 18.05$, $p < 0.001$).

Summary

In summary, profiles of sports-related injuries in young people may best be provided in multi-agency profiles. Over-use injuries and growth-related conditions were more frequently seen at specialist practices but acute injuries were more prevalent at the emergency departments. Knowledge of paediatric sporting injury presentations is also useful for justifying modifications to existing medical education programmes relevant to different types of medical practices.

Acknowledgement

We are indebted to the New South Wales Sporting Injury Committee for their support in funding this project.

References

Baquie, P. and Brukner, P., 1997, Injuries presenting to an Australian sports medicine centre: A 12–month study. *Clinical Journal of Sports Medicine*, **7**, pp. 28–31.

Browne, G.J. and Lam, L.T., 2006, Concussive head injury in children and adolescents related to sports and other leisure physical activities. *British Journal of Sports Medicine*, **40**, pp. 163–168.

Finch, C.F. and Mitchell, D.J., 2002, A comparison of two injury surveillance systems within sports medicine clinics. *Journal of Science and Medicine in Sport*, **5**, pp. 321–335.

Finch, C.F., Valuri, G. and Ozanne-Smith, J., 1999, Injury surveillance during medical coverage of sporting events – Development and testing of a standardised data collection form. *Journal of Science and Medicine in Sport*, **2**, pp. 42–56.

Lam, L.T., 2005, Hospitalisation due to sports-related injuries among children and adolescents in New South Wales, Australia: An analysis on socioeconomic and geographic differences. *Journal of Science & Medicine in Sport*, **8**, pp. 433–440.

McMahon, K.A., Nolan, T., Bennett, C.M. and Carlin, J., 1993, Australian Rules football injuries in children and adolescents. *Medical Journal of Australia*, **159**, pp. 301–306.

Michaud, P.-A., Renaud, A. and Narring, F., 2001, Sports activities related to injuries? A survey among 9–19-year-olds in Switzerland, *Injury Prevention*, pp. 41–45.

Powell, J.W. and Barber-Foss, K.D., 1999, Injury patterns in selected high school sports: A review of the 1995–1997 seasons. *Journal of Athletic Training*, **34**, pp. 277–284.

Radelet, M.A., Lephart, S.M., Rubinstein, E.N.and Myers, J.B., 2002, Survey of the injury rate for children in community sports. *Pediatrics*, **110**, p.e28.

Skokan, E.G., Junkins, E.P. and Kadish, H., 2003, Serious winter sports injuries in children and adolescents requiring hospitalization. *The American Journal of Emergency Medicine*, **21**, pp. 95–99.

15 Osteopenia of prematurity

The role of exercise in prevention and treatment

D. Nemet and A. Eliakim

Child Health and Sports Center, Pediatric Department, Meir Medical Center, Sackler School of Medicine, Tel-Aviv University, Israel

Introduction

Despite a steady decline in live birth rates in the United States over the past two decades, the incidence of preterm births (infants born at less than 37 weeks of gestation) had increased to 12.5 per cent in 2005 (Hamilton *et al.*, 2003). Furthermore, advances in perinatal care, such as the increased use of assisted ventilation in the delivery room and surfactant therapy, have improved the chances for survival of low gestational age and low birth weight infants (Hack *et al.*, 2000). The rising incidence of preterm births, coupled with their improved survival as a result of highly evolving technologies, has placed an increased need to develop more innovative and cost-effective treatment modalities for the consequences of prematurity during the neonatal period and later in life.

One of these consequences is osteopenia of prematurity. Osteopenia of prematurity (OOP) occurs because of both limited accretion of bone and muscle mass in utero and due to the greater need for bone nutrients compared to infants delivered at term (Ziegler *et al.*, 1976). An infant born at term has a total body Ca content of approximately 30 g, while the total Ca content of a 24-weeks born infant is only 10–15 per cent of this value (Demarini *et al.*, 1997). The rate of osteopenia is inversely related to birth weight and gestational age, and severe morbidity during the neonatal period (e.g. bronchopulmonary dysplasia – BPD), and chronic drug therapy (diuretics, steroids) increase further the risk of bone demineralization.

The last trimester of pregnancy is characterized by a crescendo of physical activity in which the fetus must work in a viscous milieu, and as it grows, it encounters the elastic resistance of an increasingly limited intrauterine environment. The prematurely born infant is deprived of this crucial period of intrauterine growth and development and 'physiological exercise training'. This, together with the prolonged hospitalization of premature infants in neonatal intensive care units (weeks or even months) without sensory and physical stimulation may be another reason for bone demineralization in the preterm infant.

Diagnosis of osteopenia

Currently, the diagnosis of osteopenia is based on clinical and radiological signs and measurements of biochemical markers. The relatively new development of assays for circulating biochemical markers of bone turnover (Delmas, 1995) allows us to gain greater mechanistic insight into the effects of prematurity on bone development.

Another major progress in the evaluation of bone metabolism in preterm infants was made by the use of quantitative ultrasound measurements (QUS) of tibial bone speed of sound (SOS). QUS was developed, in recent years, for the diagnosis and treatment of osteoporosis (Foldes *et al.*, 1995). In addition to bone density, it assesses other bone properties such as cortical thickness, elasticity and micro-architecture, thus providing a more complete picture of bone strength (Njeh *et al.*, 1999). QUS is an inexpensive, portable method, and free of ionizing radiation. Therefore, it was suggested that this method may be an important tool in the diagnosis, management and follow-up of osteopenia in premature infants.

We used QUS measurements of bone SOS to determine bone strength in a group of preterm and full-term infants (Nemet *et al.*, 2001). Tibial bone SOS was successfully measured in all infants. There was a significant correlation between tibial SOS and gestational age (Figure 15.1), but a significant inverse correlation between tibial SOS and postnatal age.

Bone SOS was significantly higher in full-term infants compared to premature infants, and compared to a sub-group of the premature infants who reached corrected age of full-term. Furthermore, we recently demonstrated that bone strength continues to decrease in premature infants during the first eight postnatal weeks.

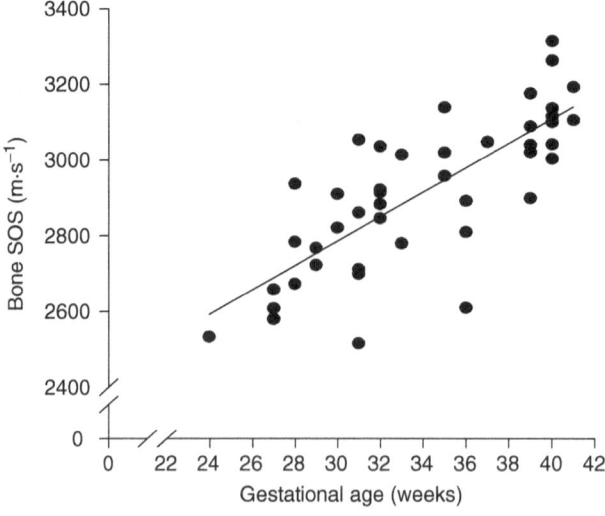

Figure 15.1 Correlation between tibial speed of sound and gestational age.

Prevention and treatment

Since the major cause of osteopenia of prematurity was thought to be inadequate calcium and phosphorus intake compared to the physiological accretion of these minerals during the last trimester of pregnancy (Demarini *et al.*, 1997), most of the efforts to prevent osteopenia of prematurity have been focused on nutritional changes.

In addition to the major efforts to increase the calcium and phosphorus supply by the use of fortified human milk and/or neonatal enriched special formula, simultaneous efforts are made to reduce other possible causes of osteopenia in premature infants such as to reduce the use of systemic corticosteroids and calcium loosing diuretics (e.g. furosamide) in preterm infants with lung disease, and to decrease the content of aluminum in TPN solutions. However, despite the nutritional goal to provide optimal support for growth (as similar as possible to the growth in utero during the last trimester), nutritional interventions were only partially successful in improving premature infants' bone mineralization.

Spontaneous physical activity

Mechanical strain is one of the most powerful stimulators of bone formation and growth. Several studies have demonstrated that physical activity increases bone mass in children, adolescents and adults (Eliakim *et al.*, 1997; Slemenda *et al.*, 1991), while inactivity results in bone resorption and decreased bone mineral density.

This may be particularly important for premature infants since, during prolonged hospitalization in the NICU (i.e. in small incubators and cradles), the traditional standard of care involves minimal sensory and/or tactile stimulation. The limited physical activity of hospitalized premature infants may play an important role in the development of bone demineralization and osteopenia. Therefore, in order to avoid that, efforts are now made to understand the mechanisms that link physical activity and bone metabolism in preterm infants, and to develop strategies to increase physical activity in this unique population.

Attempts to measure the effects of assisted exercise (termed 'kinesthetic stimulation' by some investigators) in human infants were first reported by White and Labarba in 1976. They studied 12 (six control) preterm infants born at 34 weeks and showed significant increases in body weight in the treatment group after a 10-day intervention, beginning on the second day of life. In 1995, Moyer-Mileur *et al.* studied the effects of a single daily session of passive range of motion movement with gentle compression of the upper and lower limbs in 13 intervention and 13 control preterm infants (born at 28 weeks). The intervention started at an average post natal age of two weeks and lasted four weeks, and resulted in significant increases in body weight (by 33 per cent) and bone density (by 34 per cent, measured by single photon absorptiometry) in the exercise group compared to control preterm infants. In 2000, the same group of investigators repeated this study using DEXA and corroborated their original observations in 16 intervention and 16 control preterm infants (Moyer-Mileur *et al.*, 2000). The authors concluded that when premature infants perform daily physical activity in addition to the consumption of the recommended energy and nutrient intake, bone mass accretion is similar to the increase in bone indexes in utero during the last trimester. This enhancement of bone mass by physical activity was not accompanied by changes in circulating levels of calcium, phosphate, alkaline phosphatase, parathyroid hormone, or vitamin D. Therefore, the mechanism for the exercise-induced increased bone density in premature infants was unknown. Recently, we (Nemet *et al.*, 2002) assessed in randomized, prospective studies the effects of daily assisted exercise on weight gain, serum leptin, and insulin-like growth factor-I (IGF-I), and bone markers in preterm infants (Eliakim *et al.*, 2002). The exercise protocol started at the fourth week of life (corrected age 32 weeks).

The assisted exercise training led to:

1   A significant increase in weight gain in the exercising group (784 ± 51 vs 608 ± 26 g in exercise and controls, respectively, $p < 0.05$) – namely, an almost 50 g week^{-1} difference between the groups (Figure 15.2).
2   An increase in circulating IGF-I (an increase of 16.7 ± 3.1 vs 9.2 ± 4.1 ng mL^{-1} in training and controls, respectively).
3   A significant increase in leptin (0.60 ± 0.19 vs 0.13 ± 0.06 ng mL^{-1} in training and controls, respectively).
4   An increase in bone formation marker (i.e. BSAP), and to a significant decrease in the bone resorption marker compared to the control subjects (Figure 15.3).

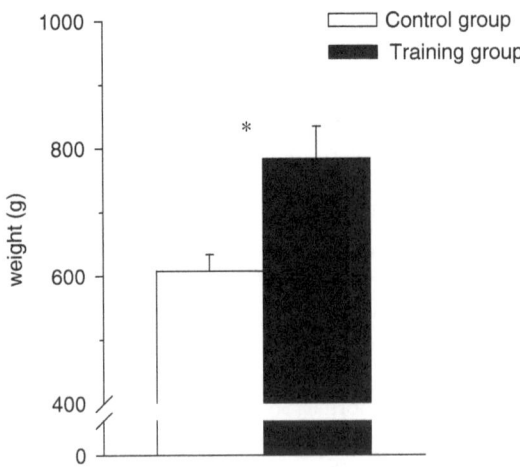

Figure 15.2 The effects of passive range of motion exercise on changes in body weight in premature infants.

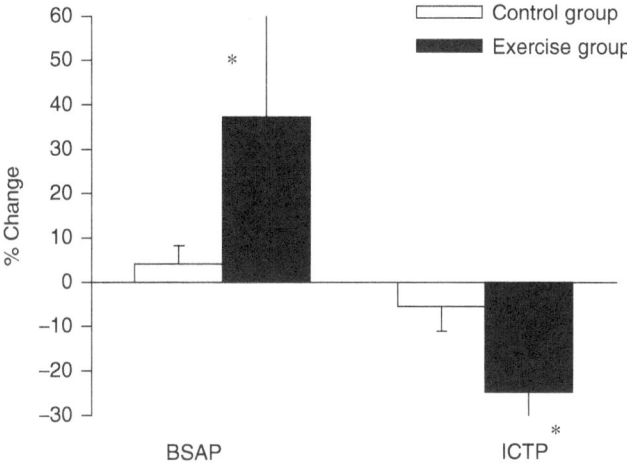

Figure 15.3 The effects of passive range of motion exercise on markers of bone metabolism.

The changes in leptin correlated with the changes in body weight. The mechanism for the exercise-induced weight gain in premature infants is not clearly understood. Moyer-Mileur *et al.* (1995) suggested that part of the exercise-induced weight gain is related to increased bone mineralization. Interestingly, several studies (Kume *et al.*, 2002 ; Reseland *et al.*, 2001) indicated that leptin is secreted from human osteoblasts and promotes bone mineralization. Therefore, our finding of an increase in circulating leptin using the same daily exercise protocol may also explain the exercise induced increase in bone mineral density in premature infants. The significant increase in circulating leptin, and the correlation between these changes and the changes in body weight may also suggest that at least part of the increase in body weight was due to an increase in adipose tissue.

The increase in circulating IGF-I in the exercise group subjects was greater than the increase in the control subjects, but this difference was not statistically significant ($p < 0.09$). Interestingly, the exercise-associated increase in IGF-I was statistically significant in a subgroup of premature infants with BPD. It is not clear whether this suggests that daily movement exercise has a stronger effect in the more catabolic premature infants (i.e. BPD). Increased IGF-I may play an important role in brain protection and normal retinal development (Hellstrom *et al.*, 2002). Therefore, beneficial effects of an exercise-associated increase in IGF-I levels may not be limited to the bone and muscle tissue.

The exercise intervention studies in premature infants were started mainly at postnatal age of two to five weeks after the critical period of the first days of life, and when all preterm infants were stable. Recently, in a prospective randomized study, we used the same exercise protocol to evaluate the effect of early exercise training (i.e. first week of life) on bone strength, and turnover in VLBW premature infants

(Litmanovitz *et al.*, 2003). The major finding of this study was that bone SOS decreased during the first four postnatal weeks in the control infants, and that the relatively brief, daily, passive range of motion physical activity attenuated this decrease. Consistent with previous reports the results of this study suggest again that exercise has an important role in bone development during the neonatal period, and may contribute to the prevention of osteopenia of prematurity.

Finally, in contrast to exercise interventions that started at a postnatal age of four to five weeks, early exercise was not associated with a greater increase in weight gain. This observation is in agreement with Moyer-Miller *et al.* (1995), who also found that the increase in weight gain was significant only when the premature infants reached body weight of 1.8–2 kg. This suggests that the accelerated weight gain occurs only when exercise training is introduced later in the neonatal course (four to five weeks vs first week). The early exercise-associated bone effects without differences in weight gain suggest that the positive bone effects were not related to the increased weight gain.

Summary

All together these studies demonstrate that exercise training for premature infants results in favorable effects on bone metabolism. Collectively, these studies suggest that both duration and timing of the intervention influence the overall beneficial effect of assisted exercise in preterm infants. It is still unclear if the positive bone effects are related just to the brief range of motion exercise, or to longer metabolic changes following the brief exercise. Moreover, whether this degree and frequency of exercise is the optimal for bone development in premature infants still needs to be determined.

A large prospective study is now in process to try and evaluate both the structural aspects and the underlying growth mediator/inflammatory mechanisms leading to improved growth and bone strength following assisted exercise in the preterm infants.

References

Delmas, P.D., 1995, Biochemical markers of bone turnover. *Acta Orthopedica Scandinavica*, **266**, pp. 176–182.

Demarini, D., Mimouni, F.B. and Tsang, R.C., 1997, Rickets of prematurity. In: *Neonatal-perinatal Medicine – Diseases of the Fetus and Infant*, edited by Fanaroff, A.A., Martin, R.J., 6th edn, Vol. 2. St Louis: Mosby, pp. 1473–1476.

Eliakim, A., Dolfin, T., Weiss, E., Shainkin-Kestenbaum, R., Lis, M. and Nemet, D., 2002, The effects of exercise on body weight and circulating leptin in premature infants. *Journal of Perinatology*, **22**, 7, pp. 550–554.

Eliakim, A., Raisz, L.G., Brasel, J.A. and Cooper D.M., 1997, Evidence for increased bone formation following a brief endurance-type training intervention in adolescent males. *Journal of Bone and Mineral Research*, **12**, pp. 1708–1713.

Foldes, A.J., Rimon, A., Keinan, D.D. and Popovtzer M.M., 1995, Quantitative ultrasound of the tibia: A novel approach for assessment of bone status. *Bone*, **17**, pp. 363–367.

Hack, M. and Fanaroff, A.A., 2000, Outcomes of children of extremely low birthweight and gestational age in the 1990s. *Seminars in Neonatology*, **5**, pp. 89–106.

Hamilton, B.E., Martin, J.A. and Sutton, P.D., 2003, Births: Preliminary data for 2002. *National Vital Statistic Report*, **51**, pp. 1–20.

Hellstrom, A., Carlsson, B., Niklasson, A., Segnestam, K., Boguszewski, M., de Lacerda, L., Savage, M., Svensson, E., Smith, L., Weinberger D., Albertsson, W.K. and Laron, Z., 2002, IGF-I is critical for normal vascularization of the human retina. *Journal of Clinical Endocrinology and Metabolism*, **87**, pp. 3413–3416.

Kume, K., Satomura, K., Nishisho, S., Kitaoka, E., Yamanouchi, K., Tobiume, S. and Nagayama, M., 2002, Potential role of leptin in endochondral ossification. *Journal of Histochemistry and Cytochemistry*, **50**, pp. 159–169.

Litmanovitz, I., Dolfin, T., Friedland, O., Arnon, S., Regev, R., Shainkin- Kestenbaum, R., Lis, M. and Eliakim, A., 2003, Early physical activity intervention prevents decrease of bone strength in very low birth weight infants. *Pediatrics*, **112**, 1, Pt 1; pp. 15–19.

Moyer-Mileur, L.J., Luetkemeier, M., Boomer, L. and Chan, G.M., 1995, Effect of physical activity on bone mineralization in premature infants. *Journal of Pediatrics*, **127**, pp. 620–625.

Moyer-Mileur, L.J., Brunstetter, V., McNaught, T.P., Gill G. and Chan, G.M., 2000, Daily physical activity program increases bone mineralization and growth in preterm very low birth weight infants. *Pediatrics*, **106**, pp. 1088–1092.

Nemet, D., Dolfin, T., Litmanowitz, I., Shainkin-Kestenbaum, R., Lis, M. and Eliakim, A., 2002, Evidence for exercise-induced bone formation in premature infants. *International Journal of Sports Medicine*, **23**, pp. 82–85.

Nemet, D., Dolfin, T., Wolach, B. and Eliakim, A., 2001, Quantitative ultrasound measurements of bone speed of sound in premature infants. *European Journal of Pediatrics*, **160**, pp. 736–740.

Njeh, C.F., Hans, D., Wu, C., Kantorovich, E., Sister, M., Fuerst T. and Genant, H.K., 1999, An in vitro investigation of the dependence on sample thickness of the speed of sound along the specimen. *Medical Engineering and Physics*, **21**, pp. 651–659.

Reseland, J.E., Syversen, U., Bakke, I., Qvigstad, G., Eide, L.G, Hjertner, O., Gordeladze, J.O. and Drevon, C.A., 2001, Leptin is expressed in and secreted from primary cultures of human osteoblasts and promotes bone mineralization. *Journal of Bone and Mineral Research*, **16**, pp. 1426–1433.

Slemenda, C.W., Miller, J.Z., Hui, S.L., Reister, T.K. and Johnston, C.C. Jr., 1991, Role of physical activity in the development of skeletal mass in children. *Journal of Bone Mineral Research*, **6**, pp. 1227–1233.

White, J.L. and Labarba, R.C., 1976, The effects of tactile and kinesthetic stimulation on neonatal development in the premature infant. *Developmental Psychobiology*, **9**, pp. 569–577.

Ziegler, E.E., O'Donnell, A.M., Nelson, S.E. and Fomon S.J., 1976, Body composition of the reference fetus. *Growth*, **40**, pp. 329–341.

16 Children's psychological well-being, habitual physical activity and sedentary behaviour

T.G. Pavey, G. Parfitt and A. Rowlands
University of Exeter, Exeter, UK

Introduction

Parfitt and Eston (2005) was the first study to use pedometers to objectively measure activity and investigate the relationship between children's habitual activity levels and psychological well-being. Correlation analyses revealed that habitual physical activity had a strong positive association with global self-esteem ($r = 0.66$, $p < 0.01$), and negative associations with depression ($r = -0.60$, $p < 0.01$) and anxiety ($r = -0.48$, $p < 0.01$). When groups were created based upon activity level, children achieving $>12,000$ steps/day had more positive psychological profiles than children achieving <9200 steps/day. There were limitations in the Parfitt and Eston (2005) study as only global self-esteem was measured. There was an inability to measure and discuss the intensity of the accrued physical activity and the recorded results could be accounted for by factors not assessed, including, socio-economic status.

This cross-sectional study aims to replicate and extend Parfitt and Eston (2005) and forms part of a larger study (Parfitt *et al.*, submitted). To overcome previous limitations, accelerometry was used to assess physical activity and intensity, and a more chronic measure of physical activity was adopted. Socio-economic status was also accounted for and the measure of self-esteem was expanded to incorporate Harter's (1985) five esteem domains, as well as global self-esteem, physical self-worth, and its four sub-domains.

Method

During the first meeting with the children, anthropometric data were collected; the children's age, height, sitting height, mass and body fat percentage were recorded and the children were each given an RT3 accelerometer and shown how to wear it. The accelerometers were worn by the children for two seven-day periods (one during the autumn and one during the spring). Activity counts were converted into MET equivalents which provided the following cut-off points for the intensity levels: <1.9 METS = sedentary, 1.9–3 METS = light, 3–6 METS = moderate and >6 METS = vigorous. Following the second seven-day period, the children completed three psychological well-being inventories to assess trait anxiety, depression and global, domain and sub-domain measures of self-esteem. Pearson's correlations (r) and 2 (sex) × 3 (activity/intensity groups) analyses of variance were used to assess the relationships between the psychological well-being constructs and physical activity/intensity.

Results

A total of 57 participants (23 boys, 34 girls) provided adequate data for analysis. Girls accumulated significantly more minutes in light intensity activity ($t(55) = 2.678, p = 0.010$) and significantly fewer minutes in vigorous intensity activity ($t(55) = 2.218, p = 0.031$) than boys. No further sex differences were present.

As indicated in Table 16.1, sedentary behaviour was positively associated with measures of anxiety and depression ($r > 0.345, p < 0.009$), and negatively associated with measures of global self-worth, physical self-worth, appearance, attractive body and scholastic competence ($r > -0.297, p < 0.025$). Light intensity activity was negatively associated with global self-worth, physical self-worth, appearance and attractive body ($r > -0.297, p < 0.025$) and moderate intensity activity ($r = -0.315, p = 0.017$) was negatively associated with behaviour. Finally, vigorous intensity activities were negatively associated with anxiety ($r = -0.310, p = 0.019$) and positively associated with measures of scholastic, social, athletic competence and stamina ($r > 0.281, p < 0.034$). All significant relationships remained after controlling for socio-economic status and body fat.

ANOVA analyses revealed there were no sex by tertile (low, mid and high minutes) group interactions. However, as shown in Table 16.2, there were main effects for sedentary behaviour on anxiety ($F(2,51) = 4.86, p < 0.05$), global self-worth ($F(2,51) = 4.56, p < 0.05$), physical self-worth ($F(2,51) = 6.31, p < 0.01$), appearance ($F(2,51) = 6.73, p < 0.01$), attractive body ($F(2,51) = 4.80, p < 0.05$) and scholastic competence ($F(2,51) = 3.21, p < 0.05$). Post hoc tests show

Table 16.1 Correlations: activity, intensity and psychological well-being

	Overall activity	Sedentary	Light	Moderate	Vigorous
Anxiety	−0.195	0.384**	0.173	−0.110	−0.310**
Depression	−0.014	0.345**	0.202	0.103	−0.177
Global self-worth	−0.032	−0.385**	−0.345*	−0.132	0.121
Scholastic competence	0.081	−0.341**	−0.225	−0.119	0.281*
Social acceptance	0.248	−0.118	0.002	0.018	0.338**
Behavioural competence	−0.359**	−0.067	−0.229	−0.315*	−0.273*
Physical appearance	−0.050	−0.385**	−0.345*	−0.132	0.121
Physical self-worth	−0.055	−0.388**	−0.301*	−0.139	0.115
Athletic competence	0.242	−0.133	−0.056	0.090	0.335*
Stamina	0.258	−0.184	−0.053	0.122	0.324*
Attractive body	−0.103	−0.297*	−0.297*	−0.188	0.066
Strength	0.025	−0.085	−0.103	0.039	0.066

Table 16.2 Well-being scores by time spent in sedentary activity

Psychological well-being	Sedentary		
	Low group (197 Minutes)	Mid group (225 Minutes)	High group (262 Minutes)
Anxiety	29.3[a](1.5)	31.1 (1.7)	36.1[a](1.6)
Global self-worth	19.2[a](.8)	20.2[b] (.9)	16.5[a,b](.9)
Physical self-worth	18.9[a](1.0)	19.6[b] (1.1)	14.8[a,b](1.0)
Appearance	17.7[a](.8)	19.7[b] (1.1)	14.1[a,b](.8)
Attractive body	19.0[a](1.1)	17.3 (1.0)	14.3[a](1.0)
Scholastic competence	18.5[a](.9)	16.2 (1.0)	15.4[a](1.0)

[a] = high sedentary group significantly different from low sedentary group.
[b] = high sedentary group significantly different from mid sedentary group.

that measures of anxiety were significantly lower in the low minutes group (mean = 29.30 ± 1.58) than the high minutes group (mean = 36.13 ± 1.61), while measures of global self-worth, physical self-worth, appearance, attractive body and scholastic competence were significantly lower in the high minutes group (mean < 16.76, ± > 0.86) compared to the low minutes group (mean > 17.76, ± < 1.14).

Discussion

This confirms previous cross-sectional research concerning the relationship between habitual physical activity and psychological well-being in children, using a mechanical measure of physical activity (Parfitt and Eston, 2005). Time spent in sedentary and light intensity activities were negatively associated with primarily the physical self-esteem domains. Further, time spent in sedentary activities had positive associations with both anxiety and depression. Time spent in vigorous activity was positively associated with the physical self-esteem domains, and negatively associated with anxiety. Measures of global and physical self-esteem, appearance, attractive body and scholastic competence were significantly lower in the high minute sedentary group compared to the low minute sedentary group. This was also apparent for anxiety, with significantly lower anxiety scores for the low minute sedentary group.

Although this study was cross-sectional in nature, previous intervention research has highlighted the positive effects of physical activity on psychological well-being constructs (Mutrie and Parfitt, 1998; Ekeland et al., 2005). Given the current findings from the tertile group analyses, data for the anxiety, global self-esteem, physical self-worth and various sub-domains suggest that a reduction of around 60 mins a day of sedentary intensity activities should help to improve the psychological well-being profiles for children of this age group.

The domains of physical self-esteem, in particular, are associated with physical activity intensity. These domains are negatively associated with sedentary and light activity, and positively associated with vigorous activity. These associations are represented further with children in the accumulated low minute sedentary intensity group having more positive psychological well-being profiles. This suggests that less time in sedentary behaviour should be promoted in order to improve psychological well-being for this age group. The ongoing longitudinal research may help to clarify this and the potential causal links.

References

Ekeland, E., Heian, F. and Hagen, K.B., 2005, Can exercise improve self-esteem in children and young people? A systematic review of randomised controlled trials. *British Journal of Sports Medicine*, **39**, p. 792.

Harter, S., 1985, *Manual for the Self-perception Profile for Children*. Denver, CO: University of Denver.

Mutrie, N. and Parfitt, G., 1998, Physical activity and its link with mental health, social and moral and moral health in young people. In: *Young and Active? Young People and Health-enhancing Physical Activity: Evidence and Implications*, edited by Biddle, S.J.H., Cavill, N. and Sallis, J.F., London: Health Education Authority, pp. 49–68.

Parfitt, G. and Eston, R.G., 2005, The relationship between children's habitual activity level and psychological well-being. *Acta Paediatrica*, **94**, pp. 1791–1797.

Parfitt, G., Pavey, T.G. and Rowlands, A.V., The relevance of intensity level when assessing physical activity and psychological well-being in children. Acta paediatrica (submitted).

17 Epidemiological study of scoliosis and postural faults of Romanian schoolchildren

C. Serbescu,[1,4] D. Ianc,[1,4] O. Straciuc,[2] G. Carp[3] and D. Courteix[4]

[1]Faculty of Physical Education and Sport, Oradea, Romania; [2]County Clinic Hospital Oradea, Romania; [3]Paediatric Clinic Hospital Oradea, Romania; [4]Universite Blaise Pascal, France

Introduction

Orthostatic posture and movement functions are very complex adaptive and integrative functions of the child in today's sedentary environment. The lack of physical activity (Juskeliene et al., 1996) associated with prolonged sitting periods (Linton et al., 1994) are implicated in the appearance of poor postures and/or functional deformities of children. Scoliosis may appear during childhood and aggravate during the pubertal growth spurt, but importantly, it may also determine pain syndromes and stress pathologies later in life.

Screening programmes can be effective in identifying postural disorders and structural scoliosis, providing opportunity for early diagnosis, treatment, and education (Mirtz et al., 2005). Physical education teachers and physiotherapists should integrate health promotion into their work, and teach preventive measures for a healthy posture and to detect faulty posture. The aim of this study was to assess the prevalence and correlates of scoliosis and posture in Romanian children aged 8–11.

Methods

A total of 113 boys (9.5± 0.8 y, 34.7 ± 9.7 kg, 137.7 ± 8 cm) and 139 girls (9.5 ± 0.8 y, 32.8 ± 7.3 kg, 136.6 ± 7.2 cm) from Oradea city entered the study. Body mass index (BMI) was derived from stature and body mass. Body composition was assessed through sum of four skinfolds according to the method described by Durnin and Rahaman (1967). Skeletal maturation was assessed using a radiographic scan of the left hand and wrist (Greulich, 1960), and pubertal development was evaluated according to the method of Marshall and Tanner (1975). A screening test for poor posture and for scoliosis was realized by the physical examination of the whole body and forward bending test (Adams, 1882). The Cobb methods (1948) were used to measure the curve angles and transversal plane vertebral rotation on the posterior-anterior radiographs of the spine in the standing position. Comparison between parameters was examined using analysis of variance (ANOVA). Statistical significance was established at $p < 0.05$.

Results

Subjective assessment

During clinical examination subjects were assessed for postural faults. 94.4 per cent presented one or more postural faults as follows: hypercyphosis 49.2 per cent [50.9 per cent, boys (B) and 47.8 per cent girls (G)], hyperlordosis 29 per cent (33.3 per cent B, 25.4 per cent G); pelvic deviations 10.3 per cent (5.3 per cent B, 14.5 per cent G) ; thoracic impairments 21.4 per cent (29 per cent B, 15.2 per cent G); shoulder imbalance 35.3 per cent (42 per cent B, 29.7 per cent G); knee deviations 20.2 per cent (20.2 per cent B, 20.3 per cent G); functional flat feet 50 per cent (44.7 per cent B, 49.6 per cent G). 46.4 per cent (40.8 per cent B, 39.5 per cent G) of children presented at forward-bending test a rib-hump or lumbar-hump.

Objective assessment

Radiological measurements revealed that 16.8 per cent of all subjects, 22 girls (mean Cobb angle 12.4° ± 2.7) and 20 boys, (12.9° ± 1.8) presented structural scoliosis. The cutting point used to differentiate between functional and structural scoliosis was: Cobb angle value > or = 10° + vertebral rotation. Girl to boy ratio was 1.1:1 for functional scoliosis and 0.89:1 for structural scoliosis, increasing with age. Prevalence rates of structural scoliosis were 18 per cent for boys and no case for girls at seven to eight years of age, 6 per cent for boys and 9 per cent for girls at 8–9 years of age, 12 per cent for boys and 5 per cent for girls at 9–10 years of age and 4 per cent for boys and 14 per cent for girls at 10–11 years of age. Mean Cobb angle values were 10.5° at 7–8 years old, 12.6° at 8–9 years old, 13.9° at 9–10 years old and 11.7° at 10–11 years old, but there was no significant difference ($p > 0.05$) between values of Cobb angle of the four age groups. The most prevalent curve was left thoracic 49.3 per cent followed by left-thoracic-right lumbar 1.13 per cent and left-lumbar 0.8 per cent. The differences between characteristics of girls presenting functional scoliosis and those with structural scoliosis are shown in Table 17.1.

Discussion

Postural faults and asymmetrical posture are very frequent in the studied population, but the prevalence remains within the reported data for the same age populations. The prevalence rate of structural scoliosis tends to increase with age as in reported screening studies (Smyrnis *et al.*, 1987; Stirling *et al.*, 1996).

Table 17.1 Comparison between characteristics of girls presenting functional scoliosis and those with structural scoliosis (n total = 126)

Characteristics of the subjects	Functional scoliosis (n = 97)	Structural scoliosis (n = 29)	Difference
Age (y)	9.5 ± 0.8	9.8 ± 0.8	ns
Bone age (y)	10.2 ± 1.2	10.2 ± 1.4	ns
Stature (cm)	137 ± 7.1	134.5 ± 7.4	ns
Body mass (kg)	33.4 ± 7.2	29.7 ± 7.1	$p < 0.05$
BMI (kg·m^{-2})	17.7 ± 3.0	16.2 ± 2.4	$p < 0.05$
Body fat %	25.8 ± 9.0	19.6 ± 8.0	$p < 0.01$

There is a tendency for a higher prevalence of scoliosis in girls than boys of 9 to 11 years old but the difference is not significant ($p > 0.05$).

In girls the scoliosis incidence increased rapidly up to the 11-year-old group, whereas in boys there was a decreased prevalence up to 11 years of age.

Epidemiological data show an increased tendency toward 11–12 and 12–13 years old in boys and in girls (Penha *et al.*, 2005, Wong *et al.*, 2005). Thoracic curves, the most frequent in our study, are considered typical in epidemiological data on scoliosis, with the greatest aggravating potential risk (Marty and Duval-Beaupère, 1999), whereas the left oriented curvature showed low progressive potential (Soucacos *et al.*, 1998). Scoliotic girls in our study are thinner, and they have a lower BMI and body fat than the normal population of the same age. Our findings confirm the data in the literature (LeBlanc *et al.*, 1998; Sugita, 2000; Siu King Cheung *et al.*, 2003).

Conclusions

This study showed a high incidence of postural faults, asymmetrical posture and structural scoliosis in children from Oradea, Romania. The prevalence rate of structural scoliosis was more marked than reported epidemiological data even though angular values were smaller than 20 degrees. Girls presenting scoliosis have a different morphotype than the normal population. This could be a valuable indicator for preventive measures and a subsequent therapeutic strategy. It could also be valuable information for specialists involved in sport selection, especially for those searching for this specific morphotype in girls (e.g. rhythmic gymnastics).

References

Adams, W., 1882, *Lectures on the Pathology and Treatment of Lateral and other Forms of Curvature of the Spine*, London: Churchill & Sons.

Cobb, J., 1948, Study of scoliosis. In: *American Academy of Orthopedic Surgeons Instructional Course*, pp. 261–275.

Durnin, J.V. and Rahaman, M.M., 1967, The assessment of the amount of fat in the human body from measurements of skinfold thickness. *British Journal of Nutrition*, **3**, pp. 681–689.

Greulich, W.W., 1960, Value of X-ray films of hand and wrist in human identification. *Science*, pp. 155–156.

Juskeliene, V., Magnus, P., Bakketeig, L.S., Dailidiene, N. and Jurkuvenas, V., 1996, Prevalence and risk factors for asymmetric posture in preschool children aged 6–7 years. *International Journal of Epidemiology*, **5**, pp. 1053–1059.

LeBlanc, R., Labelle, H., Forest, F. and Poitras, B., 1998, Morphologic discrimination among healthy subjects and patients with progressive and nonprogressive adolescent idiopathic scoliosis. *Spine*, **10**, pp. 1109–1115; discussion 1115–1106.

Linton, S.J., Hellsing, A.L., Halme, T. and Akerstedt, K., 1994, The effects of ergonomically designed school furniture on pupils' attitudes, symptoms and behaviour. *Applied Ergonomics*, **5**, pp. 299–304.

Marty, C. and Duval-Beaupère, G., 1999, Scoliose idiopathique juvénile et de l'adolescent. Les éléments de décision de traitement des scolioses idiopathiques mineures reconnues en cours de croissance. *Lettre de Médecine physique et de Réadaptation*.

Mirtz, T.A., Thompson, M.A., Greene, L., Wyatt, L.A. and Akagi, C.G., 2005, Adolescent idiopathic scoliosis screening for school, community, and clinical health promotion practice utilizing the PRECEDE-PROCEED model. *Chiropractic & Osteopathy*, p. 25.

Penha, P. J., Joao, S. M., Casarotto, R. A., Amino, C. J. and Penteado, D. C., 2005, Postural assessment of girls between 7 and 10 years of age. *Clinics*, **1**, pp. 9–16.

Siu King Cheung, C., Tak Keung Lee, W., Kit Tse, Y., Ping Tang, S., Man Lee, K., Guo, X., Qin, L. and Chun Yiu Cheng, J., 2003, Abnormal peri-pubertal anthropometric measurements and growth pattern in adolescent idiopathic scoliosis: A study of 598 patients. *Spine*, **18**, pp. 2152–2157.

Smyrnis, T., Antoniou, D., Valavanis, J. and Zachariou, C., 1987, Idiopathic scoliosis: Characteristics and epidemiology. *Orthopedics*, **6**, pp. 921–926.

Soucacos, P.N., Zacharis, K., Gelalis, J., Soultanis, K., Kalos, N., Beris, A., Xenakis, T. and Johnson, E.O., 1998, Assessment of curve progression in idiopathic scoliosis. *European Spine Journal*, **4**, pp. 270–277.

Stirling, A.J., Howel, D., Millner, P.A., Sadiq, S., Sharples, D. and Dickson, R.A., 1996, Late-onset idiopathic scoliosis in children six to fourteen years old. A cross-sectional prevalence study. *Journal of Bone and Joint Surgery*, **9**, pp. 1330–1336.

Sugita, K., 2000, Epidemiological study on idiopathic scoliosis in high school students. Prevalence and relation to physique, physical strength and motor ability. *Nippon Koshu Eisei Zasshi*, **4**, pp. 320–325.

Wong, H.K., Hui, J.H., Rajan, U. and Chia, H.P. 2005, Idiopathic scoliosis in Singapore schoolchildren: A prevalence study 15 years into the screening program. *Spine*, **10**, pp. 1188–1196.

18 Health related fitness in 10–15-year-old boys and girls

S.R. Siegel

California State University, San Bernardino, CA, USA

Introduction

Health related physical fitness (HRF) is composed of five components: cardio-respiratory endurance, body composition, muscular strength and endurance, and flexibility. While all five components are important when looking at overall fitness, cardiovascular function and body composition are of particular import due to their immediate impact on children and youth as well as their future risk factors for adult health.

Fitnessgram® is a national HRF test battery used primarily for youth in the United States (US). It was developed by The Cooper Institute in 1982 in response to the need in physical education programmes for a comprehensive assessment protocol (Welk *et al.*, 2002). The objective was to increase parental awareness of children's fitness levels by developing an easy tool for physical education teachers to use when reporting the results of physical fitness assessments. Many states in the US use the Fitnessgram® to assess HRF. Based on the results of their fitness testing, students are either in the Healthy Fitness Zone (HFZ), or in the Needs Improvement category.

In addition to the apprehension regarding current levels of aerobic fitness in American children and youth, concern also exists for the trend of lower fitness in these groups since the 1970s (Freedman *et al.*, 2006; Wang and Zhang, 2006; Malina, 2007). While secular trend has been assessed in the BMI, and for the most part it is consistently higher than in the past, results for the other components of health related fitness vary (Malina, 2007).

In general, the current prevalence of individuals in the Fitnessgram® healthy fitness zone needs to be assessed, as does the actual fitness within each of the health related components. As the legislation of California (CA) is making it possible to use the passing of the Fitnessgram® to alleviate the need for PE in high school youth, it is particularly timely that current data are available.

Purpose

Many aspects of the fitness paradigm exist; the analysis of the Fitnessgram® data set will lend itself to a better understanding of the current overall fitness levels of

California students. The purpose of this preliminary assessment is twofold. First, to describe the characteristics of CA state youth aged 10–15 years, and second, to determine whether differences exist in HRF score by grade level.

Methods

Male and female students in the fifth, seventh, and ninth grade (10–11 y, 12–13 y, and 14–15 y, respectively) who attended school in the state of CA in the 2005–2006 school year were tested with the Fitnessgram®. The testing was usually performed by each school's PE instructors, who then submitted the data to the CA Department of Education.

The HRF test battery options for the Fitnessgram® can vary. For aerobic capacity, the schools had a choice of the PACER (progressive aerobic capacity endurance run), the one-mile run/walk, or a mile walk. The majority used the one-mile run/walk time. Body composition was gauged via the body mass index (BMI), bioelectrical impedance analysis, or the sum of the triceps and calf skinfold; most practitioners used the BMI. Abdominal strength was estimated using curl-ups, and upper body strength/endurance was estimated with either the push-up, pull-up, modified pull-up, or flexed arm hang. Trunk extension strength was assessed using the trunk lift, and flexibility was evaluated using the modified sit and reach. HFZ cutoffs are age and sex specific.

The Fitnessgram® data set for the state of CA contains data for 1.43 million students. Students in the fifth ($N_{boys} = 247,024$ and $N_{girls} = 237,269$), seventh ($N_{boys} = 241,703$, and $N_{girls} = 242,753$), and ninth ($N_{boys} = 230,551$, and $N_{girls} = 230,847$) grade were assessed for this study. Data analyzed included time for the mile run, the BMI, curl-ups, trunk lift, push-ups, and modified sit and reach for the right (Right S & R) and left leg (Left S & R).

Basic descriptive statistics were calculated for the data set, including means and standard deviations. In addition, sex-specific univariate ANOVAs were used to analyze differences by grade, with a Scheffé post hoc to determine where the differences lie.

Results

Boys and girls significantly differed by grade in their mile run time, the BMI, curl-ups, push-ups, and the modified left and right sit and reach ($p < 0.001$ for all variables, Table 18.1). There was little difference in the trunk lift by grade level. Although the data are all cross-sectional, and thus cannot show a trend with age, in general, males and females fitness scores were higher in the older age groups. However, on average, the right and left sit and reach was slightly lower in the ninth grade for both males and females.

Discussion

Despite the quicker mile run times from grades 5 to 7 to 9, the actual percentage of students in the HFZ for aerobic capacity only ranges from 52–60 per cent.

Table 18.1 Descriptive statistics for selected variables from Fitnessgram®

Variable	Mile run time (mins) M ± SD	BMI (kg m⁻²) M ± SD	Curl-ups (#) M ± SD	Trunk lift (cm) M ± SD	Push-ups (#) M ± SD	Right S & R (cm) M ± SD	Left S & R (cm) M ± SD
Girls							
5th grade	11.4 ± 4.0	20.5 ± 5.3	30.2 ± 20.9	28.4 ± 6.9	11.2 ± 9.9	20.8 ± 11.9	20.6 ± 12.2
7th grade	10.9 ± 3.7	21.9 ± 5.3	37.9 ± 22.0	28.4 ± 6.9	11.5 ± 9.0	23.4 ± 11.4	23.1 ± 11.4
9th grade	10.5 ± 4.2	23.0 ± 5.2	40.8 ± 23.0	28.2 ± 7.1	12.5 ± 9.6	22.4 ± 13.2	22.1 ± 13.2
Boys							
5th grade	10.6 ± 4.0	20.9 ± 5.3	32.8 ± 22.2	27.9 ± 7.1	14.1 ± 11.3	18.8 ± 11.2	18.5 ± 11.7
7th grade	9.7 ± 3.8	21.9 ± 5.4	43.5 ± 22.6	27.9 ± 6.4	17.1 ± 11.6	20.1 ± 10.7	19.8 ± 10.7
9th grade	8.9 ± 4.2	23.2 ± 5.4	48.5 ± 22.7	27.9 ± 7.9	22.2 ± 13.4	19.6 ± 12.4	19.3 ± 12.5

Summary results for the 2005–2006 CA Physical Fitness Report show the percentage of students in the HFZ (Table 18.2). The results vary by age; however, fewer CA students in the ninth grade are in the HFZ for aerobic capacity compared to either fifth or seventh grade. This is also the case with trunk extension strength. The percentage of students in the HFZ increases slightly in the higher grades for body composition and upper body strength.

Table 18.2 Percentage of CA students in the Healthy Fitness Zone (HFZ)

Physical fitness task	Grade 5 % in HFZ	Grade 7 % in HFZ	Grade 9 % in HFZ
Aerobic capacity	60.2	60.5	52.4
Body composition	67.4	67.0	68.0
Abdominal strength	80.6	83.1	82.6
Trunk extension strength	88.2	89.3	86.3
Upper body strength	67.1	68.7	69.5
Flexibility	66.6	72.4	70.3

(California Dept. of Education, 2007).

Table 18.3 Percentage of CA students achieving fitness standards

Number of fitness standards achieved	Grade 5	Grade 7	Grade 9
6 of 6 fitness standards	25.6	29.6	27.4
5 of 6 fitness standards	26.4	26.1	26.4
4 of 6 fitness standards	20.5	19.2	19.4
3 of 6 fitness standards	14.0	12.9	12.7
2 of 6 fitness standards	8.2	7.3	6.8
1 of 6 fitness standards	3.7	3.1	3.3
0 of 6 fitness standards	1.5	1.9	4.0

(California Dept. of Education, 2007).

Another relevant variable in the equation is the percentage of CA students in fifth, seventh, and ninth grade who passed the fitness standards for multiple HRF components. Roughly a quarter of students are achieving at least five of the six standards of the six fitness tests. Naturally, improving the passing rate is a key aspect for improving the overall fitness of students in CA.

Conclusion

The students' scores are higher in the older age groups; nevertheless, the overall fitness levels of these youths need to be examined further. Given that, at most, 60 per cent of these students are in the HFZ for aerobic capacity, further attention needs to be directed at the cardiorespiratory fitness of youths in CA. Of additional concern is the dire state of physical education in CA; further steps must be taken to ensure that children and youths in CA are allowed to optimize their physical activity in the school setting.

References

California Department of Education, 2007, *2005–06 California Physical Fitness Report Summary of Results*. http://data1.cde.ca.gov

Freedman, D.S., Khan, L.K., Serdula, M.K., Ogden, C.L. and Dietz, W.H., 2006, Racial and ethnic differences in secular trends for childhood BMI, weight, and height. *Obesity*, **14**, pp. 301–308.

Malina, R.M., 2007, Physical fitness of children and adolescents in the United States: status and secular change. *Medicine and Sports Science*, **50**, pp. 67–90.

The Cooper Institute, Fitnessgram®/ActivityGram® information. http://www.cooperinst. org/products/grams/index.cfm

Wang, Y. and Zhang, Q., 2006, Are American children and adolescents of low socioeconomic status at increased risk of obesity? Changes in the association between overweight and family income between 1971 and 2002. *American Journal of Clinical Nutrition*, **84**, pp. 707–716.

Welk, G.J., Morrow, J.R.J. and Falls, H.B. (eds.) 2002, *Fitnessgram Reference Guide*. Dallas, TX: The Cooper Institute.

19 Effects of a three-week recreational health programme on 14-year-old obese boys

E. Szczepanowska,[1] D. Umiastowska[2] and M. Bronikowski[3]

[1] The Almamer University of Economics, Faculty of Tourism and Recreation, Warsaw, Poland; [2] University of Szczecin, Faculty of Natural Sciences, Institute of Physical Culture, Szczecin, Poland; [3] University School of Physical Education, Poznań, Poland

Introduction

Considering causes of obesity in humans there is no clear explanation of the civilization phenomenon. Research designed by Deutsche Sporthochschule in Köln (Germany) and carried out in various countries of Europe has shown that, even if the level of life is very poor and there is a lack of access to modern technical media, the percentage of obesity in this kind of population is almost equal to the mean value of the whole of Europe – about 6–7 per cent (International Research Seminar, 2007). It is now commonly known that to diminish the percentage of obesity it is most important to achieve a high economic level of the population or country to increase in a direct way access to education in the field of healthful life, health promotion and health care. Thus, an aspiration after getting to know metabolic causes of obesity and effects of some elements of life conditions such as the amount of physical activity, an applied diet or nutrition limitations is very important in widening a range of knowledge possible to transmit healthful education. The role of tourist and recreational elements in this process is not possible to overstate. Throughout a three-week health programme (HP) in the case of obese children these natural and enjoyable elements can make a necessary high amount of physical activity more attractive and less depressive as a result of physiological stress (energy expenditure) during exercises.

The aim of this study was to observe metabolic and somatic results of an HP with exercise and elements of tourism and recreation in a group of Polish obese boys from a central part of the country.

Methods

A group ($n = 13$) of obese boys (age 14.6 y; SD 0.96 y; body height 172.2 cm; SD 4.95 cm) were examined before and after a three-week special health camp at a clinic. The place is located in beautiful countryside, far from big cities, near to a great forest, with a lake very close to the clinic and a small village with very interesting pieces of historical architecture and an indoor swimming pool. The obese boys participated in the specially designed HP. A proper diet with limited fat and a decreased amount of energy substrates to the level of $1600\,kcal.d^{-1}$ was applied (Maffiuletti *et al.*, 2004). The boys performed a 30-min aerobic exercise three times a week on a cycle ergometer with an adequate for age heart rate measured using a Sport-Tester (Sartorio *et al.*, 2003). They also swam for one hour once a week in an indoor swimming pool and walked every day during the one-hour excursion into the surrounding countryside.

Before and after the HP three-week period the boys performed an incremental exercise test monitored by continuous computer analysis (AVL Inc.) until the intensity reached the anaerobic threshold (Wong and Harber, 2005). Anthropological measurements, together with body composition (BodyStat 1500), were made at rest before an incremental exercise test twice: at the beginning and at the end of the HP. In blood drawn from a fingertip Hb resting level (Hbrest) was determined. In venous blood from an elbow flexure the following hormones were measured by radioimmunoassay in serum: insulin (I), growth hormone (hGH), cortisol (C), oestradiol (E_2), progesterone (Prg), testosterone (T) and prolactin (Prl). In venous blood the concentration of glucose (GLU), total cholesterol (CHOL), HDL fraction (HDL), and triglycerides (TG) were assayed using enzymatic kits. Data were analyzed using one-way ANOVA and MRA (Multiple Regression Analysis) in regard to haemoconcentration. All participants gave their informed consent to enroll in the examination. The research was approved by the Regional Commission for Research Ethics.

Results

One of the groups of metabolic determinants, besides hormones influencing body somatic-morphological changes as a result of physical activity, were glucose-lipid parameters (G-LP). These parameters are examined in this work.

During the HP with exercise and elements of tourism and recreation a decrease of all body mass components was manifested. The decrease in BMI and per cent of fat was statistically significant ($p \leq 0.05$) (Table 19.1). The concentration of Hbrest was increased (Table 19.1). Changes of resting values of G-LP (rest) and their exercise increases (Δ) were not statistically significant, but the tendency to decrease levels of CHOL and TG, and to increase HDL, is clear (Table 19.2).

In an analysis of selected determinants the most important status of each parameter was a resting status and exercise increase. In the MRA analysis (Tables 19.3 and 19.4) G-LP were independent variables and hormone changes were dependent variables. In Table 19.3 among G-LP changed during the exercise test before the HP the greatest significances for all selected hormones were TG, GLU and CHOL, and surprisingly, not HDL. After the HP the same three parameters were repeated. The R^2 percentage coefficient showed relatively

Table 19.1 ANOVA results of anthropometrical profile of examined subjects before and after the HP

$n = 13$	Before		After		
	X	SD	X	SD	p
Body mass [kg]	87.7	15.51	80.3	16.02	0.08
BMI [kg·m^{-2}]	29.4	3.77	27.0	3.95	**0.02**
LBM [kg]	57.4	7.42	55.7	8.22	0.33
Fat [%]	34.3	4.84	30.0	5.40	**0.02**
Water contents [kg]	42.0	5.42	40.9	5.80	0.33
Hbrest [g·dL^{-1}]	13.7	0.74	14.4	0.95	0.05

Note: bold = $p \leq 0.05$.

Table 19.2 ANOVA results of metabolic G-LP profile of examined subjects before and after the HP

$n = 13$	Before		After		
	X	SD	X	SD	p
GLUrest [g·dL^{-1}]	82.5	7.52	84.5	8.88	0.56
ΔGLU [g·dL^{-1}]	−0.5	5.13	2.0	6.60	0.30
CHOLrest [g·dL^{-1}]	162.9	26.58	156.4	24.80	0.54
ΔCHOL [g·dL^{-1}]	0.2	8.23	−5.8	14.05	0.21
HDLrest [g·dL^{-1}]	52.9	8.65	56.1	6.11	0.31
ΔHDL [g·dL^{-1}]	0.1	5.99	−0.8	3.01	0.64
TGrest [g·dL^{-1}]	71.4	13.36	75.0	14.77	0.54
ΔTG [g·dL^{-1}]	3.8	4.98	1.2	5.36	0.22

Table 19.3 G-LP–MRA coefficients for obese boys in an incremental exercise test before the HP

Hormone	$R^2\%$	p	Variable in a model	p for MRA coefficients
ΔI	49.74	**0.03**	**TGrest**, ΔTG, HDLrest, CHOLrest, ΔCHOL	**0.03**, 0.77, 0.10, 0.10, 0.25
ΔhGH	25.76	0.05	TGrest, HDLrest	0.06, 0.14
ΔC	43.62	**0.01**	HDLrest, **ΔGLU**, ΔCHOL	0.11, **0.04**, 0.08
ΔE$_2$	30.51	0.16	CHOLrest, HDLrest	0.07, 0.14
ΔPrg	73.31	0.12	**CHOLrest**, GLUrest, ΔGLU, **ΔCHOL**, ΔTG, ΔHDL	**0.01**, 0.32, 0.10, **0.04**, 0.06, 0.32
ΔT	44.02	0.14	CHOLrest, GLUrest, TGrest	0.08, 0.08, 0.26
ΔPrl	25.80	0.08	ΔCHOL	0.08

Table 19.4 G-LP–MRA coefficients for obese boys in an incremental exercise test
after the HP

Hormone	$R^2\%$	p	Variable in a model	p for MRA coefficients
ΔI	25.56	**0.00**	ΔGLU, HDLrest	**0.03**, 0.12
ΔhGH	27.61	0.07	CHOLrest	0.07
ΔC	62.33	**0.03**	HDLrest, CHOLrest, GLUrest	0.27, 0.09, 0.12
ΔE₂	42.09	0.16	CHOLrest, ΔHDL, ΔGLU	0.05, 0.07, 0.26
ΔPrg	26.36	0.22	GLUrest, CHOLrest	0.18, 0.19
ΔT	63.93	0.06	**CHOLrest**, GLUrest, **ΔCHOL**, ΔTG	**0.01**, 0.31, **0.04**, 0.08
ΔPrl	70.18	**0.03**	HDLrest, **ΔTG**, **CHOLrest**, TGrest	0.58, **0.01**, **0.03**, 0.11

high relations between G-LP and Prg before the HP (Table 19.3) and C, T and
Prl after the HP (Table 19.4). The R^2 percentage coefficient should be as high
as possible.

Discussion

In this study it was assumed that the term before the HP three-week period
provided a control group for the term after the HP. This kind of assumption
was in agreement with general principles of scientific research. The decrease of
all body mass components and proper changes in G-LP proved the tendency to
normalization of the whole metabolic profile in examined obese boys during the
HP with elements of tourism and recreation. Many other studies have shown the
same phenomenon (Rudolph *et al.*, 2006; Maffiuletti *et al.*, 2004; Szczepanowska,
2001). The increased level of Hbrest could be a result of both determinants:
a restricted diet and an applied amount of physical activity. The Hbrest was
an indicator of performance improvement in examined boys and could allow
increasing oxygen intake during the resting status and exercise. The tendency
to normalization was clear, first of all, in the decrease of body mass components
(Table 19.1), and in the decrease of CHOL and TG resting concentrations after
the HP (Table 19.2). A great influence of Prg before the HP, especially on CHOL,
proved the role of this hormone in fat mobilization (Viru *et al.*, 1996). Then, the
increased influence of C, T, and particularly Prl after the HP shows the specific
hormonal regulation of metabolism in obese subjects who represent impaired
neuroendocrine secretion of Prl through hypothalamus-pituitary disorders (Gillis
et al., 2006).

In conclusion, the three-week HP with exercise and elements of tourism and
recreation caused a decrease of all body mass components and appropriate changes
in G-LP parameters in 14-year-old obese boys. It also demonstrated a tendency to
normalization of the whole metabolic profile in these obese boys.

References

Gillis, L.J., Kennedy, L.C. and Bar-Or, O., 2006, Overweight children reduce their activity levels earlier in life than healthy weight children. *Clinical Journal of Sports Medicine*, **16**, pp. 51–55.

International Research Seminar, 2007, Children's lifestyles, June 21–24, 2007, Deutsche Sporthochschule, Köln, author's materials.

Maffiuletti, N.A., De Col, A., Agosti, F., Ottolini, S., Moro, D., Genchi, M., Massarini, M., Lafortuna, C.L. and Sartorio A., 2004, Effect of a 3-week body mass reduction program on body composition, muscle function and motor performance in pubertal obese boys and girls. *Journal of Endocrinology Investigation*, **27**, pp. 813–820.

Rudolph, M., Christie, D., McElhone, S., Sahota, P., Dixey, R., Walker, J., Wellings, C., 2006, WATCH IT: A community-based programme for obese children and adolescents. *Archives of Diseases of Children*, **91**, pp. 736–739.

Sartorio, A., Lafortuna, C.L., Silvestri, G., Narici, M.V., 2003, Effects of short-term, integrated body mass reduction program on maximal oxygen consumption and anaerobic alactic performance in obese subjects. *Diabetes Nutrition and Metabolism*, **16**, pp. 24–31.

Szczepanowska, E., 2001, Odpowiedzi hormonów glukostatycznych i plciowych na wysilek fizyczny organizmu czlowieka, *Monografie AWF w Poznaniu* Nr 345, Poznań: Wydawn. Naukowe AWF, Poznań.

Viru, A., Smirnova, T., Karelson, K., Snegovskaya, V., Viru M., 1996, Determinants and modulators of hormonal responses to exercise. *Biologija Sporta*, **13**, pp. 169–187.

Wong, T. and Harber V., 2005, Lower excess postexercise oxygen consumption and altered growth hormone and cortisol responses to exercise in obese men. *Journal of Clinical Endocrinology and Metabolism*, **91**, pp. 678–686.

20 Respiratory gas exchange and metabolic responses during exercise in children and adolescents with achondroplasia

T. Takken, M. van Bergen, R. Sakkers,
P.J.M. Helders and R.H Engelbert
Department of Pediatric Physical Therapy and Exercise Physiology,
Wilhelmina Children's Hospital, University Medical Center, Utrecht,
The Netherlands

Introduction

Skeletal dysplasias consist of a large group of different, rare skeletal disorders, which often express themselves in disproportionate short stature. Classification is not always possible (Savarirayan and Rimoin, 2002). The disturbed growth related to achondroplasia may influence functional ability and exercise capacity. Little research has been performed concerning the functional ability of achondroplastic dwarfs. Exercise intolerance and exercise induced fatigue is an often heard complaint in children with achondroplasia. The most commonly found and well-known skeletal dysplasia is achondroplasia with an incidence of 1 in 25,000 to 40,000 births (Savarirayan and Rimoin, 2002). This type of dwarfism is characterized by rhizomelic shortening of the limbs in combination with an almost normal trunk length. Little research has been performed concerning the exercise response in subjects with achondroplasia. The aims of the present study were to determine whether subjects with achondroplasia have a different response to exercise and gas exchange compared to reference values of healthy peers, and whether VO_{2peak} might be associated with anthropometric measurements or daily physical activity levels.

Methods

Seventeen patients (seven boys and ten girls; mean age 11.8 $\pm$ 3.3; range 6.9–19.4) diagnosed with achondroplasia participated in this study. Body weight, standing height, sitting height, arm span and head circumference were measured in a standardized manner. A three-day Bouchard physical activity record was used to estimate daily physical activity (Bouchard *et al.*, 1983). The subjects performed a maximal graded treadmill exercise test using a modified Bruce protocol (Bruce *et al.*, 1963) to assess the response to exercise. Heart rate (HR) and gas exchange variables (peak oxygen uptake: VO_{2peak}, $VO_{2peak/kg}$, respiratory gas exchange ratio: RER, and minute ventilation: VE) during the test were measured using a heart-rate monitor (Polar) and a calibrated mobile gas analysis system (Cortex Metamax B3, Cortex Medical GmbH, Leipzig, Germany). All analyses were performed in SPPS 12.0. Z-scores were calculated using reference values for healthy children and adolescents (Binkhorst *et al.*, 1992). Independent samples t-tests were used to test differences between patients and the reference values. Correlations were calculated using Pearson's correlation coefficient.

Results

All anthropometrical measurements differed significantly from age and sex specific reference values. Mean standing height was -5.77 ± 0.98 ($p < 0.0001$) standard deviations lower compared to normal values. Physical activity levels were significantly lower in subjects with achondroplasia compared to reference values, and correlated significantly with $\dot{V}O_{2peak}$ ($r = 0.594$, $p = 0.05$).

All subjects were able to perform the maximal exercise test without complications. HR_{peak} of the patients was 178.6 ± 14.9 (range 151–201) beats $\cdot$ min^{-1} and RER_{peak} was 1.15 ± 0.1 (range 1.0–1.41). Z-scores for $\dot{V}O_{2peak}$ (-3.23 ± 0.66), $\dot{V}O_{2peak}$ peak per kg (-2.59 ± 0.70), and VE (-2.20 ± 0.73) were significantly lower compared to reference values for age and gender ($p < .001$). Peak ventilatory equivalent for $\dot{V}O_2$ ($VE_{peak}/\dot{V}O_{2peak}$) was higher in subjects with achondroplasia (45.25 ± 5.9) compared with reference values (37.9 ± 2.8 ($p < 0.001$). Peak O_2 pulse ($HR_{peak}/\dot{V}O_{2peak}$) was significantly lower in subjects with achondroplasia (5.9 ± 1.9 mL$\cdot$beat^{-1}) compared to reference values (9.3 ± 2.3 mL$\cdot$beat^{-1}; $p < 0.0001$). Also, when the values for $\dot{V}O_{2peak}$ were scaled to the two-thirds, three-quarters or seven-eights power of body mass, $\dot{V}O_{2peak}$ was still significantly reduced in subjects with achondroplasia.

Discussion

The exercise capacity of the subjects with achondroplasia, $\dot{V}O_{2peak}$ and in $\dot{V}O_{2peak/kg}$, was significantly lower compared to age and sex-matched reference values from the general population. Due to a lower weight for age, the mean Z-score of $\dot{V}O_{2peak/kg}$ was less pronounced than $\dot{V}O_{2peak}$. Remarkably, their reduced exercise capacity cannot be explained by their smaller standing height, because no significant correlation was found between these two variables. In fact these children showed a significantly higher exercise capacity, with a mean Z-score of $+1.77$ when compared with height-matched reference values, which could be the result of a higher muscle mass for a given height compared to healthy subjects. The $\dot{V}O_{2peak}$ and $\dot{V}O_{2peak/kg}$ in our subjects was 56 and 70 per cent of predicted for age, which is lower compared to children with other growth disturbances. Hinkel *et al.* (1985) found a $\dot{V}O_{2peak}$ and $\dot{V}O_{2peak/kg}$ between 57–77 per cent and 79 and 108 per cent of predicted respectively, in a heterogeneous group of 139 patients with growth disturbances. They found a normalisation of $\dot{V}O_{2peak/kg}$ in their patients (Hinkel *et al.*, 1985), which was not observed in the current study, most likely because of the higher weight for standing height in subjects with achondroplasia.

The increased ventilatory equivalent for oxygen uptake showed that subjects with achondroplasia have to ventilate more (higher breathing frequency) for the uptake of 1 litre of oxygen, compared to age- and sex-matched reference values. This might be caused by the reduced vital capacity (Stokes *et al.*, 1990). A lower tidal volume is thus compensated with a higher breathing frequency and thus a higher ventilation of alveolar death space, and thus a lower ventilatory efficiency.

Moreover, the reduced oxygen pulse of the patients showed that they have a higher heart rate for a given oxygen uptake, compared to age- and gender-matched reference values. This implies that they have a reduced cardiac stroke volume during exercise as a result of their smaller thoracic volume, as can be concluded from the Fick equation ($\dot{V}O_2$ = heart rate × stroke volume × peripheral oxygen extraction) (Fick, 1870).

One of the challenges we faced during this study was the choice of an appropriate comparison group. In this study age- and gender-matched reference values were used. Hinkel *et al.* (1985) used standing height related reference values for their growth retarded patients. However, because of the disproportion in patients with achondroplasia matching is very difficult. Standing height-matched subjects will have a lower body mass, and weight-matched subjects will be taller. This means that patients with achondroplasia are a population with an unique physique and provide a challenge for scaling outcomes in relation to body size (Schmidt-Nielsen, 1984). Clinicians should review the energy balance of subjects with achondroplasia regularly because of the frequently occurring obesity in this patient group (Hecht *et al.*, 1988). An appropriate activity programme with acceptable physical activities should be developed to increase energy expenditure (Trotter and Hall, 2005) and improve exercise capacity. A future study should determine the effects of a life-style intervention (eating and physical activity habits) in subjects with achondroplasia.

In conclusion, cardiopulmonary exercise capacity in subjects with achondroplasia was reduced compared to age and sex matched reference values. Subjects with achondroplasia seem to possess a unique physique and response to exercise. Clinicians should take these differences into account when the exercise capacity of subjects with achondroplasia is being tested.

References

Binkhorst, R.A., van't Hof, M.A. and Saris, W.H.M., 1992, Maximale inspanning door kinderen; referentiewaarden voor 6–18 jarige meisjes en jongens [maximal exercise in children; reference values girls and boys, 6–18 years of age]. Den-Haag, Nederlandse Hartstichting.

Bouchard, C., Tremblay, A., LeBlanc, C., Lortie, G. and Savard, R., 1983, A method to assess energy expenditure in children and adults. *American Journal of Clinical Nutrition*, **37**, pp. 461–467.

Bruce, R.A., Blackmon, J.R., Jones, J.W. and Strait, G., 1963, Exercise testing in adult normal subjects and cardiac patients. *Pediatrics*, **32**, pp. 742–756.

Fick, A., 1870. Ueber die messung des blutquantums in den herzventrikeln. Sitx. der Physik-Med. Ges. Wurzburg, **2**, p. 16.

Hecht, J.T., Hood, O.J., Schwartz, R.J., Hennessey, J.C., Bernhardt, B.A. and Horton, W.A., 1988, Obesity in achondroplasia. *American Journal of Medical Genetics*, **31**, pp. 597–602.

Hinkel, G.K., Damme, M., Leupold, W. and Lorenz, K., 1985. [Performance capacity of children with growth retardation]. *Kinderarztlichen Praxis*, **53**, pp. 27–32.

Savarirayan, R. and Rimoin, D.L., 2002, The skeletal dysplasias. *Best Practice in Research and Clinical Endocrinology and Metabolism*, **16**, pp. 547–560.

Schmidt-Nielsen, K., 1984. Scaling: Why is animal size so important? Cambridge: Cambridge University Press.

Stokes, D.C., Wohl, M.E., Wise, R.A., Pyeritz, R.E. and Fairclough, D.L., 1990, The lungs and airways in achondroplasia. Do little people have little lungs? *Chest*, **98**, pp. 145–152.

Trotter, T.L. and Hall, J.G., 2005, Health supervision for children with achondroplasia. *Pediatrics*, **116**, pp. 771–783.

21 Sensitivity to change of aerobic exercise parameters in patients with juvenile myositis

T. Takken, R.H. Engelbert, S. Pater, P.J.M. Helders and J. van der Net

Department of Pediatric Physical Therapy and Exercise Physiology, Wilhelmina Children's Hospital, University Medical Center Utrecht, Utrecht, The Netherlands

Introduction

Juvenile myositis (JM) is a rare disease in which the immune system targets the microvasculature of the skeletal muscle and skin, leading to significant muscle weakness and exercise intolerance, though the precise aetiology is unknown.

Generally the symptoms of muscle weakness and stiffness follow the skin manifestations. JM patients often experience strong exercise intolerance, especially during a period of active disease (Takken *et al.*, 2003). Since cardiac or pulmonary involvement is uncommon in JM (Constantin *et al.*, 2006), the major contributor to the impaired exercise capacity is the pathological change in muscle tissue. The main pathological changes found in muscle biopsies are muscle fiber degeneration and necrosis with inflammatory infiltration in perivascular, perimysial and endomysial areas. Atrophied fibres, particularly in perifascicular areas, and fibres with an abnormal architecture may be found as well. A previous study reported a significant association between exercise capacity (i.e. $\dot{V}O_{2peak}$ and W_{peak}) and disease activity/damage score (T1-weighted MRI muscle score and physicians global assessment) which indicated the validity of exercise capacity as an indicator for physical function in patients with JM (Hicks *et al.*, 2002). Another study found very low measurement errors in both $\dot{V}O_{2peak}$ and peak work load, suggesting a good reliability of maximal exercise testing in JM patients (Takken *et al.*, 2005). Takken *et al.* found in a cross-sectional study a lower $\dot{V}O_{2peak}$ in patients with an active JM compared to patients with a JM in remission (Takken *et al.*, 2003). Since longitudinal data are lacking in children with JM, the sensitivity to change (responsiveness) of exercise testing to evaluate treatment has never been established in this population. In this study we sought to investigate firstly the differences in exercise capacity between patients with juvenile inflammatory myositis during an active and inactive disease period, and secondly to determine the sensitivity to change of several exercise parameters.

Methods

In this study 13 children with JM participated. Subjects performed two maximal exercise tests using an electronically-braked cycle ergometer and a calibrated respiratory gas analysis system (Jaeger Oxycon Pro). Exercise parameters were analyzed, including peak oxygen uptake ($\dot{V}O_{2peak}$), peak work rate (W_{peak}), peak heart rate (HR_{peak}), and ventilatory anaerobic threshold (VAT)(see Table 21.1). All children were tested once during an active period of the disease and once during a remission period. Two children were tested first during a remission period, 11 children were first tested during an active disease period. From these exercise data four different responsiveness statistics were calculated: standardized response mean, Cohen's effect size, *t*-tests and percentage change from the test during active disease.

Results

The mean age of exercise testing during active disease was 11.19 ± 2.6 years and 11.98 ± 3.1 years when they were in remission. The children performed significantly better during the remission period compared to a period of active disease ($p < 0.05$). Most exercise parameters showed a very large responsiveness

Table 21.1 Responsiveness statistics and ranking of responsiveness of the exercise parameters

	SRM (rank)	Cohen ES (rank)	% change (rank)	P-value t-test (rank)	Overall ranking
W_{peak} (Watt)	−1.75 (1)	−2.15 (1)	81.01 (2)	0.00004 (1)	1
W_{peak} (% pred)	−0.88 (5)	−1.83 (2)	70.47 (3)	0.0040 (4)	2
$\dot{V}O_2/HR$ (mL·beat^{-1})	−1.25 (2)	−1.29 (4)	32.58 (5)	0.0007 (2)	3
$\dot{V}O_{2peak}$ (mL)	−1.06 (3)	−1.63 (4)	34.45 (3)	0.00238 (4)	4
PAT (Watt)	−0.79 (8)	−1.11 (5)	95.48 (1)	0.0208 (8)	5
$\dot{V}O_2$ VAT (mL)	−0.83 (7)	−0.93 (6)	27.56 (6)	0.0112 (7)	6
$\dot{V}O_{2peak}$/kg (mL·kg^{-1}·min^{-1})	−0.92 (4)	−0.75 (7)	25.36 (7)	0.0062 (5)	7
$\dot{V}O_{2peak}$ (% pred)	−0.85 (6)	−0.73 (8)	23.09 (8)	0.0095 (6)	8
VAT (% pred $\dot{V}O_{2peak}$)	−0.59 (9)	−0.47 (9)	17.11 (9)	0.0560 (9)	9
$\Delta\dot{V}O_2/\Delta W$($\dot{V}O_2$/Watt)	−0.45 (10)	−0.25 (10)	7.29 (10)	0.2570 (11)	10
VAT (% $\dot{V}O_{2peak}$)	0.42 (11)	0.41 (11)	−8.35 (11)	0.1594 (10)	11

Legend: SRM: standardized response mean; Cohen ES: Cohen's Effect Size; $\dot{V}O_{2peak}$: peak oxygen uptake; W_{peak}: peak power; $\dot{V}O_{2peak}$/kg: $\dot{V}O_{2peak}$ per kg; $\dot{V}O_2/HR$: $\dot{V}O_{2peak}$ per heart beat; $\Delta\dot{V}O_2/\Delta W$: slope of oxygen/power relationship; VAT: ventilatory anaerobic threshold; PAT: work rate at VAT; $\dot{V}O_2AT$: $\dot{V}O_2$ at VAT; pred: predicted.

(Table 21.1). The five most responsive parameters were W_{peak}, W_{peak} percentage of predicted, oxygen pulse ($\dot{V}O_{2peak}/HR_{peak}$), $\dot{V}O_{2peak}$ and power output at the VAT.

Discussion

The purpose of this study was twofold: first to investigate whether exercise capacity increases in children with JM when the disease goes into remission, and second to determine the responsiveness of exercise parameters.

We found that children with an active JM had reduced exercise parameters when compared to an inactive disease period. The five most responsive parameters were W_{peak}, W_{peak} percentage of predicted, oxygen pulse, $\dot{V}O_{2peak}$ and PAT. The effect sizes were between $-.1$ and -2.2 standard deviations, which suggest very large improvements in these variables when the disease goes into remission. The different responsiveness statistics yielded quite similar results, as indicated by the significant correlations between the four statistics. The improvement in exercise capacity when disease goes into remission can be explained from improvements in pathological changes in muscle tissue. One of the first manifestations in muscle biopsies of patients with active dermatomyositis is the increased muscle fibre area served per capillary (Jerusalem *et al.*, 1974). Thus muscle hypoxia during exercise is an important contributor to the reduced exercise capacity. A recent study found a significantly increased neovascularization in muscle biopsies of patients with dermatomyositis (Nagaraju *et al.*, 2006). The neovascularization will improve the oxygen delivery from blood to the muscle.

Another part of the improvement is a result of physiological development of the child when it becomes older (Cooper *et al.*, 1984). Correcting for development resulted in somewhat lower responsiveness values, however the improvements were still highly statistically significant (i.e. $\dot{V}O_{2peak}$ (percentage predicted) and W_{peak} (percentage predicted)). This indicates that the changes in exercise capacity through disease (and rigorous treatment with steroids) are larger than the changes through growth and development. The $\dot{V}O_{2peak}$ and W_{peak} were approximately 70 per cent during the inactive state, suggesting still an incomplete recovery as well, although the latter two were more sensitive to change. However, data from Magnetic Resonance Imaging studies in patients with dermatomyositis have shown that deficient muscle bioenergetics persist after the resolution of inflammation as well (Park *et al.*, 1994). It is not yet known if full recovery from JM is possible. Maybe exercise training might help to improve further in exercise capacity after a disease episode. The VAT (percentage $\dot{V}O_{2peak}$) suggests that not only the oxygen uptake above the VAT is impaired, but also that the oxygen uptake below the VAT is impaired. This means that not the central circulation but the peripheral circulation is affected in patients with JM. Even at low exercise intensities oxygen delivery from the capillaries to the muscle is impaired in patients with JM. Drinkard *et al.* (2003) analyzed the oxygen uptake work rate slope below the VAT and found reduced values compared to healthy children, which supports this hypothesis.

In conclusion, we found in our longitudinal study that children with inflammatory myositis when in remission had significantly improved exercise parameters compared to an active disease period. Moreover, we found that several parameters had a very good sensitivity to change. With a previously established validity and reliability, exercise testing has shown to be an excellent non-invasive instrument in the longitudinal follow-up of children with inflammatory myositis and might be of use in clinical trials.

References

Constantin, T., Ponyi, A., Orban, I., Molnar, K., Derfalvi, B., Dicso, F., Kalovics, T., Muller, J., Garami, M., Sallai, A., Balogh, Z., Szalai, Z., Fekete, G. and Danko, K., 2006, National registry of patients with juvenile idiopathic inflammatory myopathies in Hungary – Clinical characteristics and disease course of 44 patients with juvenile dermatomyositis. *Autoimmunity*, **39**, pp. 223–232.

Cooper, D.M., Weiler-Ravell, D., Whipp, B.J. and Wasserman, K., 1984, Aerobic parameters of exercise as a function of body size during growth in children. *Journal of Applied Physiology*, **56**, pp. 628–634.

Drinkard, B.E., Hicks, J., Danoff, J. and Rider, L.G., 2003, Fitness as a determinant of the oxygen uptake/work rate slope in healthy children and children with inflammatory myopathy. *Canadian Journal of Appied Physiology*, **28**, pp. 888–897.

Hicks, J.E., Drinkard, B., Summers, R.M. and Rider, L.G., 2002, Decreased aerobic capacity in children with juvenile dermatomyositis. *Arthritis Rheumatology*, **47**, pp. 118–123.

Jerusalem, F., Rakusa, M., Engel, A.G. and MacDonald, R.D., 1974, Morphometric analysis of skeletal muscle capillary ultrastructure in inflammatory myopathies. *Journal of Neurological Sciences*, **23**, pp. 391–402.

Nagaraju, K., Rider, L.G., Fan, C., Chen, Y.W., Mitsak, M., Rawat, R., Patterson, K., Grundtman, C., Miller, F.W., Plotz, P.H., Hoffman, E. and Lundberg, I.E., 2006, Endothelial cell activation and neovascularization are prominent in dermatomyositis. *Journal of Autoimmune Dieases*, **3**, p. 2.

Park, J.H., Vital, T.L., Ryder, N.M., Hernanz-Schulman, M., Partain, C.L., Price, R.R. and Olsen, N.J., 1994, Magnetic resonance imaging and P-31 magnetic resonance spectroscopy provide unique quantitative data useful in the longitudinal management of patients with dermatomyositis. *Arthritis Rheumatology*, **37**, pp. 736–746.

Takken, T., Spermon, N., Helders, P.J., Prakken, A.B. and van der Net, J., 2003, Aerobic exercise capacity in patients with juvenile dermatomyositis. *Journal of Rheumatology*, **30**, pp. 1075–1080.

Takken, T., van der Net, J. and Helders, P.J., 2005, The reliability of an aerobic and an anaerobic exercise tolerance test in patients with juvenile onset dermatomyositis. *Journal of Rheumatology*, **32**, pp. 734–739.

22 Initiatives related to childhood obesity and inactivity in Canada

Year 2007 in review

M. S. *Tremblay*
Children's Hospital of Eastern Ontario Research Institute, Ottawa, Ontario, Canada

Introduction

Dramatic increases in childhood obesity in Canada were observed several years ago (Tremblay and Willms, 2000) and have since been confirmed (Tremblay *et al.*, 2002; Shields, 2006). Accurate measures of the physical activity (PA) level of Canadian children have been lacking and suggest both increases (Eisenmann *et al.*, 2004) and decreases (Tremblay *et al.*, 2005) over time. In recent years Canada has received failing grades with respect to childhood PA and obesity (Active Healthy Kids Canada (AHKC), 2007). This issue is important and requires attention, adaptations and resources of all sectors. The purpose of this short review is to highlight ten initiatives in Canada in 2007 that demonstrate the breadth and depth of efforts directed towards this issue in Canada.

Ten Canadian initiatives in 2007

1 The 2006 federal budget proposed to create a children's fitness tax credit to cover eligible fees up to $500 for enrolment in PA programmes. Background research was completed in 2006 to provide guidance and recommendations related to eligible programmes, special considerations for children with disabilities, implementation logistics and future considerations (Leitch *et al.*, 2006). In January 2007, the Canadian Government implemented a Children's Fitness Tax Credit to reimburse parents for expenses related to eligible fitness activities.

2 In February 2007, the Canadian Fitness and Lifestyle Research Institute released the first national direct measures data on PA levels of Canadian children and youth (2007). These data were based on seven-day pedometer measurements from a national sample of approximately 6000 children aged 5–19 years. The results indicate that 73–91 per cent of Canadian children do not accumulate sufficient daily steps.

3 In February 2007, Canada resurrected the internationally renowned PA social marketing and communications organization 'ParticipACTION' (ParticipACTION, 2004). ParticipACTION has an adult brand awareness of approximately 85 per cent in Canada (Bauman *et al.*, 2004). The federal

government committed $5 million for the first 14 months to assist the organization in getting re-established, formulate a social marketing strategy, partner with stakeholder groups, initiate funding partnerships within the private sector and develop a business plan.

4 In March 2007, after nearly a year of study, the Standing Committee on Health of the House of Commons released its report on Healthy Weights for Healthy Kids (House of Commons Canada, 2007). The Committee heard from over 100 witnesses and received briefs from over 60 organizations. The report includes 13 specific recommendations that the federal government should act upon to increase PA, improve eating behaviors, and reduce childhood obesity in Canada.

5 In March 2007, Statistics Canada launched the Canadian Health Measures Survey, the most comprehensive, national direct health measures survey ever conducted in Canada (Tremblay et al., 2007). Direct measures of health, including anthropometry, blood pressure, spirometry, PA, physical fitness and oral health will be obtained on approximately 5000 Canadians aged 6–79 years. Blood and urine specimens are also being collected for measures of general health, chronic disease, infectious disease, nutrition and environmental biomarkers. These data should be available in 2009–2010.

6 In April of 2007, Canadian researchers published the first clinical practice guidelines (CPG) on the management and prevention of obesity in adults and children (2006 Canadian CPG, 2007). The 26 papers and executive summary published in the Canadian Medical Association Journal supplement are all evidence-based and include eight papers specific to children and youth. CPG specific to children are provided in papers related to the classification of overweight and obesity; clinical evaluation; dietary interventions; PA and exercise therapy; combined diet and exercise treatment; pharmacotherapy and bariatric surgery; prevention through PA; and prevention through nutrition.

7 In April 2007, Canada's food and beverage industry announced three significant initiatives affecting food advertising and marketing directed to children <12 years (Food and Consumer Products of Canada (FCPC), 2007). The initiative is a partnership with the FCPC, Concerned Children's Advertisers and Advertising Standards Canada and includes a social marketing program called 'Long Live Kids', the Canadian children's food and beverage advertising initiative and a strengthening of the framework for regulating advertising to children.

8 Canada hosted the International Conference on PA and Obesity in Children (ICPAOC) in Toronto on June 24–27, 2007 with over 1000 delegates from around the world. The short-term goal of the conference was to assimilate, interpret and share the evidence with key stakeholders to develop recommendations concerning effective physical activity policies and programmes at the community level to address obesity in children and youth.

The long-term aim of the conference is to inform the development of a scientifically-based community strategy to reduce the incidence of childhood and youth obesity through increased sport and PA participation (ICPAOC, 2007).

9   On June 27 2007, AHKC released the third Annual Report Card on PA for Children and Youth (AHKC, 2007). The AHKC Report Card provides comprehensive, evidence-informed assessments of the 'state of the nation' with respect to PA for Canadian children and youth. The preparation and distribution of the report card is meant to serve as an accountability index for all Canadians, a surveillance mechanism, an advocacy tool for PA leaders and organizations, a policy driver and a process for identifying research and surveillance needs. The 2007 Report Card indicated a failing grade of 'D' for the third consecutive year and provided recommendations for action to 'improve the grade'.

10 In November 2006, the Canadian Society for Exercise Physiology (CSEP), in partnership with the Public Health Agency of Canada, the First Nations and Inuit Health Branch of Health Canada, and the Canadian Institutes of Health Research initiated a project titled 'Advancing the Future of Canada's PA Measurement and Guidelines' (CSEP, 2007). The project involved an expert think tank, a research retreat, and the preparation of 14 scientific background papers designed to inform Canada's PA guides (Public Health Agency of Canada, 2007) including papers specifically addressing PA guidelines and measurement concerns for pre-school children, and school-aged children and youth. The papers will be published in a special supplement of the *Canadian Journal of Public Health* and *Applied Physiology, Nutrition and Metabolism* in November 2007.

Conclusion

The diversity and intensity of activities surrounding the childhood obesity and inactivity 'epidemic' in Canada is encouraging. To achieve success, and have a positive influence on the health of Canadian children and the environments where they live, learn and play, interventions and policy changes will need to be developed, implemented, monitored and evaluated; recommendations will need to be acted upon; ongoing research and surveillance will be required; and clinical practice will require adaptations. All sectors (governments, industry, health care, media, communities, schools and families) must participate in an aggressive, informed and sustained movement to recalibrate the behaviors of Canadian children to achieve sustained and pervasive healthy living outcomes.

Note

This paper is an adaptation of a manuscript prepared for the *Canadian Journal of Public Health* 98 (6), 457–459, 2007.

References

Active Healthy Kids Canada, 2007, *Canada's Report Card on Physical Activity for Children and Youth.* Available at: www.activehealthykids.ca/Ophea/ActiveHealthyKids_v2/programs_2006reportcard.cfm

Bauman, A., Madill, J., Craig, C.L. and Salmon, A., 2004, ParticipACTION: This mouse roared, but did it get the cheese? *Canadian Journal of Public Health,* **95** (suppl. 2), pp. S14–S19.

2006 Canadian clinical practice guidelines on the management and prevention of obesity in adults and children, 2007. *Canadian Medical Association Journal,* **176** (suppl. 8), pp. (Online) 1–117.

Canadian Fitness and Lifestyle Research Institute, 2007, *2005, Physical Activity Monitor – Physical Activity and Sport: Encouraging Children to Be Active.* Ottawa: CFLRI.

Canadian Society for Exercise Physiology, 2007, Pre-conference think tank to advance the future of physical activity measurement and guidelines. Available at: www.csep.ca/main.cfm?cid=574&nid=6260

Eisenmann, J.C., Katzmarzyk, P.T. and Tremblay, M.S., 2004, Leisure-time physical activity among Canadian adolescents, 1981–1998. *Journal of Physical Activity and Health,* **1**, pp. 154–162.

Food and Consumer Products of Canada, 2007, Canada's food and beverage industry unveils integrated children-focused initiatives. Press release. Available at: www.fcpmc.com/mediaroom/releases/2007/ca041607-eng.pdf

House of Commons Canada, 2007, *Healthy Weights for Healthy Kids: Report of the Standing Committee on Health.* Ottawa: Communication Canada.

International Conference on Physical Activity and Obesity in Children, 2007, Available at: www.obesityconference.ca

Leitch, K.K., Bassett, D. And Weil, M., 2006. *Report of the Expert Panel for the Children's Fitness Tax Credit.* Ottawa: Department of Finance Canada.

ParticipACTION, 2004, The mouse that roared: A marketing and health communications success story. *Canadian Journal of Public Health,* **95** (suppl. 2), pp. S1–S44.

Public Health Agency of Canada, 2007, *Canada's Physical Activity Guides for Children and Youth.* Available at: http://www.phac-aspc.gc.ca/pau-uap/paguide/child_youth/index.html

Shields, M., 2006, Overweight and obesity among children and youth. *Health Reports* (Statistics Canada Cat. No. 82-003), **17**, pp. 27–42.

Tremblay, M.S. and Willms, J.D., 2000, Secular trends in body mass index of Canadian children. *Canadian Medical Association Journal,* **163**, pp. 1429–1433; erratum 2001, 164, 970.

Tremblay, M.S., Katzmarzyk, P.T. and Willms, J.D., 2002, Temporal trends in overweight and obesity in Canada, 1981–1996. *International Journal of Obesity and Related Metabolic Disorders,* **26**, pp. 538–543.

Tremblay, M.S., Barnes, J.D., Copeland, J.L. and Esliger, D.W., 2005, Conquering childhood inactivity: Is the answer in the past? *Medicine and Science in Sports and Exercise,* **37**, pp. 1187–1194.

Tremblay, M.S., Wolfson, M. and Connor Gorber, S., 2007, Canadian Health Measures Survey: Background, rationale and overview. *Health Reports* (Statistics Canada, Catalogue 82-003), **18** (Suppl.), pp. 7–20.

23 Active Healthy Kids Canada report card on physical activity for children and youth

M.S. Tremblay,[1,2,3] M. Brownrigg[3] and R. Deans[3]

[1]Children's Hospital of Eastern Ontario Research Institute; [2]Statistics Canada, Ottawa, Ontario, Canada; [3]Active Healthy Kids Canada, Toronto, Ontario, Canada

Introduction

Active Healthy Kids Canada was established as a charitable organization in 1994 to advocate the importance of physical activity for children and youth. As a national leader in this area, Active Healthy Kids Canada advocates an increase in quality, accessible, enjoyable physical activity participation experiences for all children and youth where they live, learn and play. Its vision is a nation of active healthy kids and it is focused on making physical activity a major priority in the everyday lives of Canadian families. Active Healthy Kids Canada has embarked upon a strategy to provide 'The Power to Move Kids™' through a variety of public education, communications and advocacy activities. The primary activity of this strategy is the establishment of an annual 'report card' that assesses physical activity behaviors and opportunities for children and youth in Canada. The first report card was released in 2005. Each year a concise summary report card is produced (in English and French) in addition to a more detailed 'long-form' report card containing the detailed research and statistical information informing the grades. An overall failing grade of 'D' was assessed on the 2005 and 2006 report cards (AHKC, 2005a, 2006). The purpose of this paper is to describe the process and outcome of the 2007 Report Card on Physical Activity for Children and Youth.

Methods

The first step in the development of the report card was a National Physical Activity Symposium (AHKC, 2005b), involving academic experts across various disciplines of child and youth physical activity, who came together to identify a preliminary set of indicators for the report card. Based on the symposium, the following categories were identified as important to 'grade' (pending available information) to provide a comprehensive assessment of the physical activity of children and youth in Canada: leisure-time physical activity and inactivity measures; health implications of physical inactivity; family indicators; school indicators; community opportunities and built infrastructure; socio-economic and cultural factors; and government policy. Custom analyses and findings from multiple sources, including the National Longitudinal Survey of Children and Youth (Statistics Canada, 2006); Health Behavior in School-Aged Children Survey (Currie *et al.*, 2001; www.hbsc.org); Canadian Community Health Survey (Béland, 2002; www.statcan.ca/english/concepts/hs/index.htm); Tell Them From Me school evaluation system (www.thelearningbar.com/ttfm/student.php); Ontario SHAPES surveys (www.shapes.uwaterloo.ca); various surveys from the Canadian Fitness and Lifestyle Research Institute (e.g. CFLRI, 2007; www.cflri.ca); and other smaller research studies and reports were used to inform the 'grades' assigned on the report card. A survey of key stakeholders and an 'improving the grade' on-line teleconference also contributed to the 2007 report card content and messaging.

An expert committee of researchers met to assess the collective evidence and assign the grades guided by the following 'criteria':

A   Canadian children and youth are active enough and reaching optimal growth and development
B   Majority of Canadian children and youth are active enough and reaching optimal growth and development; however, children who are obese, physically or mentally challenged may not have appropriate physical activity opportunities provided
C   Insufficient appropriate physical activity opportunities and programmes available to large segments of Canadian Children and youth
D   Insufficient appropriate physical activity opportunities and programmes available to the majority of Canadian children and youth
E   Canadian children and youth have a sedentary lifestyle.

Recommendations for action were developed based on the report card grades and consultations with key stakeholders (non-governmental organizations, researchers, government officials, corporate representatives, and others).

Results

The 2007 report card was released at the International Conference on Physical Activity and Obesity in Children in Toronto on June 27 (www.obesityconference.ca). An overall failing grade of 'D' was assigned for the third consecutive year (AHKC, 2007). The grades for each of the specific categories below were assigned based on empirical evidence and/or expert consensus and details of the evidence informing the grades can be found at www.activehealthykids.ca.

Specific grades included: physical activity levels (F); screen time (D–); sport participation (C); overweight and obesity (F); overall physical well-being and psychosocial development (C–); family perceptions and roles regarding physical activity (D); progress on government strategies and investments (C); sector investments from research, industry, foundations (too little evidence to grade);

physical activity programming at school (C); social support for physical activity at school (B–); training of school personnel (C–); community facilities and programmes access and use (C); community parks and outdoor spaces access and use (C+).

The media and advocacy impact of the report cards (2005–2007) has been extensive with approximately 170 million media impressions through print, radio, television and Internet; with an approximate advertising value of $2,000,000.

Discussion, recommendations and conclusion

The report card is a research-based communications and advocacy document designed to provide insight into Canada's 'state of the nation' each year on how, as a country, Canada is being responsible in providing physical activity opportunities for children and youth. Data from multiple sources were used to inform the 'grades' assigned on the report card. To improve the grade, the 2007 AHKC Report Card recommends to:

1   engage and empower youth to direct and design motivating, socially stimu-lating and enjoyable physical activity opportunities
2   transform the after school hours from screen time to active time in partner-ship with schools, community agencies, programme delivery organizations, neighbourhoods, parents and children and youth
3   demand and employ more robust measures for programme and policy evaluation, research and surveillance.

Scholarly dialogue and critiques of this process are encouraged to facilitate the evolution and refinement of the annual report card. The preparation and distribution of this report card is meant to serve as an accountability index for all Canadians, a surveillance mechanism, an advocacy tool for physical activity leaders and organizations, a policy driver, a process for identifying research and surveillance needs and a challenge to other countries and juris-dictions to implement similar processes to allow comparisons and facilitate improvements.

The report card indicates substantial room for improvement and provides recommendations for action to 'improve the grade'. The report card is a powerful advocacy instrument that can help to provide 'The Power to Move Kids™'.

Acknowledgments

The authors are indebted to Cora Craig, Ian Janssen, Peter Katzmarzyk, Steve Manske, Louise Masse and Doug Willms who served on the expert committee of researchers. The preparation and development of the 2007 Report Card was supported by the Canadian Institutes of Health Research, Institute of Population and Public Health; Heart and Stroke Foundation of Canada; Kellogg Canada; and The Lawson Foundation.

References

Active Healthy Kids Canada, 2005a, *Canada's Report Card on Physical Activity for Children and Youth – 2005*. Available at: www.activehealthykids.ca/Ophea/ActiveHealthyKids_v2/programs_2005reportcard.cfm

Active Healthy Kids Canada, 2005b, *Proceedings of the Canadian Physical Activity Symposium*. November 30–December 3, 2004. Available at: www.activehealthykids.ca/Ophea/ActiveHealthyKids_v2/programs_symposium.cfm

Active Healthy Kids Canada, 2006, *Canada's Report Card on Physical Activity for Children and Youth*. Available at: www.activehealthykids.ca/Ophea/ActiveHealthyKids_v2/programs_2006reportcard.cfm

Active Healthy Kids Canada, 2007, *Canada's Report Card on Physical Activity for Children and Youth*. Available at: www.activehealthykids.ca/Ophea/ActiveHealthyKids_v2/programs_2007reportcard.cfm

Béland, Y., 2002, Canadian Community Health Survey – Methodological overview. *Health Reports*, **13**, pp. 9–14.

Canadian Fitness and Lifestyle Research Institute, 2007, *2005 Physical Activity Monitor – Physical Activity and Sport: Encouraging Children to Be Active*, Ottawa: CFLRI.

Currie, C., Samdal, O., Boyce, W., Smith, B. (eds), 2001, *Health Behaviour in School-aged Children: A World Health Organization Cross-national Study (HSBC)*. *Research Protocol for the 2001/2002 Survey*. Edinburgh: Child and Adolescent Health Research Unit, University of Edinburgh.

Statistics Canada, 2006, *National Longitudinal Survey of Children and Youth (NLSCY) 2004–2005 (Cycle 6)*. Available at: www.statcan.ca/cgibin/imdb/p2SV.pl?Function=getSurvey&SDDS=4450&lang=en&db=IMDB&dbg=f&adm=8&dis=2

24 Applying the new WHO child growth standards in Canada

What is our prevalence of obesity?

M.S. Tremblay[1,2] and M. Shields[2]

[1]Children's Hospital of Eastern Ontario Research Institute, Ottawa;
[2]Statistics Canada, Ottawa, Ontario, Canada

Introduction

Dramatic increases in childhood obesity in Canada have been observed in recent years (Tremblay and Willms, 2000; Tremblay et al., 2002; Shields, 2006) but the prevalence of childhood obesity is not clear. Different cut-points (Tremblay and Willms, 2000; Tremblay et al., 2002) and different measurement methodologies (Shields, 2006) produce different results. The 95th percentile of recognized normative growth curves (e.g. U.S. Centers for Disease Control; Kuczmarski et al., 2002) or the International Obesity Task Force (IOTF) age- and sex-specific cut-points established by Cole et al. (2000) are typically used to determine the prevalence of obesity, but the two methods yield different results (Flegal et al., 2001). In contrast to the CDC curves, the IOTF curves predict a trajectory which is forced to intersect with established health-related cut-points (85th percentile to intercept a body mass index (BMI) of 25 and 95th percentile at 30 kg/m^2) for adults at 18 years of age. The new Canadian clinical practice guidelines on the management and prevention of obesity in children recommend using the IOTF cut-points for establishing the prevalence of childhood obesity (Katzmarzyk et al., 2007).

Recently, the World Health Organization (WHO) published child growth standards that included BMI growth curves (WHO, 2006). The new WHO curves were generated from the Multicentre Growth Reference Study (MGRS; de Onis et al., 2006) which gathered data on children five years of age and younger from six countries (Brazil, Ghana, India, Norway, Oman, United States). All children were exposed to healthy living conditions (e.g. breastfed, transition to good diet, non-smoking mother, adequate access to health care and immunizations) resulting in standards that represent how children should grow. The application of the cut-offs generated from these new curves will result in different prevalences of obesity that are believed to result in better predictions of future health outcomes and burden. The aim of this paper is to compute and compare the prevalence of early childhood obesity using the WHO Child Growth Standards released in 2006 with those using the International Obesity Task Force (IOTF) cut-points.

Methods

Directly measured height and weight data on a national sample of children aged 24–60 months from the Canadian Community Health Survey (CCHS, 2004) and parental-reported height and weight from the National Longitudinal Survey of Children and Youth (NLSCY, 2002/03) were used to calculate body mass index (BMI; $kg \cdot m^{-2}$). Overweight and obesity prevalences were determined using the WHO (85th and 95th percentile) and IOTF cut-points.

The 2004 CCHS was designed to gather information about the nutritional status of the Canadian population (see http://www.statcan.ca/english/concepts/hs/index.htm). The survey does not include residents of the three Territories, Indian reserves and some remote areas. The response rate was 76.5 per cent. Measured height and weight were obtained for 52 per cent of children aged 24–60 months for whom a response was obtained for the 2004 CCHS, a total of 1,222 children.

The NLSCY is a long-term study designed to collect information about factors influencing the social, emotional and behavioral development of children and youth. Specifically excluded from the survey's coverage are residents of three Territories and Indian reserves. The survey is conducted by Statistics Canada and is sponsored by Human Resources and Social Development Canada. In 2002/03 a cross-sectional file was produced for the NLSCY that represents all children who were zero to five years old on January 1st, 2003 (Statistics Canada, 2005). The response rate was 84 per cent. Parental-reported height and weight were obtained for 69 per cent of children aged 24–60 months for whom a response was obtained for the 2002/03 NLSCY, a total of 5,555 children.

All estimates are based on weighted data. Standard errors and coefficients of variation were estimated using the bootstrap technique, which accounts for the survey design effects.

Results

The overall prevalence of overweight (including obese) using the IOTF criteria was 21.3 per cent and 35.8 per cent for the CCHS and NLSCY respectively and 35.4 per cent and 45.4 per cent using the WHO growth standards. The overall prevalence of obesity alone using the IOTF criteria was 6.3 per cent and 20.0 per cent for the CCHS and NLSCY respectively and 19.1 per cent, and 33.5 per cent using the WHO growth standards (Figure 24.1). The prevalence of overweight and obesity was higher in boys than girls. Different results are obtained using the WHO 85th and 95th percentile standards (Figure 24.1) compared to using +2 standard deviations from the z-score curves (which produce lower prevalences).

Discussion

Monitoring trends in childhood obesity is important for public health surveillance and assessing the impact of programme and policy interventions. For example,

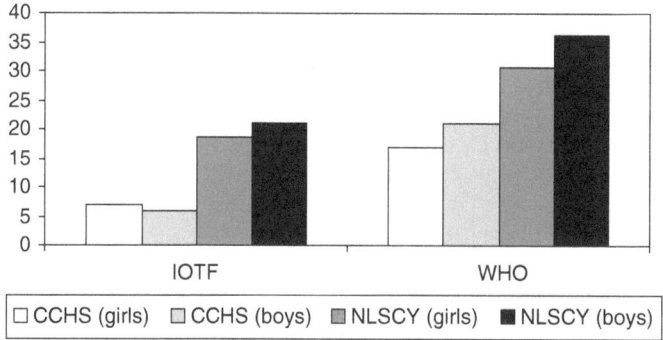

Figure 24.1 Prevalence (%) of obesity among Canadian girls and boys (aged 24–60 months) using CCHS (2004) and NLSCY (2002/03) data and IOTF and WHO cut-points.

the implementation of new recommendations by the Federal Government in Canada (House of Commons, 2007) will need to be evaluated. Clearly, standardized analytical procedures and cut-points need to be employed, but which ones? The new WHO Child Growth Standards provide criterion-based (healthy development exposures) growth data, which differ fundamentally from the quasi-norm referenced growth data used for the development of the IOTF overweight and obesity cut-points. The prevalence of childhood obesity varies by approximately sevenfold (Figure 24.1) depending on data collection methods (direct measure vs parental report) and cut-points (IOTF vs WHO). Comparing childhood obesity prevalences between countries can be very misleading if based on differing data collection methods or reference standards. The particular problems associated with self-reported measures of height and weight have been recently summarized and show consistent and often considerable bias resulting in underestimates of BMI (Connor Gorber *et al.*, 2007).

The new WHO child growth standards are based on conceptually appealing criteria; however the global acceptance of these standards is yet to be determined. In addition to the challenges associated with explaining apparent, and substantial, immediate rises in early childhood obesity prevalence, the wide-spread implementation of these standards will require significant training for public health practitioners on their development and use.

This study demonstrates that the prevalence of overweight and obesity differs significantly depending on the method of data collection used and the cut-points employed. Consequently, reporting and interpreting obesity prevalences and changes over time must be done with careful attention to the measurement and analytical methods. Future research should assess the various methods and cut-points available, and how they predict positive and negative future health outcomes.

References

Cole, T.J., Bellizzi, M.C., Flegal, K.M. and Dietz, W.H., 2000, Establishing a standard definition for child overweight and obesity worldwide: international survey. *British Medical Journal*, **320**, pp. 1240–1243.

Connor Gorber, S., Tremblay, M.S., Moher, D. and Gorber, B., 2007, A comparison of direct versus self-report measures for assessing height, weight and body mass index: A systematic review. *Obesity Reviews*, **8**, pp. 307–326.

de Onis, M., Garza, C., Onyango, A.W. and Martorell, R. (eds), 2006, WHO child growth standards. *Acta Paediatrica*, **95** (suppl. 450), pp. 5–101.

Flegal, K.M., Ogden, C.L., Wei, R., Kuczmarski, R.L. and Johnson, C.L., 2001, Prevalence of overweight in US children: Comparison of US growth charts from the Centers for Disease Control and Prevention with other reference values for body mass index. *American Journal of Clinical Nutrition*, **73**, pp. 1086–1093.

House of Commons Canada, 2007, *Healthy Weights for Healthy Kids: Report of the Standing Committee on Health*. Ottawa: Communication Canada.

Katzmarzyk, P.T., Janssen, I., Tremblay, M.S. and Morrison, K., 2007, Classification of overweight and obesity in children and adolescents. *Canadian Medica Association Journal*, **176** (8 suppl), pp. (Online) 27–32.

Kuczmarski, R.J., Ogden, C.L. and Guo, S.S., 2002, 2000 CDC growth charts for the United States: Methods and development. *Vital Health Statistics*, **11** (246), pp. 1–190.

Shields, M., 2006, Overweight and obesity among children and youth. *Health Reports* (Statistics Canada Cat. No. 82-003), **17**, pp. 27–42.

Statistics Canada, 2005, *Microdata User Guide: National Longitudinal Survey of Children and Youth, Cycle 5, September 2002 to June 2003*. Ottawa: Statistics Canada, Special Surveys Division.

Tremblay, M.S. and Willms, J.D., 2000, Secular trends in body mass index of Canadian children. *Canadian Medical Association Journal* **163**, pp. 1429-1433; erratum 2001, **164**, p. 970.

Tremblay, M.S., Katzmarzyk, P.T. and Willms, J.D., 2002, Temporal trends in overweight and obesity in Canada, 1981–1996. *International Journal of Obesity and Related Metabolic Disorders*, **26**, pp. 538–543.

World Health Organization, 2006, WHO child growth standards: length/height-for-age, weight-for-age, weight-for-length, weight-for-height and body mass index-for-age: methods and development. Geneva, Switzerland: WHO, Department of Nutrition for Health and Development.

Part III
Physical activity patterns

25 Epidemiology of the physical activity of secondary school students in Madrid

C.A. Cordente,[1] P. Garcia-Soidan,[2] J. Calderon,[1]
M. Sillero[1] and J. Dominguez[1]
[1]Faculty of Physical Activity and Sport Sciences (INEF-Madrid)
Universidad Politécnica de Madrid, Spain; [2]Faculty of Social
Sciences and Communication, Universidad de Vigo, Spain

Introduction

Over the past decades, scientific studies have demonstrated that regular physical activity provides health benefits (Boreham et al., 1997; Richardson et al., 2004; Cordente, 2006; Cordente et al., 2007). In recent years in Spain the effect of physical activity on health has been acknowledged to be of much importance. This trend is influenced by the increased prevalence of cardiovascular diseases and the increased support of preventive medicine in an effort to reduce the cost of traditional curative medicine. As a result what is believed to constitute a healthy lifestyle has now changed (Boreham et al., 1997). The aim of our study was to assess the physical activity level (PAL) of adolescents in Madrid (Spain) and to examine its relationship with some demographic (gender), sociologic (socio-economic level, tobacco use, alcohol use and screen time – TV, computer and videogames) and anthropometric (body fat) factors.

Methods

The subjects were (after written consent of their parents) 554 students (266 boys and 288 girls) from 35 (18 public and 17 private) randomly chosen secondary schools from 16 of the 21 districts of Madrid. Table 25.1 shows the distribution of the subjects by age and gender. The adolescents completed a survey including questions regarding their socio-demographic and behavioural details and their PAL measured by the Modifiable Physical Activity questionnaire for adolescents (Aaron and Kriska, 1997), previously validated for its use in Spain. The classification of subjects as a function of the PAL was identical to that used in the Amsterdam Longitudinal Growth and Health Study (Van Mechelen et al., 2000). The intensity of physical activity was categorized as moderate (4–7 METs), vigorous (7–10 METs) and very vigorous (>10 METs). To assess the volume of the physical activity, we followed the recommendations of the English Health

Table 25.1 Distribution of the subjects by age (years) and gender

		Gender				Total	
		Boys		Girls			
		n	%	n	%	n	%
	12	1	0.2	3	0.5	4	0.7
	13	60	10.8	57	10.3	117	21.1
	14	79	14.3	94	17.0	173	31.2
Age	15	80	14.4	83	15.0	163	29.4
	16	36	6.5	32	5.8	68	12.3
	17	9	1.6	15	2.7	24	4.3
	18	1	0.2	4	0.7	5	0.9
Total		266	48.0	288	52.0	554	100

Education Authority (Pate *et al.*, 1998). At least one hour per day of moderate physical activity was recommended to improve the health of adolescents and young people.

The percentage of body fat (BF) was measured following the recommendations of the International Working Group of Kinanthropometry (Aragonés *et al.*, 1993). Classification of the subjects according to their BF defined by Carter's equations was made as proposed by Porta *et al.* (1993).

Compiled data were processed with the statistical programme SPSS. The association between variables was checked by using either the chi-squared test of independence or, in case of normality, the ANOVA test.

Results

Of the subjects 45.1 per cent had a high or very high PAL and 25.3 per cent were inactive or sedentary. In addition there was a significant difference ($\chi^2 = 79.913$; $p > 0.05$) between the PAL of boys and girls. Boys who were active or very active totalled 64.2 per cent, whilst 13.2 per cent were sedentary (the rest were moderately active) in comparison; for the girls these values were 27.4 per cent and 36.4 per cent respectively. We found also that the socio-economic level (SEL) was a determinant of the PAL of the girls ($\chi^2 = 14.010$; $p < 0.05$).

Tobacco consumption (TC) was significantly higher in girls than boys ($\chi^2 = 16.492$; $p < 0.05$). 22.5 per cent of the boys and 34 per cent of the girls were smokers, whilst 68 per cent of the boys and 55.9 per cent of the girls never smoked. We also observed a significant inverse relationship between the TC and the PAL for boys ($\chi^2 = 14.202$; $p < 0.05$). It was found that the greatest proportion of boys in all of the groups were active. Regarding sedentary behaviour, however, 23.3 per cent of the smokers were sedentary in comparison to 10.5 per cent of the boys that never smoke. No significant relationship between TC and PAL was observed for the girls.

Abusive alcohol consumption (AC) (after the point of alcoholic intoxication) was significantly higher in girls than in boys ($\chi^2 = 16.245$; $p < 0.05$).

Table 25.2 Relative level of body weight as a function of body fat

Relative body weight	All		Boys		Girls	
	n	%	*n*	%	*n*	%
Slim	34	6.14	29	10.9	5	1.74
Optimal weight	345	62.27	201	75.56	144	50.00
Slightly overweight	123	22.2	32	12.03	91	31.6
Overweight	47	8.48	4	1.5	43	14.93
Obese	5	0.9	0	0	5	1.74
Total	554	100	266	100	288	100

Nevertheless, for both girls and boys no relation between AC and PAL level existed.

The screen time (ST) was excessive (more than $2\ h\,d^{-1}$) in more than 70 per cent of the subjects. The most worrying values were noted in the boys ($225\ min\,d^{-1}$) and the subjects of the lower SEL ($248\ min\,d^{-1}$) for the boys and 188 for the girls). We did not find any relationship between PAL and SC.

There was a significant difference in the BF of boys and girls ($F = 704, 34$; $p = 0.000$). We found mean values of 11.15 per cent (± 3.30) for boys and 20.47 per cent (± 4.76) for girls. Classification of the subjects was made following the guidelines given in Pacheco (1996), as can be seen in Table 25.2. Using this classification we found an inverse relationship between the PAL and the BF in girls ($\chi^2 = 21.159$; $p = 0.007$). Of the slim and optimally sized girls 7.6 per cent were sedentary in comparison to 20.5 per cent of those that were classified as between slightly overweight and obese.

Discussion

Of subjects, 25.3 per cent were found to be inactive or sedentary. This is worrying at this age due to the repercussions that may occur to middle- and long-term health. Moreover it should be noted that after adolescence, physical activity levels tend to fall very significantly in boys and girls (Nelson *et al.*, 2006).

The comparison of our work with other similar studies confirms that tobacco consumption and alcohol abuse of Spanish adolescents has changed from being a predominantly male problem to being a predominantly female one, however, there is still a problem amongst males. We hypothesize that this is due to significant changes in Spanish society over the last decades.

Screen time is a relevant variable due to the current proliferation of multimedia entertainment means (Cordente, 2006). In our study we did not find any relationship between ST and PAL, however, the time spent in front of a screen reduces significantly the time available for physical activity.

With respect to the significant difference found between the body fat of boys and girls, our results are very similar to those found in the literature (Boreham *et al.*, 2002; Cordente *et al.*, 2007). Metabolic or genetic factors are considered to cause only a few of the cases (De Vito *et al.*, 1999) of overweight or obese adolescents; usually the main cause is an energy imbalance produced by a high caloric intake which is not compensated for by an adequate energy expenditure.

We recommend that girls and subjects from the low socio-economic level should receive high-priority attention regarding health-related habits. In order to increase the physical activity level and reduce alcohol consumption, activities for adolescents and young people in public sport facilities should be promoted, especially during afternoons and nights of the weekend.

References

Aaron, D.J. and Kriska, A.M., 1997, Modifiable activity questionnaire for adolescents. *Medicine and Science in Sports and Exercise*, **29** (1 Suppl. 2), pp. 79–82.

Aragonés, M.T., Casajús, J.A., Rodríguez, F. and Cabañas, M.D., 1993, Protocólo de medídas antropométricas. In: *Manual de Cineantropometría. Monografías FEMEDE*, edited by Esparza Ros, F. Madrid: FEMEDE, pp. 35–66.

Boreham, C.A., Twisk, J. and Savage, M.J., 1997, Physical activity, sports participation, and risk factors in adolescents. *Medicine and Science in Sports and Exercise*, **29**, pp. 788–793.

Boreham, C., Twisk, J., Neville, C., Savage, M., Murray, L. and Gallagher, A., 2002, Associations between physical fitness and cardiovascular risk factors in young adulthood: The Northern Ireland young hearts project. *International Journal of Sports Medicine*, **23** (1 Suppl. 2), pp. 22–26.

Cordente, C.A., 2006. *Doctoral dissertation*. http://www.cafyd.com/tesis12cordente.pdf

Cordente, C.A., García, P., Sillero, M. and Domínguez, J., 2007, Relationship of the degree of physical activity, blood pressure and body fat among teenagers in Madrid. *Revista Española de Salud Pública*, **81**, pp. 307–317.

De Vito, E., La Torre, G., Langiano, E., Berardi, D. and Ricciardi, G., 1999, Overweight and obesity among secondary school children in central Italy. *European Journal of Epidemiology*, **15**, pp. 649–654.

Nelson, M.C., Neumark-Stzainer, D., Hannan, P.J., Sirard, J.R. and Story M., 2006, Longitudinal and secular trends in physical activity and sedentary behavior during adolescence. *Pediatrics*, **118**, pp. 1627–1634.

Pacheco DelCerro, J.L., 1996, Valoración anthropométrica de la masa qrasa en atletas de elite. In Metodos de Estuilio de Composición Corporal en Deportistas. Edited by Consejo Superior de Desportes, Madrid: Ministerio de Educación y cultura, pp. 27–54.

Pate, R.R., Trost, S.M. and Williams, C., 1998, Critique of existing guidelines for physical activity in young people. In: *Young and Active? Young People and Health Enhancing Physical Activity: Evidence and Implication*, edited by Biddle, S., Sallis, J., Cavill, N. London: Health Education Authority, pp. 162–176.

Porta, J., Galiano, D., Tejedo, A. and González, J.M., 1993, Valoración de la composición corporal. Utopías y realidades. In: *Manual de Cineantropometría*, edited by Esparza Ros F. Madrid: FEMEDE, pp. 113–170.

Richardson, C.R., Kriska A.M., Lantz P.M. and Hayward R.A., 2004, Physical activity and mortality across cardiovascular disease risk groups. *Medicine and Science in Sports and Exercise*, **36**, pp. 1923–1929.

Van Mechelen, W., Twisk, J.W.R., Post G.B., Snel J. and Kemper H.C.G., 2000, Physical activity of young people: The Amsterdam longitudinal growth and health study. *Medicine and Science in Sports and Exercise*, **32**, pp. 1610–1617.

26 Tracking the relationship between motor proficiency and BMI over a 24-month period among Canadian schoolchildren

J. Hay,[1] *S. Veldhuizen*[2] *and J. Cairney*[2]
[1]Brock University; [2] University of Toronto, Canada

Introduction

The prevalence of overweight and obesity among children is increasing at an alarming pace throughout the world (Haslam and James, 2005). There is a clear association between physical inactivity and obesity (Martínez-González *et al.*, 1999). As such, factors that influence physical activity, either as barriers to or promoters of, are worthy of investigation in order to inform both clinical and public health interventions. Motor ability, while clearly a fundamental factor in movement and complex play, is typically not considered as a risk factor for either physical inactivity or overweight/obesity in children. A small but growing body of literature has examined children with significant difficulties in motor coordination in relation to participation in active play (Hay and Missiuna, 1998; Wrotniak *et al.*, 2006), perceptions of self-efficacy toward physical activity (Cairney *et al.*, 2005a), physical fitness (Faught *et al.*, 2005) and overweight/obesity (Cairney *et al.*, 2005b). However, we are unaware of any work that has examined the full range of motor proficiency/ability and its impact on overweight and obesity over time in children. This study examines the effect of motor ability on body mass over a 24-month period among a large cohort of children aged 9–11 at baseline.

Methods

We obtained ethics approval for this study from the district school board and Brock University. Our target population consisted of children enrolled in grade 4 in the public school system in the Niagara Region of Ontario, Canada in 2004. Testing and training protocols were established and baseline testing was completed in 2004–2005. Data collection occurred during the school years from 2005 to 2007. A total of 1281 students (640 male, 641 female), from 50 schools, completed motor coordination testing and form the sample used in the present study. This represents 95 per cent of all eligible students in these schools. Children with known physical, intellectual, or medical impairments that prevented completion of the assessments were excluded. Students were assessed in the spring of 2004 and fall of 2004 and again in the spring and fall of 2005, for a total of four assessments over 24 months. Most students were age 9 (46 per cent) or 10 (52 per cent) at baseline, with a small number age 11 (2 per cent).

Measurements

Motor proficiency (MP) was assessed using the short form of the Bruininks-Oseretsky Test of Motor Proficiency (BOTMP-SF) the most commonly used standardized test to diagnose motor difficulties in North America (Crawford et al., 2001) The short form has been validated against the full scale with intercorrelations between 0.90 and 0.91 for children in the 8 to 14 age range (Bruininks, 1978). Height and weight were measured using SECA stabilometers and precise Tanita electronic weight scales. Children wore light clothing without footwear for anthropometric measurements and gym clothes and running shoes for the BOTMP-SF. All testing was conducted by trained research assistants and took place privately in the school gymnasium.

Analysis

To identify basic patterns in the data, we examined correlations between BMI and MP within time points and plotted trends in BMI for each decile of MP. To formally test for differences over time in BMI while taking into account the nesting of observations within schools, we then constructed a mixed-effects model with time, baseline age, and MP as fixed effects and school as a random effect. We included gender and gender interactions in initial models, but these proved non-significant and were removed. We also explored the possibility of a non-linear trend by adding additional polynomial terms for time, but these also proved non-significant and were dropped. We used an unstructured covariance matrix, which, possibly because of seasonal effects that increased the correlations between non-consecutive waves, proved to fit the data better than autoregressive or other options. We used SPSS version 14.0 for all analyses.

Results

MP and BMI and MP were significantly correlated cross-sectionally ($r = -0.3$ and $r = -0.3$; $p < 0.001$), and an analysis by MP deciles (Figure 26.1) revealed that children with poorer MP have higher BMIs at each of the five measurement points and that they demonstrate greater increases over time than their peers.

The mixed effects model confirmed these results (Table 26.1). As expected, BMI increased for all students, but this increase was significantly greater for those with lower motor proficiency (time by MP interaction, $B = -0.002$, $df = 1235.5$, $t = 4.2$, $p < 0.001$). Predicted values (estimated marginal means; Figure 26.2) for BMI for children scoring at the 5th percentile on the BOTMP-SF were 20.7 at baseline, rising to 22.1 at last follow-up. This represents an increase of 7.1 per cent. For children with high MP (95th percentile on the BOTMP-SF),

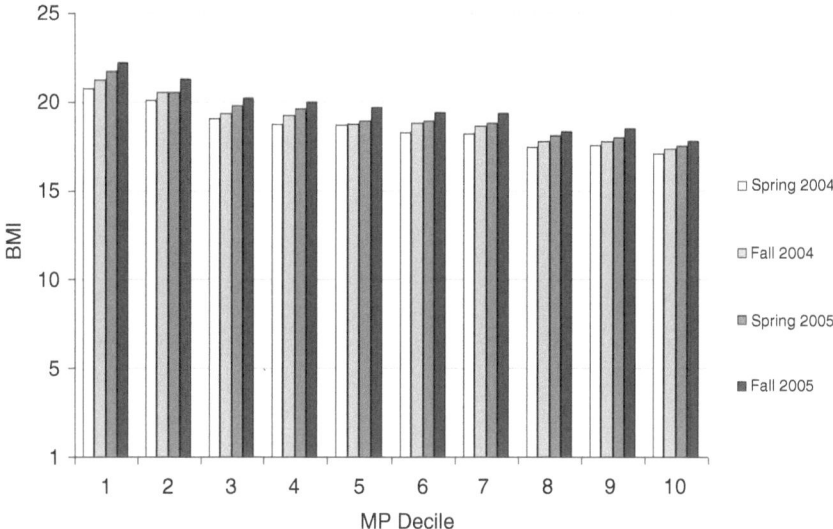

Figure 26.1 BMI at each measurement point by MP.

Table 26.1 Results of mixed effects model predicting change in BMI over time

	B	SE	df	t	p	L95%	U95%
Intercept	19.65	0.45	1467.9	43.6	< 0.001	18.76	20.53
Time (months)	0.07	0.01	1103.1	14.0	< 0.001	0.06	0.09
BOTMP percentile	−0.03	0.003	1592.1	−11.9	< 0.001	−0.04	−0.03
Age at baseline (centred)	0.76	0.24	1597.2	3.1	0.002	0.28	1.23
Time (months) *BOTMP percentile	0.0003	0.00007	1102.6	−4.0	< 0.001	−0.0004	−0.0001

the corresponding values were 17.6 and 18.5, an increase of 5.3 per cent. Accepted BMI cut-points for overweight in this age range fall between 20.2 and 21.2 for both sexes.

Discussion

It is evident that motor proficiency (MP) is associated with changes in BMI over time. Among children in Grade Four with below average MP, mean BMI scores are already significantly higher than their peers with average or above average MP. It is troubling that this gap between the bottom and the top groups (deciles)

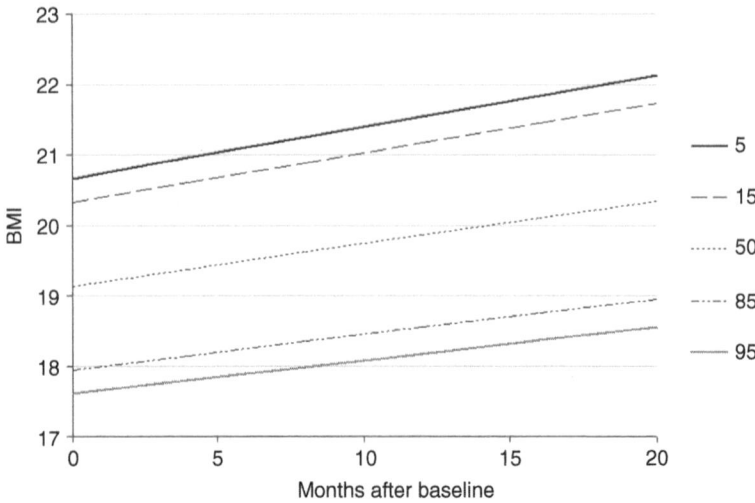

Figure 26.2 Predicted increases in BMI over time for various levels of MP.

seems to widen with time. This is of particular concern since this cohort had yet to reach adolescence, a developmental period where physical activity levels decline.

This analysis does not report the contribution of motor performance to physical activity, aerobic fitness, or perceived self-efficacy which have all been established as interacting together in the development of overweight. It is plausible that poor motor proficiency leads to poor self-efficacy that, in turn, leads to reduced physical activity, and increased overweight in a self-fueled cycle (Cairney *et al.*, 2005b). The lack of import provided to motor performance is clear and the consequences apparent as those children in the lowest 5 per cent were already well above average BMI at ages eight and nine and even more so at ages 10 and 11. These children alone account for a sizeable minority of all overweight children found in this sample. Whatever the mechanism the relationship between motor proficiency and body weight is clear. This finding provides strong support for arguments that motor proficiency testing should be commonplace among young children in order to allow teachers, parents, and public health programme planners to provide acceptable activity choices to children of differing levels of motor ability. This is commonplace for intellectual and sensory capacities and may prove equally important for the physical domain.

References

Bruininks, R.H., 1978, *Bruininks-Oseretsky Test of Motor Proficiency: Examiner's Manual.* Circle Pines, MN: American Guidance Service.

Cairney, J., Hay, J., Faught, B. and Hawes, R., 2005a, Developmental coordination disorder and overweight and obesity in children aged 9 to 14 years. *International Journal of Obesity*, **29**, 369–372.

Cairney, J., Hay, J.A., Faught, B.E., Wade, T.J., Corna, L. and Flouris, A., 2005b, Developmental coordination disorder, generalized self-efficacy toward physical activity and participation in organized and free play activities. *Journal of Pediatrics*, **147**, 515–520.

Crawford, S.G., Wilson, B.N. and Dewey, D., 2001, Identifying developmental coordination disorder: Consistency between tests. *Physical and Occupational Therapy*, **20**, 29–50.

Faught, B.E., Hay, J.A., Cairney, J. and Flouris, A., 2005, Increased risk for coronary vascular disease in children with developmental coordination disorder. *Journal of Adolescent Health*, **37**, pp. 376–380.

Haslam, D.W. and James, W.P., 2005, Obesity, *Lancet*, **366**, 1197–1209.

Hay, J.A. and Missiuna, C. A., 1998, Motor proficiency in children reporting low levels of participation in physical activity. *Canadian Journal of Occupational Therapy*, **65**, 64–71.

Hay, J.A., Cairney, J., Faught, B.E. and Flouris, A., 2003, The contribution of clumsiness to risk factors of coronary vascular disease in children. *Rev. Port. Ciencias Desporto [Port. J. Sports Sci.]*, **3**, 127–129.

Martínez-González, M.A., Martínez, J.A., Hu, F.B., Gibney, M.J. and Kearney, J. 1999, Physical inactivity, sedentary lifestyle and obesity in the European Union. *International Journal of Obesity* **23**, 1192–1201.

Wrotniak, B., Epstein, L., Dorn, J.M., Jones, K.E. and Kondilis, V., 2006, The relationship between motor proficiency and physical activity in children. *Pediatrics*, **118**, pp. e1758–e1765.

27 Seasonal variation in objectively measured physical activity in 3- and 4-year-old children

D.P. McKee,[1] *C.A.G. Boreham,*[2] *G. Davison,*[3] *M.H. Murphy*[3] *and A.M. Nevill*[4]

[1]Stranmillis University College, Belfast, Northern Ireland; [2]Institute for Sport and Health, University College Dublin, Ireland; [3]School of Sports Studies, University of Ulster, Newtownabbey, Northern Ireland; [4]Research Institute for Health Care Sciences, University of Wolverhampton, Wolverhampton, England

Introduction

The accurate assessment of physical activity (PA) in young children has been identified as a research priority (Fulton et al., 2001). However, PA is a multifaceted behaviour, which is difficult to assess accurately (Wareham and Rennie, 1998). Further, there appears to be a relationship between the validity of a measure, the invasiveness of the assessment and the cost of the method (Montoye et al., 1996). Traditionally research interest has tended to focus on the concurrent validity of instruments to assess PA. To this end there is a consensus emerging that accelerometers (Finn and Specker, 2000; Pfeiffer et al., 2006), heart rate monitors (Sirrard and Pate, 2001), direct observation (Puhl et al., 1990) and pedometers (McKee et al., 2005; Hands et al., 2006) have acceptable validity for assessing PA in young children and that four to five days of monitoring yields valid information about weekly activity patterns (Trost et al., 2000). However, what is less clear is the validity of an individual four- or five-day assessment of PA as an indication of typical PA and the seasonal variation of PA in young children. Using cross-sectional analysis with measurements of PA in different cohorts of children in the various seasons researchers have found children to be more active in Autumn than in Winter (Burdette et al., 2004), slight difference across seasons with Spring lower than Summer, Autumn or Winter (Fisher et al., 2005) or a trend towards a seasonal difference (Goran et al., 1998). This cross-sectional approach to assessing seasonal effects in the PA of children is beset with difficulties as it has been shown that there is high variability in the PA of young children (McKee et al., 2005) which is likely to mask the influence of seasonal variation. Using a more robust prospective design Baranowski et al. (1993) conducted a study of seasonal variation in the PA of young Texan children and found PA tended to fall during the Summer months, possibly influenced by a reduction in the amount of time spent outside. The purpose of the current study was to employ a prospective design to examine the influence of season on PA in young Irish children.

Methods

Mean daily activity was assessed using an electronic pedometer (Digiwalker™ DW-200, Yamax, Tokyo, Japan) in 85 (33 F) 3–4-year-old children over a six-day period (four weekdays and two weekend days) in Winter (December or January) and Spring (April). Pedometers have been shown to have validity for assessing PA in this age group (Mckee *et al.*, 2005; Hands *et al.*, 2006). Parents who agreed to their child's participation were sent a pack containing a pedometer, a recording sheet for the pedometer scores, cable ties to seal the pedometer and detailed instructions as to the placement and use of the pedometers. Parents were requested to ensure their child wore the pedometer for six consecutive days (including two weekend days), recording the scores on a daily basis, together with the time the pedometer was fitted and removed and any times during the day when the instrument was removed (i.e. for bathing or swimming). All participants were requested to fit the pedometer as soon as practical in the morning and to wear the device until going to bed that evening. Children were recruited from Nursery Schools in the greater Belfast area of Northern Ireland. Data included in the analysis had a minimum of 9.5 hours monitoring per day and included at least three week days and one weekend day. The effect of season and gender on PA was assessed via a between-within subjects ANOVA. Gender differences in PA in winter and spring were evaluated with t-tests. A Spearman rank order correlation (SRO) was calculated between Winter and Spring measures to assess the stability of PA ranking in children. Statistical analysis was carried out using SPSS v.14 for Windows. Alpha level was set at $p \le 0.05$. Institutional ethical approval and parental written informed consent were obtained.

Results

There was no difference in the seasonal effect on weekdays and weekend days, therefore the results were analysed and presented on the basis of average daily counts over six days. The PA results (Table 27.1) indicate a high degree of variability in the PA levels of young children. There was no gender difference in the PA levels of the current sample while the ANOVA results showed a main effect for season ($p = 0.0001$) but this was not differentiated by gender. The SRO correlation between winter and spring PA was $r = 0.397$ ($p = 0.0001$).

Table 27.1 Mean (SD) daily pedometer counts by gender and season

Group	Mean daily pedometer counts	
	Winter	*Spring*
Male (n = 52)	9780 (2979)	11417 (3374)
Female (n = 33)	8655 (2104)	11064 (2856)
Total (n = 85)	9349 (2717)	11280 (3170)

Discussion

In contrast with most (Burdette *et al.*, 2004; Hands *et al.*, 2006), but not all (Goran *et al.*, 1998; Roemmich *et al.*, 2006), other studies examining young children there was no gender difference in PA in the current sample. The reason for this finding is not clear and may be attributable to sampling error. However, a small number of studies have indicated that gender differences in PA may emerge after the age of three years (Buss *et al.*, 1980; Reilly *et al.*, 2004). The current study indicates that the stability of PA as assessed by rank order is modest and that young children take just under 2000 or approximately 20 per cent fewer steps per day in Winter. In contrast Fisher *et al.* (2005) found Scottish children to be approximately 11 per cent less active in Spring. This is surprising, as Fisher's sample was drawn from a similar setting with a comparable climate. However, Fisher's measurements were cross-sectional and the assessment of PA in Spring and Winter occurred almost a year apart. Additionally their analysis showed age to be a factor for PA.

The results of this study indicate that researchers need to try to control for seasonal effects when assessing PA in young children and that one 4–5-day assessment of PA is unlikely to be representative of a child's activity over a year. The current results need to be interrupted with caution as the sample size was modest and therefore may not be representative of Irish children. Furthermore, the measurements occurred sequentially (Winter then Spring) for all the children. The strengths of the study are that the same children were assessed in both seasons using the same methods and procedures.

References

Baranowski, T., Thompson, W.O., DuRant, R.H., Baranowski, J. and Puhl, J., 1993, Observations on physical activity in physical locations: Age, gender, ethnicity, and month effects. *Research Quarterly in Exercise and Sport*, **64**, pp. 127–133.

Burdette, H.L., Whitaker, R.C. and Daniels, S.R., 2004, Parental report of outdoor play time as a measure of physical activity in preschool-aged children. *Archives of Pediatrics and Adolescent Medicine*, **158**, pp. 353–357.

Buss, D.M., Block, J.H. and Block, J., 1980, Preschool activity level: Personality correlates and developmental implications. *Child Development*, **51**, pp. 401–408.

Finn, K.J. and Specker, B., 2000, Comparison of Actiwatch activity monitor and the children's activity rating scale in children. *Medicine and Science in Sports and Exercise*, **32**, pp. 1794–1797.

Fisher, A., Reilly, J.J., Montgomery, C., Kelly, L.A., Williamson, A., Jackson, D.M., Paton, J.Y. and Grant, S., 2005, Seasonality in physical activity and sedentary behaviour in young children. *Pediatric Exercise Science*, **17**, pp. 31–40.

Fulton, J.E., Burgeson, C.R., Perry, G.R., Sherry, B., Galuska, D.A. and Alexander M.P., 2001, Assessment of physical activity and sedentary behavior in preschool-age children: Priorities for research. *Pediatric Exercise Science*, **13**, pp. 113–126.

Goran, M.I., Nagy, T.R., Gower, B.A., Mazariegos, M., Solomons, N., Hood, V. and Johnson, R., 1998, Influence of sex, seasonality, ethnicity, and geographic location on the components of total energy expenditure in young children: Implications for energy requirements. *American Journal of Clinical Nutrition*, **68**, pp. 675–682.

Hands, B., Parker, H. and Larkin, D., 2006, Physical activity measurement methods for young children: A comparative study. *Measurement in Physical Education and Exercise Science*, **10**, pp. 203–214.

McKee, D.P., Boreham, C.A.G., Murphy, M.H. and Nevill A.M., 2005, Validation of the Digiwalker™ Pedometer for measuring physical activity in young children. *Pediatric Exercise Science*, **17**, pp. 345–352.

Montoye, H.J., Saris, W.H.M. and Kemper, H.C.G., 1996, *Measuring Physical Activity and Energy Expenditure*. Champaign, IL: Human Kinetics.

Pfeiffer, K.A., McIver, K.L., Dowda, M., Almeida, M.J.C.A. and Pate, R.R., 2006, Validation and calibration of the Actical accelerometer in preschool children. *Medicine and Science in Sports and Exercise*, **38**, pp. 152–157.

Puhl, J., Greaves, K., Hoyt, M. and Baranowski, T., 1990, Children's activity rating scale (CARS). Description and calibration. *Research Quarterly for Exercise and Sport*, **61**, pp. 26–36.

Reilly, J.J., Jackson, D.M., Montgomery, C., Kelly, L.A., Slater, C., Grant, S. and Paton, J.Y., 2004, Total energy expenditure and physical activity in young Scottish children: Mixed longitudinal study. *The Lancet*, **363**, pp. 211–212.

Roemmich, J.N., Epstein, L.H., Raja, S., Yin, L., Robinson, J. and Winiewicz, D., 2006, Association of access to parks and recreational facilities with physical activity of young children. *Preventive Medicine*, **43**, pp. 437–441.

Sirard, J.R. and Pate, R.R., 2001, Physical activity assessment in children and adolescents. *Sports Medicine*, **31**, pp. 439–454.

Trost, S.G., Pate R.R., Freedson P.S., Sallis, J.F. and Taylor, W.C., 2000, Using objective physical activity measures with youth: How many days of monitoring are needed? *Medicine and Science in Sports and Exercise*, **32**, pp. 426–431.

Wareham, N.J. and Rennie, K.L., 1998, The assessment of physical activity in individuals and populations: Why try to be more precise about how physical activity is assessed. *Journal of Obesity and Related Metabolic Disorders*, **22**, pp. S30–S38.

28 Contribution of recess to habitual physical activity levels in boys and girls

The A-CLASS project

N.D. Ridgers and G. Stratton
Liverpool John Moores University, Liverpool, UK

Introduction

Physical activity is an integral component of a healthy lifestyle. There is concern that children are not engaging in sufficient physical activity to benefit health (Anderson *et al.*, 2006). Recently, empirical attention has focused on different time segments of the day where children can engage in physical activity, and identifying which segments may play an important role in the accumulation of daily physical activity. However, little attention has focused on the contribution of specific segments of the day to children's physical activity levels. During the school day, recess represents the main opportunity for children to be active on a daily basis (Ridgers *et al.*, 2006). As such, the contribution of recess to daily activity is an important consideration.

The aim of the study was to determine the contribution of recess towards boys' and girls' daily physical activity levels.

Methods

Participants and settings

Fifty-eight boys and 87 girls (9.7 ± 0.3 years, 46 per cent overweight) selected from eight primary schools in one large city in the North West of England returned signed parental consent to participate in the study. All children were part of the Active City of Liverpool, Active Schools and SportsLinx (A-CLASS) Project, which is a multi-disciplinary project investigating the effects of after school clubs and a lifestyle intervention on markers of health, fundamental movement skills and daily physical activity levels. The research protocol received ethical approval from the University Ethics Committee.

Procedures

Anthropometry

Measurements of body mass (to the nearest 0.1 kg) and stature (to the nearest 0.1 cm) were recorded using analogue Seca scales (Seca Ltd, Birmingham, UK) and the Leicester Height Measure (Seca Ltd, Birmingham, UK) using standardised procedures.

Recess

All schools participating in the project had one playground that children accessed during recess in all weather conditions except for heavy rain. The playgrounds had existing playground markings, and while not identical, common features included hopscotch, snakes and ladders, number squares and targets. Small pieces of sports equipment such as soccer balls, jump rope and tennis balls were available for use during recess in all schools throughout the study. Recess duration was defined as the time that the school bell rang to start recess to the time it rang to conclude recess. This time was used to identify and extract children's physical activity levels during recess in subsequent analyses.

Physical activity

Physical activity was objectively monitored over seven consecutive days using a uni-axial accelerometer (GT1M, Actigraph, Florida, USA). Epoch length was set at five seconds. Children were asked to wear the monitor, which was positioned on the midaxillary line of the right hip using a tightly fitted elastic belt, during all waking hours except when swimming or bathing.

Data reduction and analysis

Data were analysed using a customised data reduction programme which determined the amount of time children spent in moderate, high and very high physical activity using activity cut-points of 163–479, 480–789, and ≥ 790 counts per five-second epoch respectively (Nilsson *et al.*, 2002). Sustained 20-minute periods of zero counts were deemed to indicate that the accelerometer had been removed. Children were required to have produced successful recordings on a minimum of three weekdays for 10 hours a day to be included in the analyses (Anderson *et al.*, 2006).

The outcome variables extracted from the customised macros were daily moderate-to-vigorous physical activity (MVPA) levels (min), and the relative (percentage) and absolute (min) time children engaged in MVPA during recess. The relative contribution of recess to daily MVPA was calculated for each as a proportion using (time in MVPA during recess/total time in MVPA during the day * 100). Gender differences in daily and recess physical activity levels, and in the relative contribution of recess to daily physical activity, were analysed using analyses of variance. All analyses were conducted using the Statistical Package for Social Sciences version 14 (SPSS Inc., Chicago, IL, USA). The alpha level was set at $p < 0.05$.

Results

Descriptive data

No significant differences were found between boys' and girls' age, stature, body mass and body mass index. The mean daily recess time available for children to engage in physical activity on the school playground was 85 ± 10 min (range 75 to 105 min).

Daily physical activity

Boys (73.4 ± 21 min) engaged in significantly more daily MVPA than girls (62.8 ± 16.6 min; $p < 0.01$).

Recess physical activity

Boys ($25.2 \pm 8.5\%$) engaged in significantly more MVPA during recess than girls ($17.1 \pm 5.1\%$; $p < 0.001$). This equated to 22.3 min and 15 min of MVPA for boys and girls respectively during recess.

Contribution of recess to daily physical activity

Recess contributed significantly more MVPA towards weekday physical activity for boys ($30.4 \pm 7.6\%$) than for girls ($24 \pm 7.6\%$; $p < 0.01$).

Discussion

The finding that boys are more physically active than girls both daily and during recess is consistent with previous research that has used a range of objective measures to quantify physical activity (Mota *et al.*, 2005; Flohr *et al.*, 2006; Ridgers *et al.*, 2006). Within a recess context, the underlying reasons for the gender difference have not been established. However, recess behavioural studies have suggested that boys are more likely to engage in ball games, whilst girls are more likely to engage in sedentary play, conversation and skipping (Blatchford *et al.*, 2003). It should be noted, however, that recess is a salient opportunity for children to engage in physical activity on a daily basis (Ridgers *et al.*, 2005).

The contribution of discrete segments of the school day, including physical education and extra-curricular activities, has begun to receive empirical attention. However, only two studies have assessed the contribution of recess to daily physical activity (Mota *et al.*, 2005; Tudor-Locke *et al.*, 2006). This present study found that recess contributed more towards daily physical activity levels for boys (5.6–24 per cent) and girls (0.3–16 per cent) compared to the previous two studies. The importance of recess is further emphasised when compared to the contribution of physical education to daily physical activity. Research has indicated that physical education contributes approximately 8–20 per cent for boys and 11–17 per cent for girls towards daily activity on physical education days (Flohr *et al.*, 2006; Tudor-Locke *et al.*, 2006).

Recess provides an opportunity for children to engage in physical activity on a daily basis that could benefit health. The reduction and removal of daily recess time may have a negative impact on children's daily physical activity levels. Overall, the results highlight that recess is an important non-curriculum school-based context for boys and girls to accumulate at least moderate intensity physical activity on a daily basis.

References

Andersen, L.B., Harro, M., Sardinha, L.B., Froberg, K., Ekelund, U., Brage, S. and Anderssen, S.A., 2006, Physical activity and clustered cardiovascular risk in children: A cross-sectional study (The European Youth Heart Study). *Lancet*, **368**, pp. 299–304.

Blatchford, P., Baines, E. and Pellegrini, A.D., 2003, The social context of school playground games: Sex and ethnic difference, and changes over time after entry to junior school. *British Journal of Developmental Psychology*, **21**, pp. 481–505.

Flohr, J.A., Todd, M.K. and Tudor-Locke, C., 2006, Pedometer-assessed physical activity in young adolescents. *Research Quarterly in Exercise and Sport*, **77**, pp. 309–315.

Mota, J., Silva, P., Santos, M.P., Ribeiro, L.C., Oliveira, J. and Duarte, J.A., 2005, Physical activity and school recess time: Differences between the sexes and the relationship between children's playground physical activity and habitual physical activity. *Journal of Sports Sciences*, **23**, pp. 269–275.

Nilsson, A., Ekelund, U., Yngve, A. and Sjöström, M., 2002, Assessing physical activity among children with accelerometers using different time sampling intervals and placements. *Pediatric Exercise Science*, **14**, pp. 87–96.

Ridgers, N.D., Stratton, G. and Fairclough, S.J., 2005, Assessing physical activity during recess using accelerometry. *Preventive Medicine*, **41**, pp. 102–107.

Ridgers, N.D., Stratton, G. and Fairclough, S.J., 2006, Physical activity levels of children during playtime. *Sports Medicine*, **36**, pp. 359–371.

Tudor-Locke, C., Lee, S.M., Morgan, C.F., Beighle, A. and Pangrazi, R.P., 2006, Children's pedometer-determined physical activity during the segmented school day. *Medicine and Science in Sports and Exercise*, **38**, pp. 1732–1738.

29 Frequency, intensity and duration of activity bouts in children

A.V. Rowlands, E.L. Pilgrim, M.R. Stone and R.G. Eston
School of Sport and Health Sciences, University of Exeter, UK

Introduction

Accelerometers are increasingly used to assess physical activity as they are objective, unobtrusive and measure movement directly. However, until recently the memory capacity has limited the assessment of habitual activity patterns to a minute-by-minute resolution. As children's activity is typically sporadic – consisting of frequent short bouts of activity – (Bailey *et al.*, 1995; Berman *et al.*, 1998) – this has limited understanding of the pattern of activity.

The transitory nature of children's physical activity was highlighted by Bailey *et al.* (1995) in an observation study of fifteen 6–10-year-old children from the US. The median duration of low and medium intensity activities was found to be only 6 s, and of high intensity activities only 3 s. Later spectral analysis of the data set showed the frequency of activity bouts to be over 80 per hour, with a mean duration of approximately 20 s (Berman *et al.*, 1998). The latest version of the uniaxial ActiGraph (GT1M) accelerometer has a memory size of 1 MB, enabling the objective assessment of habitual activity using high-frequency accelerometry monitoring. Results using this technology have shown very similar patterns of activity to the earlier observation studies (Baquet *et al.*, 2007). However, to date, there are few data on the variability of the activity pattern between sexes, across days and between high- and low-active children. Therefore, the aim of this study was to characterise the temporal pattern of activity in boys and girls across weekdays and weekend days. A secondary aim was to investigate how the pattern differed across high- and low-active children.

Methods

Eighty-four 9–11-year-old children (45 boys [age (mean ± SD): 9.9 ± 0.3 y; height: 1.38 ± 0.06 m; mass: 34.3 ± 7.4 kg] and 39 girls [age: 9.8 ± 0.3 y; height: 1.39 ± 0.05 m; mass: 34.4 ± 6.2 kg]) were recruited from two schools in the South West of England. The School Ethics Committee granted approval for this study. Parents or guardians provided written informed consent and children gave verbal assent.

Physical activity was assessed for six days with uniaxial accelerometry (GT1M ActiGraph, Monrovia, CA) during term time in January and February 2007. Each child wore an accelerometer on the hip for up to four weekdays and two weekend days during waking hours. The accelerometer epoch was set at 2 s as this was the lowest epoch that would allow data to be stored for the entire measurement period without download. For inclusion in the weekday analyses, a child needed a minimum of 10 hours wearing time within this period for each of three weekdays. For inclusion in the weekend analyses, a child needed a minimum of eight hours wearing time within this period for at least one weekend day. This resulted in the exclusion of two boys from analyses including weekend days.

Output measures were: total daily activity; frequency of bouts of at least light ($\geq$LIGHT), moderate ($\geq$MOD), vigorous ($\geq$VIG) intensity; mean duration and intensity of bouts above each intensity threshold. A bout was defined as a minimum of two consecutive epochs (i.e. 4 s) above each intensity threshold ($\geq$4 s bouts). To determine activity intensity, published threshold values (Trost *et al.*, 1998) relating counts min^{-1} to intensity in METs were divided by 30 to provide thresholds for the 2 s epoch data. A lower threshold of 10 counts s^{-1} (300 counts min^{-1}) was used to differentiate sedentary activity from whole body movement. Children were described as high-, medium- or low-active based on a sex-specific tertile split of the total activity data. These data are part of a larger ongoing study.

Results

The frequency of bouts of $\geq$LIGHT intensity did not differ by sex or day. However, both the duration ($p < 0.001$) and intensity of these bouts were greater in boys than girls ($p < 0.05$), and the duration of the bouts was greater on weekdays than weekend days ($p < 0.001$) (Figure 29.1a and b). High-active children experienced more frequent (941 vs 775 per day, $p < 0.001$) and intense (66.5, vs 60.7 counts 2s^{-1}, $p < 0.001$) daily bouts of $\geq$LIGHT activity.

Boys experienced a similar number of daily $\geq$MOD bouts on weekdays and weekends. However, girls experienced fewer bouts than boys irrespective of day

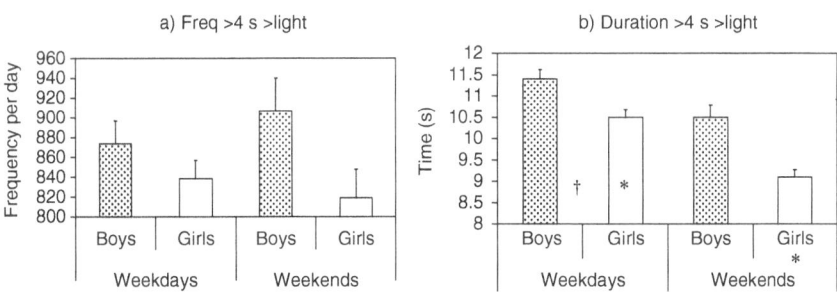

Figure 29.1 Frequency (a) and duration (b) of $\geq$LIGHT activity bouts by sex and type of day. (*Girls lower than boys. †Weekdays greater than weekend days.)

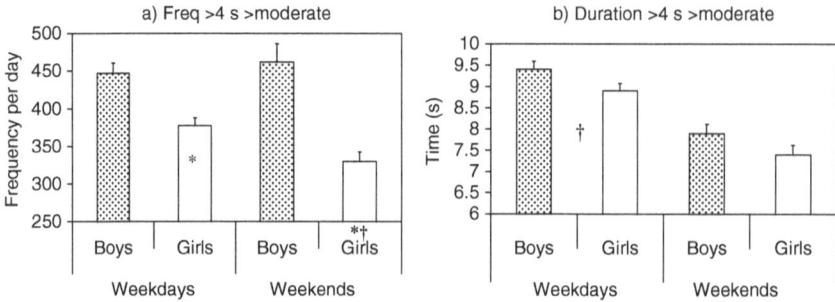

Figure 29.2 Frequency (a) and duration (b) of ≥MOD activity bouts by sex and type of day. (*Girls lower than boys. †Weekdays greater than weekend days.)

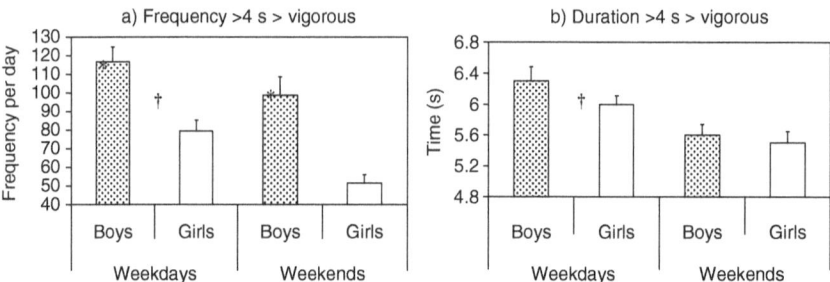

Figure 29.3 Frequency (a) and duration (b) of ≥VIG activity bouts by sex and type of day. (*Girls lower than boys. †Weekdays greater than weekend days.)

and fewer bouts on weekend days than weekdays ($p < 0.05$). The duration of bouts was also greater on weekdays than weekends ($p < 0.001$) (Figure 29.2a and b). The frequency, intensity and duration of ≥MOD bouts did not differ between high- and low-active children.

Boys experienced more bouts of ≥VIG intensity ($p < 0.001$) than girls. Weekday bouts were more frequent ($p < 0.001$) and longer ($p < 0.001$) than weekend bouts (Figure 29.3a and b). High-active children experienced more frequent (138 vs 66 per day, $p < 0.001$) and intense (267.4 vs 257.0 counts $2\,s^{-1}$, $p < 0.001$) daily bouts of ≥VIG activity in comparison with low-active children.

Discussion

The duration and frequency of weekday activity bouts is comparable to research using both observation and accelerometry protocols (Baquet *et al.*, 2007; Berman *et al.*, 1998). Children were more active on weekdays than weekends, consistent with some (Chu *et al.*, 2006), but not all (Wilkin *et al.*, 2006) previous research. The decrease in both frequency and duration of activity bouts at the weekends supports findings in Hong Kong Chinese children (Chu *et al.*, 2006).

In accordance with previous findings, boys were more active than girls (Wilkin, *et al.*, 2006). Assessment of activity patterns revealed that sex differences were largely due to the intensity of the most frequent bouts and the frequency of the more intense bouts. The frequency of the high intensity bouts was 65 per cent greater in boys than girls, and 100 per cent greater in high-active than low-active children.

Highlighting differences in the activity patterns of high- and low-active children could inform activity interventions, perhaps increasing adherence. In addition to characterising the pattern of activity in children, it is important to know which aspects of activity are related to health. It is not clear whether it is necessary to accumulate sustained bouts of activity, or whether short frequent bursts are just as important. This will differ according to the aspect of health of interest. However, the ability to characterise the activity pattern using high-frequency accelerometry monitoring will allow these questions to be addressed.

References

Bailey, R.C., Olson, J., Pepper, S.L., Porszasz, J., Barstow, T.J. and Cooper, D.M., 1995, The level and tempo of children's physical activities: An observational study. *Medicine and Science in Sports and Exercise*, **27**, pp. 1033–1041.

Baquet, G., Stratton, G., Van Praagh, E. and Berthoin, S., 2007, Improving physical activity assessment in prepubertal children with high-frequency accelerometry monitoring: A methodological issue. *Preventive Medicine*, **44**, pp. 143–147.

Berman, N., Bailey, R., Barstow, T.J. and Cooper, D.M., 1998, Spectral and bout detection analysis of physical activity patterns in healthy, prepubertal boys and girls. *American Journal of Human Biology*, **10**, pp. 289–297.

Chu, E.Y.W., Hu, Y., Tsang, A.M.C. and McManus, A.M., 2006, The influence of the distinguished pattern of locomotion to fitness and fatness in prepubertal children. *Children and Exercise XXII*, 23rd Pediatric Work Physiology Meeting Conference Book, P-B-39, 2006.

Trost, S.G., Ward, D.S., Moorehead, S.M., Watson, P.D., Riner, W. and Burke, J.R., 1998, Validity of the computer science and applications (CSA) activity monitor in children. *Medicine and Science in Sports and Exercise*, **30**, pp. 629–633.

Wilkin, T.J., Mallam, K.M., Metcalf, B.S., Jeffery, A.N. and Voss, L.D., 2006, Variation in physical activity lies with the child, not his environment: Evidence for an 'activitystat' in young children (EarlyBird 16). *International Journal of Obesity and Related Metabolic Disorders*, **30**, pp. 1050–1055.

30 Understanding the decline in physical activity of adolescent girls

L.B. Sherar,[1] *N.C. Gyurcsik,*[1] *M.L. Humbert,*[1]
D.W. Esliger[2] *and A.D.G. Baxter-Jones*[1]

[1]University of Saskatchewan, Saskatchewan, Canada; [2] University of Exeter, Devon, UK

Introduction

Physical activity (PA) declines with an increase in biological maturity (Sherar *et al.*, 2007). Girls of the same age differ considerably in their degree of physical maturity. Barriers to PA, defined as factors perceived to limit or hinder PA participation, differ across grade level (Gyurcsik *et al.*, 2006), but little is known about whether barriers differ by physical maturity. Understanding the relationship between physical maturity status (i.e. early, average or late) and barriers to PA would be important to understand when designing appropriately tailored interventions aimed at alleviating salient barriers. The objective of this research is to explore the PA behaviours and barriers to PA between early, average and late maturing adolescent girls. It was hypothesized that early maturing girls would participate in less PA and experience different barriers to PA than late maturing girls.

Methods

Participants were 57 high school girls between the ages of 12.5 and 16.3 years (M = 14.6 years, SD = 1.0 years).

Measurements were taken for stature, body mass and five skinfolds (triceps, biceps, iliac crest, medial calf, subscapular). Two measurements were taken and a third measure was required if the two measures differed by more than 4 mm for standing stature, 0.4 kg for body mass and 0.4 mm for skinfolds. The average of the two closest readings was used.

Girls were asked if they had reached menarche and if so when it had occurred. Girls were grouped into maturity categories based on age at menarche tertiles.

Physical activity levels were directly measured for seven consecutive days using a hip-mounted Actical accelerometer. Participants were asked to record when the monitor was put on in the morning and removed in the evening before bed for the purpose of distinguishing between activity time and sleep time. On completion of data collection, the data were electronically downloaded, resulting in a file containing 15 s movement counts for each individual. Custom software was used to reduce the raw data into raw minutes of moderate to vigorous PA per day

(MVPA) using intensity cutpoints (i.e. counts ≥ 3 METS) established by Puyau *et al.* (2004).

Barriers to physical activity

Perceived barriers to PA over the seven-day period were assessed using a semi-structured open-ended questionnaire. Participants were asked to list the physical activities that they would have liked to have done but didn't do over the previous seven days. The girls were then encouraged to think of anything that stopped them from doing the physical activities that they had identified.

Data analysis

In order to classify the barriers to PA that the participants listed on the open-ended measure, three steps were followed. First, barriers that were similar across the data set were grouped together and labelled. Second, three researchers independently coded each of the barriers as intrapersonal, interpersonal, institutional and community. The researchers were provided with the following definitions of each barrier type, which were derived from the ecological model by McLeroy and colleagues (1988). (1) interpersonal barriers are characteristics of the individual that may prevent PA, (2) interpersonal barriers are formal and informal social networks and support systems that may prevent PA, (3) institutional barriers occur within social institutions with organizational characteristics that may prevent PA, (4) community barriers occur between organizations, institutions, and informal networks within defined boundaries that may prevent PA. (5) unclassifiable barriers (cannot be classified into any of the aforementioned groups). Third, researchers discussed all barriers that were not independently classified as the same until agreement was reached on classification.

Differences between maturity groups were obtained using ANOVA. Alpha level was set at 0.05 (SPSS version 11.5, SPSS Inc, Chicago, Illinois).

Results

Only girls who had reached menarche ($n = 51$) were retained for analysis. There were no significant differences in chronological age, stature and body mass. As expected, the girls' age at menarche differed significantly between maturity groups.

Figure 30.1 shows the average number of minutes per day early, average and late maturing girls spent in MVPA, sporadic MVPA, short MVPA and long MVPA. On average, early maturing girls engaged in 32.2 less minutes of MVPA per day compared to late maturing. Most of the difference in MVPA between maturity groups (i.e. 83 per cent or 26.8 minutes) was attributed to differences in the accumulation of sporadic minutes of MVPA. There were no significant differences in short and long minutes of MVPA between maturity groups. 119 barriers were listed by the participants and on average each participant listed 2.31 barriers (SD $= 1.16$). Interpersonal barriers were cited most often (31.1 per cent),

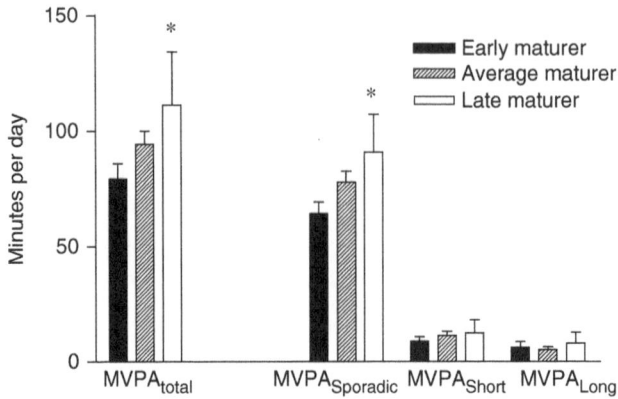

Figure 30.1 Mean (±95% CI) minutes of total MVPA and sporadic, short, and long minutes of MVPA per day between maturity groups (early, average and late) (Sporadic MVPA accumulated in bouts of 1–9 minutes; Short MVPA accumulated in bouts 10–19 minutes; Long MVPA accumulated in bouts of 20+ minutes) *= significantly different from late maturing girls.

Table 30.1 Types of barriers listed by the participants

Type of barrier	n	Type of barrier	n
Intrapersonal (n = 37)		*Institutional (n = 26)*	
Lack of motivation/lazy	9	Too much homework to do activity	14
Lack of time	9	The timing of other organized activities conflicted	7
Illness/injury	6	Other*	5
Was doing something else	5		
Other*	8		
Interpersonal (n = 36)		*Community Barriers (n = 20)*	
A person in authority (e.g. parent or older sibling) said no to activity	23	Weather is too cold/snowing	15
Friends did not want to go with me	7	Other*	5
Other*	6		

Note
Total n = 119; *Ns < 5 each

followed by intrapersonal (30.3 per cent), institutional (21.8 per cent) and community (16.8 per cent) (Table 30.1).

Early maturing girls most often cited institutional and community barriers, whereas average and late maturing girls most often cited inter- and intra- personal barriers (Table 30.2).

Table 30.2 The percentage of intrapersonal, interpersonal, institutional and community barriers cited within each maturity group (early, average and late)

Type of barrier	Maturity status		
	Early	Average	Late
Intrapersonal barriers	21.1%	29.7%	30.7%
Interpersonal barriers	21.1%	35.1%	26.9%
Institutional barriers	31.6%	16.2%	23.1%
Community barriers	26.3%	18.9%	19.2%

Conclusion

Adolescent girls identified a variety of barriers to PA. Early maturing girls participated in less MVPA than late maturing girls. Analyzing the pattern of PA accumulation suggest that sporadic MVPA is most affected by maturity status (i.e. early maturity). Early maturing girls reported more community and institutional barriers. These preliminary findings provide support for maturity targeted interventions aimed at alleviating specific type of barriers.

References

Gyurcsik, N.C., Spink, K.S., Bray, G.A., Chad, K. and Kwan, M., 2006, An ecologically-based examination of barriers to physical activity in students from grade seven through first year of university. *Journal of Adolescent Health*, **38**, pp. 704–711.

McLeroy, K.R., Bibeau, D., Steckler, A. and Glanz, K., 1988, An ecological perspective on health promotion programs. *Health Education Quarterly*, **15**, pp. 351–377.

Puyau, M.R., Adolph, A.L., Vohra, F.A., Zakeri, I. and Butte, N.F., 2004, Prediction of activity energy expenditure using accelerometers in children. *Medicine and Science in Sports and Exercise*, **36**, pp. 1625–1631.

Sherar, L.B., Esliger, D.W., Baxter-Jones, A.D. and Tremblay, M.S., 2007, Age and gender differences in youth physical activity: Does physical maturity matter? *Medicine and Science in Sports and Exercise*, **39**, pp. 830–835.

31 The use of high-frequency accelerometry monitoring to assess and interpret children's activity patterns

M.R. Stone, A.V. Rowlands and R.G. Eston
School of Sport and Health Sciences, University of Exeter, UK

Introduction

The ability to generate accurate and detailed physical activity data is essential to explore the relationship between physical activity, health, growth and development in children. Researchers must have confidence that the tool selected to measure physical activity is reliable and valid and that the data expressed are capable of characterizing and quantifying physical activity appropriately.

Accelerometers are now recognized as one of the most effective ways to obtain objective information on children's habitual physical activity. Typically, physical activity has been expressed on a minute-by-minute basis (i.e. 60 s epoch) in children (Welk, 2005). However habitual physical activity patterns in children are typically sporadic, containing short, frequent bursts of activity. Previous observational research (Bailey *et al.*, 1995) noted that 95 per cent of children's free play lasted 15 s or less. On average, low and moderate intensity activities lasted 6 s, while high intensity activities lasted 3 s. There were no bouts of vigorous physical activity longer than 10 min, and rest intervals, although longer in comparison to physical activity bouts, were < 4 min and 15 s 95 per cent of the time. Measuring physical activity in children on a minute-to-minute basis cannot appropriately describe these high-frequency activity patterns and will ultimately obscure and underestimate the intensity of accumulated physical activity (i.e. moderate and vigorous) in young populations (Nilsson *et al.*, 2002).

To properly establish links between children's unique physical activity patterns and health-related outcomes, a tool capable of assessing rapid changes in intensity and duration of activity is necessary. At present, accelerometers have sufficient memory capacity (1 MB of flash memory, rechargeable battery capable of providing power for over 14 days) to offer shorter epochs (1 s, 2 s, 5 s, 10 s) able to better identify these patterns. However, there are currently few data on the temporal patterns of activity in children assessed using these shorter epochs (i.e. high-frequency accelerometry). The aim of this study was therefore to characterize the duration and frequency of activity bouts of varying intensity and reveal discrepancies in activity data produced.

Methods

Fifty-four 8–10-year-old boys [age (mean ± SD): 9.35 ± 0.56 y; height: 1.34 ± 0.08 m; mass: 31.8 ± 7.4 kg)] were recruited from three local schools in the South West of England. The experimental protocols were approved by the Institutional Ethics Committee and written parental and child consent was attained. All assessments took place from October 2006 to March 2007.

Physical activity was assessed for seven days (five weekdays and two weekend days) with a uniaxial accelerometer (GT1M ActiGraph, Manufacturing Technologies, Inc., Fort Walton Beach, FL). Prior to data collection, all accelerometers were subjected to laboratory-based calibration during a standardized treadmill protocol to assess both quality and dependability. Coefficients of variation from the ActiGraphs were within acceptable limits (Welk, 2005; Chen and Bassett, 2005). Accelerometers were placed on the right hip of each participant and were worn all day (even when sleeping) and removed only for water activities, i.e. baths, showers, swimming, which was recorded. Accelerometers were programmed to measure activity every two seconds, as this was the lowest epoch that would store activity data over seven continuous days. Habitual activity was analyzed from 6 AM to 9 PM. Children who did not achieve a minimum of 10 hours on at least three weekdays and one weekend day were omitted from analyses. This resulted in the exclusion of activity data from three children.

Identifying the frequency and duration of activity bouts of varying intensity was the main research focus of this paper. A bout was defined as a minimum of two consecutive epochs (i.e. 4 s) above each intensity threshold ($\geq$ 4 s bouts). In order to determine activity intensity, published threshold values (counts/minute) related to intensity in METs (Trost *et al.*, 1998) were divided by 30 to provide thresholds based on 2 s epochs. Intensity thresholds for light (LPA; >10 cts 2 s^{-1}), moderate (MPA; >65 cts 2 s^{-1}), vigorous (VPA; >176 cts 2 s^{-1}) and hard (HPA; >316 cts 2 s^{-1}) activity were used. The daily number of physical activity bouts for each intensity category were calculated and expressed according to minimum bout lengths (4 s, 6 s, 8 s, 10 s, 60 s, 300 s, and 600 s). Mean bout duration(s) was also reported. These data, along with the results presented, are part of a larger ongoing study.

Results

On average children spent 105 min in LPA (range = 75–130), 70 min in MPA (range = 28–103), 16 min in VPA (range = 6–31) and 3 min in HPA (range = 1–11) each day (Figure 31.1). Mean bout durations (±SD) for LPA, MPA, VPA, and HPA was 11.6 ±1.3 s, 9.1 ± 1.2 s, 5.9 ± 0.9 s and 6.0 ± 2.0 s respectively. 95 per cent – 96 per cent of all LPA and MPA bouts and 99 per cent of all VPA and HPA bouts were 10 s or shorter (Figure 31.2a, b and c).

On an average day, children accumulated seven bouts of MPA that were 5 min or longer. However, no bouts of VPA or HPA were longer than 5 min. There were

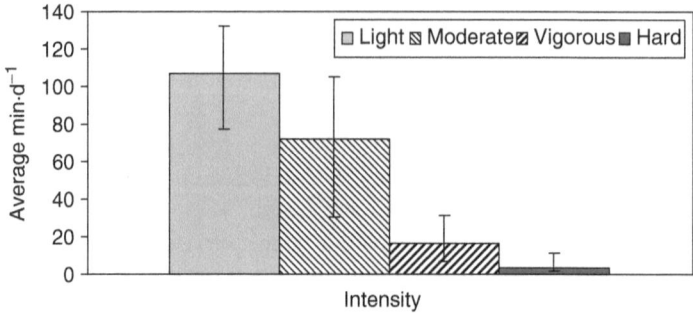

Figure 31.1 Time (min.d^{-1}; mean, range) spent in light, moderate, vigorous and hard physical activity.

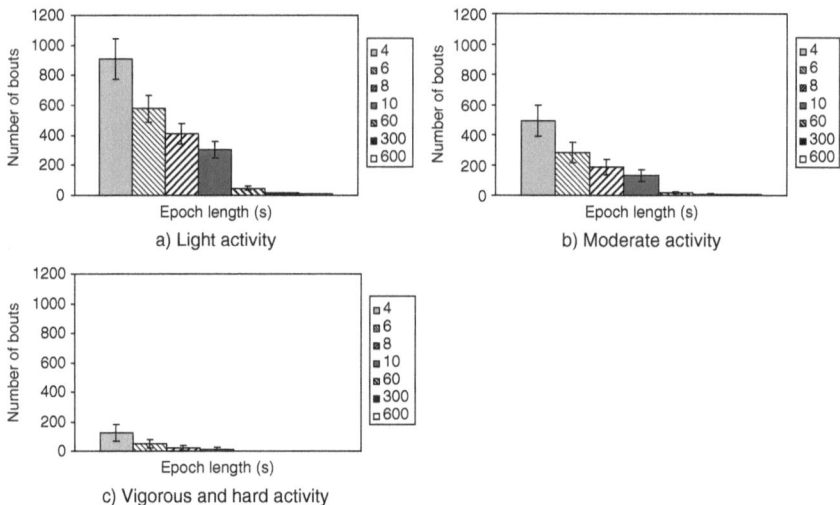

Figure 31.2 a, b and c. Frequency (±SD) of light, moderate, vigorous and hard intensity bouts according to epoch.

virtually no bouts of VPA (mean = 1; range = 0–5) or HPA (mean = 0; range = 0–2) lasting longer than 1 min.

Discussion

This study examined temporal patterns of physical activity using accelerometer data collected every 2 s. The majority of studies to date have assessed the physical activity patterns of children using 60 s sampling intervals, which can obscure and dilute the intensity of accumulated physical activity in young populations.

As the majority of children's activity bouts were found to be shorter than 10 s in this study, supporting work by Baquet and colleagues (2007), the true nature of the pattern of children's habitual activity may be masked if accelerometer epochs > 10 s are used. High-frequency accelerometer monitoring should be employed in future research to increase the validity of results and improve comparability across studies.

Physiological responses affecting the growth and development of children may vary according to activity patterns. Growth related hormones may alter their responses in response to the tempo of activity (Rowland, 1998); cardiovascular and metabolic function may be affected by rapid changes in movement and transitions from low to high intensity and/or vice-versa (Bailey *et al.*, 1995). Exploring aspects of the temporal pattern of activity using high-frequency accelerometry could uncover links to physiological health parameters. This could help clarify whether optimal ways of accumulating physical activity exist for preventing risk factors for metabolic syndrome and obesity in children today.

References

Bailey, R.C., Olson, J., Pepper, S.L., Porszasz, J., Barstow, T.J. and Cooper, D.M., 1995, The level and tempo of children's physical activities: An observational study. *Medicine and Science in Sports and Exercise*, **27**, pp. 1033–1041.

Baquet, G., Stratton, G., Van Praagh, E. and Berthoin, S., 2007, Improving physical activity assessment in prepubertal children with high-frequency accelerometry monitoring: A methodological issue. *Preventive Medicine*, **44**, pp. 143–147.

Chen, K.Y. and Bassett, D.R. Jr., 2005, The technology of accelerometry-based activity monitors: current and future. *Medicine and Science in Sports and Exercise*, **37**(11 Suppl), pp. S490–500.

Nilsson, A., Ekelund, U., Yngve, A. and Sjostrom, M., 2002, Assessing physical activity among children with accelerometers using different time sampling intervals and placements. *Pediatric Exercise Science*, **14**, pp. 87–96.

Rowland, T.W., 1998. The biological basis of physical activity. *Medicine and Science in Sports and Exercise*, **30**, pp. 392–399.

Trost, S.G., Ward, D.S., Moorehead, S.M., Watson, P.D., Riner, W. and Burke, J.R., 1998, Validity of the computer science and applications (CSA) activity monitor in children. *Medicine and Science in Sports and Exercise*, **30**, pp. 629–633.

Welk, G.J., 2005, Principles of design and analyses for the calibration of accelerometry-based activity monitors. *Medicine and Science in Sports and Exercise*, **37** (11 Suppl), pp. S501–511.

32 Short-duration patterning of physical activity and biomechanical efficiency

E.Y. Chu,[1] *A. McManus*[1] *and Y. Hu*[2]

[1]Institute of Human Performance; [2]Department of Orthopedics and Traumatology, The University of Hong Kong

Introduction

Walking is an essential daily practice and constitutes 80 per cent of children's daily physical activity (PA). Bipedal gait is a complex series of alterations in magnitude, direction, rotation and force of the body as it coordinates within space. PA has been implicated in improved kinematic and kinetic aspects of gait (Maltais *et al.*, 2005), however, despite a plethora of research investigating the metabolic cost of movement, few have directly investigated the relationship between PA and gait efficiency in children. The primary purpose of this study was to examine the variation in mechanical economy during free and paced on-ground walking as a function of short-duration PA in a group of healthy children.

Methods

Thirty-four healthy ambulatory children (mean age 11.3 ± 1.1 y), 23 of whom were boys and 11 were girls, participated in the study. Eight children were above the 90th percentile for BMI. Ethical approval was granted by the Institutional Review Board. PA was assessed using the triaxial RT3 accelerometer set at 1 s intervals. PA monitoring was scrutinized for three weekdays, only those with seven hours of data for a minimum of two weekdays were included in the final analyses. Anthropometric data were measured. Gait variables were collected using a Kistler force plate and VICON 6 camera motion analysis system. Each child completed at least three five-minute trials at a self-selected walking speed and three trials at $4 \, \text{km} \cdot \text{h}^{-1}$. Velocity was checked every ten steps. Stride length of each gait cycle was calculated and the centre of mass was also estimated. Using Kerrigan *et al.*'s (1995) geometric model, the biomechanical efficiency quotient (BEQ) was derived. The pattern characteristics of short-duration PA were identified using a cluster algorithm approach, a programme to identify and classify active and inactive clusters using population specific threshold values (Chu *et al.*, 2007). Linear regression was used to assess the relationship between BEQ, PA variables and body composition. A repeated measures analysis of variance was used to investigate the effect of walking velocity on an individual's BEQ. Alpha was set at 0.05. All analyses were performed using SPSS.

Table 32.1 Mean (SD) BEQ values at varying walking velocities

	Mean (SD)	Range
BEQ Freewalk	1.4 (0.3)	0.85 to 2.3
BEQ 4 km·h^{-1}	1.5 (0.3)	0.89 to 2.4

Results

Average body mass of the group was 38.1 (8.8) kg, whilst height was 145.6 (11.7) cm. Mean percentage body fat was 19.4 (6.7) per cent, with an average BMI of 17.3 (3.8). Walking economy (BEQ) for the on-ground walking is shown in Table 32.1. BEQ did not vary between self-paced and paced walking ($p > 0.05$).

The characteristics of short duration PA for the group are presented in Table 32.2. Significant relationships between walking economy and PA characteristics were identified. Negative associations were found between BEQ at 4 km·h^{-1}, total clusters ($r = -0.44$, $p < 0.05$) and the time spent in low-to-moderate PA ($r = -0.39$, $p < 0.05$). Positive associations were found between BEQ at 4 km·h^{-1}, the mean interval between bouts ($r = 0.50$, $p < 0.05$), as well as the total time spent being sedentary ($r = 0.38$, $p < 0.05$). The same pattern of relationships existed between PA pattern characteristics and BEQ during the free-walk, but failed to attain significance. We found no relationships between BEQ and body composition for the whole group.

Discussion

The main finding of this study suggests that biomechanical efficiency has a moderate relationship with characteristics of short-duration PA in able-bodied children. When BEQ is larger than 1.0 a decrease in biomechanical walking economy is suggested (Kerrigan *et al.*, 1995). The BEQ values found in this study show a wide variation. In the normal child, gait pattern matures and attains the adult pattern after seven years of age. The source of the wide variation

Table 32.2 Mean (SD) daily values for PA pattern characteristics

n = 35	Mean (SD)	Range
Bouts per hour	56.9 (33.9.9)	3.7 to 120.2
Mean bout duration (s)	14.3 (6.2)	6.9 to 39.2
Mean interval duration (s)	94.2 (136.5)	15.7 to 704
Mean peak amplitude of a bout (RT3 counts·s^{-1})	16.6 (3.8)	10.6 to 25.6
Daily sedentary time (h)	7.4 (1.2)	4.5 to 9.0
Daily low-to-moderate time (h)	1.7 (1.1)	0.1 to 4.4
Daily vigorous time (min)	3.5 (4.6)	0.02 to 15.2

in BEQ may relate to stature. Longitudinal work has indicated that children's average stride length is 76 per cent of their height which is not proportional to their age (Beck et al., 1981). Although velocity and stride length change with growth, the high variety in the BEQ values we found occurs in a group of children who are fairly similar in height. This would indicate that other influences play a role in mechanical efficiency. Maltais et al. (2005) speculated that variation in mechanical efficiency may relate to PA habits and substantiated this in children with cerebral palsy. The impact of low levels of PA on mechanical efficiency has also been illustrated by Chen et al. (2004). Long-term engagement in PA in theory should result in better mechanical efficiency and our data give support to this theory. The negative relationships identified between BEQ and daily clusters of activity and the amount of low to moderate intensity activity suggests that those with a lower BEQ are more active. The positive relationship between BEQ and the length of the interval between activity clusters, as well as the total time spent being sedentary, suggests those who spend more time being sedentary have reduced mechanical efficiency. The strength of these relationships is, however, somewhat weaker than that of Maltais et al. (2005), with at best 25 per cent of the variation in BEQ accounted for by PA parameters. However, the author simply looked at the total activity counts without consideration of the short-term patterning of PA. In conclusion, this study has shown evidence of a relationship between biomechanical efficiency and PA, but this is still a poorly understood relationship and future interventional work is needed.

References

Beck, R.J., Andriacchi, T.P., Kuo, K.N., Fermier, R.W. and Galante, J.O., 1981, Changes in the gait patterns of growing children. *Journal of Bone and Joint Surgery: American Volume*, **63**, pp. 1452–1457.

Chen, K.Y., Acra, S.A., Donahue, C.L., Sun, M. and Buchowski, M.S., 2004, Efficiency of walking and stepping: relationship to body fatness. *Obesity Research*, **12**, pp. 982–989.

Chu, E.Y.W., McManus, A.M. and Yu, C.C.W., 2007, Calibration of the RT3 accelerometer for ambulation and nonambulation in children. *Medicine and Science in Sports and Exercise*, **39**, pp. 2085–2091.

Kerrigan, D.C., Viramontes, B.E., Corcoran, P.J. and LaRaia, P.J., 1995, Measured versus predicted vertical displacement of the sacrum during gait as a tool to measure biomechanical gait performance. *American Journal of Physical Medicine and Rehabilitation*, **74**, pp. 3–8.

Maltais, D.B., Pierrynowski, M.R., Galea, V.A., Matsuzaka, A. and Bar-Or, O., 2005, Habitual physical activity levels are associated with biomechanical walking economy in children with cerebral palsy. *American Journal of Physical Medicine and Rehabilitation*, **84**, pp. 36–45.

Part IV

Exercise endocrinology

33 Plasma visfatin concentrations are related to metabolic parameters in physically active adolescent boys

J. Jürimäe,[1] A. Cicchella,[2] E. Lätt,[1] K. Haljaste,[1] P. Purge,[1] M. Zini,[3] C. Stefanelli[2,3] and T. Jürimäe[1]

[1]Institute of Sport Pedagogy and Coaching Sciences, Centre of Behavioural and Health Sciences, University of Tartu, Tartu, Estonia; [2]Faculty of Exercise and Sport Science; [3]Department of Biochemistry, University of Bologna, Bologna, Italy

Introduction

Visfatin is a newly identified adipocytokine in visceral adipose tissue and has insulin-like metabolic effects that may improve insulin sensitivity (Fukuhara *et al.*, 2005). Fukuhara *et al.* (2005) reported that plasma visfatin concentrations were strongly correlated with visceral fat mass among the Japanese general population. It has also been found that plasma visfatin concentrations are elevated in patients with type 2 diabetes mellitus and associated with abdominal obesity and fasting insulin in adults (Sandeep *et al.*, 2007). Visfatin has been suggested to be one of the links between intra-abdominal obesity and type 2 diabetes mellitus (Sethi and Vidal-Puig, 2005). Given that insulin sensitivity has been reported to improve with exercise training, it can be speculated that visfatin may also be involved in the regulation of insulin sensitivity under yet to be determined conditions. In this context, it is important to look at the relationships between plasma visfatin concentrations and insulin sensitivity in regularly physically active children. To our knowledge, the only published study assessing visfatin in children found that, although plasma visfatin concentrations were markedly elevated in obese children, visfatin was not associated with overall adiposity (Haider *et al.*, 2006). The aim of the present study was to examine the association of fasting plasma visfatin concentration with insulin sensitivity and body fat parameters in physically active children.

Methods

Subjects

In total, 34 healthy children (17 boys and 17 girls) aged between 13 and 16 years participated in this study. All children were swimmers recruited from local training groups and had a training history of 4.3 ± 1.2 (boys) and 4.3 ± 1.8 (girls) years. All swimmers trained for at least eight hours per week during the past two years.

During the testing period, the mean weekly training volume was 18.6 ± 5.7 km performed mainly at an aerobic pace. According to the Tanner classification (Tanner, 1962), seven boys and six girls were in pubertal stage 3, five boys and six girls in pubertal stage 4, and five boys and five girls in pubertal stage 5. This study was approved by the Medical Ethics Committee of the University of Tartu. All procedures were explained to the children and their parents who signed a consent form.

Procedures

Height (Martin metal anthropometer) and body mass (A&D Instruments, UK) of the participants were measured to the nearest 0.1 cm and 0.05 kg, respectively. Body mass index (BMI) was calculated as body mass (in kg) divided by body height^2 (in m^2). Waist circumference was also measured as a proxy measure of the amount of visceral adipose tissue (Berndt *et al.*, 2005). $\dot{V}O_{2\,peak}$ was measured on an electronically braked bicycle ergometer (Tunturi T8, Finland) using a portable open circuit system (MedGraphics VO200, St. Paul, MN, USA). Body composition was assessed by dual energy X-ray absorptiometry (DXA) using the DPX-IQ densitometer (Lunar Corporation, Madison, WI, USA) and analysed for fat and fat-free mass.

A 10 mL blood sample was obtained from the antecubital vein with the participant sitting in the upright position. The plasma was separated and frozen at $-20°$C for later analysis. Visfatin was measured with a human visfatin enzyme-linked immunosorbent assay (AdipoGen Inc., catalog no. V0523EK). Leptin was measured using an ELISA kit from DRG Instruments GmbH, Marbourg, Germany (catalog no. EIA-2395). Insulin was analysed on Immulite 2000 (DPC, Los Angeles, CA, USA). Glucose was measured using the hexokinase/ glucose 6-phosphate-dehydrogenase method with a commercial kit (Boehringer, Mannheim, Germany) and insulin resistance was calculated as fasting insulin resistance index (FIRI): [fasting glucose (mmol L^{-1}) $\times$ fasting insulin (μIU mL^{-1})]/25.

Statistical analyses were performed with SPSS 11.0 for Windows (Chicago, IL, USA). Means and standard deviations ($\pm$SD) were determined. Evaluation of normality was performed with the Shapiro-Wilk statistical method. The differences between boys and girls were compared using the Wilcoxon rank sum test. Partial correlation coefficients were used to estimate the correlations of plasma concentrations of visfatin with measured physical and blood biochemical parameters after adjustment for age in boys and girls separately. All analyses were 2-tailed and a p value <0.05 was considered statistically significant.

Results

The distribution of age and BMI was not different between boys and girls (Table 33.1). Body fat mass was significantly higher, while fat-free mass and

Table 33.1 Mean (±SD) characteristics of the study subjects

Variable	Boys (n = 17)	Girls (n = 17)
Age (y)	14.4±1.8	14.2±2.1
Height (cm)	171.2±7.7	163.0±8.9*
Body mass (kg)	57.3±12.4	53.3±9.5
BMI (kg·m^{-2})	19.4±2.8	20.0±2.8
Waist circumference (cm)	68.1±6.6	64.4±4.2
Body fat (%)	12.3±6.2	21.5±4.8*
Fat mass (kg)	6.9±4.4	11.0±3.5*
Fat free mass (kg)	47.5±11.8	39.1±6.4*
$\dot{V}O_{2\,peak}$ (L·min^{-1})	3.19±0.74	2.65±0.67*
Insulin (μU mL^{-1})	6.8±3.1	7.4±1.8
Glucose (mmol L^{-1})	4.7±0.3	4.8±0.3
FIRI	12.8±5.9	14.2±3.5
Leptin (ng·mL^{-1})	2.1±2.1	4.9±2.6*
Visfatin (ng·mL^{-1})	1.3±0.9	1.2±1.0

*Significantly different from boys; $p < 0.05$.

$\dot{V}O_{2\,peak}$ values were significantly lower in girls compared to boys. Girls presented significantly higher values for leptin compared to boys. In both sexes, visfatin concentrations were not related to height, body mass, waist circumference, fat-free mass, glucose or leptin values. Visfatin concentration was positively correlated with the markers of overall obesity (BMI, body fat percentage, fat mass) and insulin sensitivity (insulin, FIRI) only in boys. In girls, visfatin was significantly related to $\dot{V}O_{2\,peak}$ value. In boys, visfatin concentration was significantly related to BMI ($r = 0.56$), fat mass ($r = 0.53$), insulin ($r = 0.55$) and FIRI ($r = 0.52$) after adjustment for age. In contrast, no such relationships between visfatin and metabolic parameters were observed in girls.

Discussion

The main finding of the present investigation was that fasting plasma visfatin concentration was linked to metabolic and overall adiposity parameters in physically active boys but not in girls. To date, the only published study assessing visfatin in children found that visfatin was not associated with markers of metabolic and overall adiposity in nondiabetic obese and healthy control children (Haider et al., 2006). All subjects in our study were lean with relatively low body fat values and with relatively high physical activity levels. This would suggest that visfatin may contribute to enhanced insulin sensitivity in regularly physically active adolescent boys.

In contrast to our findings in boys, we observed no relationship between plasma visfatin concentration and insulin resistance parameters in girls. At present, this sex difference is difficult to explain. One possible explanation would be sex differences in the concentrations of different sex hormones. It could be speculated that further differences in sex hormones in older children may also have influenced the findings. In support of our findings, Berndt *et al.* (2005) studied the relationship between plasma visfatin concentration, BMI and body fat, and found a correlation in males only, also suggesting that there might be sex differences. As there is no clear evidence for the exact cellular role of visfatin, it has been suggested that visfatin could have autocrine and paracrine functions in the differentation of adipocytes and may also have an endocrine function in modulating insulin action at the peripheral tissues (Sethi and Vidal-Puig, 2005). The limitation of the present study is that, being cross-sectional, it cannot explain the causal relationship between visfatin and insulin resistance in physically active boys. However, our results provide some information on the relatively poorly understood relationship of visfatin with metabolic parameters in children. Further interventional studies are necessary to evaluate the relationship of plasma visfatin with different metabolic and body composition parameters in children.

In conclusion, the results of this study suggest that plasma visfatin concentrations are not different between regularly physically active boys and girls. In addition, our findings indicate that the associations between fasting plasma visafatin concentrations and metabolic and body composition parameters were sex-dependent in children. The possible mechanism underlying this sex difference should be examined in a larger cohort.

References

Berndt, J., Klöting, N., Kralisch, S., Kovacs, P., Fasshauer, M., Schön, M.R., Stumvoll, M. and Blüher, M., 2005, Plasma visfatin concentrations and fat depot-specific mRNA expression in humans. *Diabetes*, **54**, pp. 2911–2916.

Fukuhara, A., Matsuda, M., Nishizawa, M., Segawa, K., Tanaka, M., Kishimoto, K., Matsuki, Y., Murakami, M., Ichisaka, T., Murakami, H., Watanabe, E., Takagi, T., Akiyoshi, M., Ohtsubo, T., Kihara, S., Yamashita, S., Makashima, M., Funashi, T., Yamanaka, S., Hiramatsu, R., Masuzawa, Y. and Shimomura, I., 2005, Visfatin: A protein secreted by visceral fat that mimics the effects of insulin. *Science*, **307**, pp. 426–430.

Haider, D.G., Holzer, G., Schaller, G., Weghuber, D., Widhalm, K., Wagner, O., Kapiotis, S. and Wolzt, M., 2006, The adipokine visfatin is markedly elevated in obese children. *Journal of Pediatric Gastroenterology and Nutrition*, **43**, pp. 548–549.

Sandeep, S., Velmurugan, K., Deepa, R. and Mohan, V., 2007, Serum visfatin in relation to visceral fat, obesity, and type 2 diabetes mellitus in Asian Indians. *Metabolism*, **56**, pp. 565–570.

Sethi, J.K. and Vidal-Puig, A., 2005, Visfatin: the missing link between intra-abdominal obesity and diabetes? *Trends in Molecular Medicine*, **11**, pp. 344–347.

Tanner, J., 1962, *Growth at Adolescence*, 2nd edn. Oxford: Blackwell Scientific.

34 Relationships between ghrelin concentration and metabolic parameters in boys

J. Mäestu,[1] A. Cicchella,[2] V. Tillmann,[3] E. Lätt,[1] K. Haljaste,[1] P. Purge,[1] T. Pomerants,[1] J. Jürimäe[1] and T. Jürimäe[1]

[1]Institute of Sport Pedagogy and Coaching Sciences, Centre of Behavioural and Health Sciences, University of Tartu; [2]Faculty of Exercise and Sport Science, University of Bologna; [3]Department of Pediatrics, University of Tartu

Introduction

Ghrelin is an endogeneous ligand for growth hormone secretagogue receptor and its principal synthesis site is stomach (Kojima *et al.*, 1999). Plasma ghrelin levels are reduced in obese subjects and are increased in anorexic subjects (Haqq *et al.*, 2003). It has also been proposed that ghrelin could influence growth and physical development (Whatmore *et al.*, 2003). The initiation of puberty has been reported to increase leptin and decrease ghrelin (Haqq *et al.*, 2003; Whatmore *et al.*, 2003) concentrations in blood. However, knowledge of ghrelin concentrations through childhood have not yet been fully defined, especially the effect of regular high energy expenditure on ghrelin concentration during pubertal development in boys.

Accelerated growth and changes in fat, muscle and bone mass take place during puberty. These changes are mediated by many hormones, including leptin, insulin-like growth factor-I (IGF-1) and sex hormones (Yilmatz *et al.*, 2005). Therefore, the present cross-sectional study aimed to assess the influence of regular physical activity on ghrelin concentrations and the interrelationships between ghrelin and metabolic and biochemical parameters in pubertal and prepubertal boys.

Methods

Subjects

In total, 56 healthy schoolboys aged from 10 to 16 years were studied. They were divided into swimming ($n = 28$) and control ($n = 28$) group. Swimmers had a training history of 3.0 ± 1.1 years and they trained 8.4 ± 1.7 h·week^{-1}. Control subjects were not physically active, except for two physical education classes at secondary school. All participants were divided into three groups based on the method of Tanner. The groups were matched for age (± 1 years) and body mass index (BMI; ± 2 kg·m^{-2}). Group I (nine matched pairs) was prepubertal (Tanner stage 1), Group II (11 matched pairs) included pubertal stages 2 and 3, and Group III (eight matched pairs) included pubertal stages 4 and 5. The participants were not taking any medications nor had a history of bone or renal diseases. All procedures were explained to the children and their parents who signed the consent form as approved by the Medical Ethics Committee of the University of Tartu.

Procedures

Body height was measured with a Martin metal stadiometer, body mass was measured with a medical balance scale (A&D Instruments, UK) and BMI was calculated. Whole body fat and fat-free mass were measured by dual X-ray absorptiometry (DXA) using the DPX-IQ densitometer (Lunar Corporation, Madison, WI, USA).

Peak oxygen consumption was measured on an electronically braked cycle ergometer (Tunturi T8, Finland). Participants performed an initial work rate of 80 W with an increment of 20 W every 2 min. At the end of the last work rate, participants were required to sprint as fast as possible for 1 min. Gas exchange variables were measured throughout the test in a breath by breath mode and data were stored in 10 s intervals for the measurement of oxygen consumption using a portable open circuit system (MedGraphics VO2000, St Paul, MN, USA).

A 10 mL fasting blood sample was obtained from an antecubital vein at rest at 7.30 am. Ghrelin was determined in duplicate using a commercially available radioimmunoassay (RIA) kit (Linco Research, USA). Leptin was measured in duplicate by RIA (Mediagnost GmbH, Germany). Testosterone, IGF-1 and IGFBP-3 were analyzed in duplicate with an Immunolite 2000 (DPC, Los Angeles, USA).

Means and standard deviations ($\pm$SD) were calculated. The differences between the groups were tested with Friedman analyses of variance by ranks and Wilcoxon matched-pairs signed rank test was used when post hoc analysis was relevant. Spearman correlation coefficients were used to determine the relationships between the variables. Significance was set at $p < 0.05$.

Results

Physical characteristics of the subjects are presented in Table 34.1.

Resting ghrelin concentration was not different in swimmers at different maturation levels, while significant maturation effects for ghrelin were observed in control subjects (Table 34.2). Swimmers in groups II and III had significantly higher plasma ghrelin concentration compared to the controls at the same maturation level.

Leptin values were significantly lower in groups II and III compared to less mature boys in both groups. Testosterone, IGF-1 and IGFBP-3 levels increased

Table 34.1 Physical characteristics (mean $\pm$ SD) of subjects in different study groups

		Group I (9 pairs)	Group II (11 pairs)	Group III (8 pairs)
Age (y)	S	11.5 ± 0.5	13.8 ± 1.4[a]	14.4 ± 1.1[a]
	C	11.4 ± 0.5	13.2 ± 1.3[a]	14.2 ± 0.8[a]
Height (cm)	S	151.8 ± 6.9	168.1 ± 11.5[a]	171.1 ± 8.3[a,b]
	C	150.9 ± 7.5	164.7 ± 10.5[a]	174.8 ± 6.8[a,b]
Body mass (kg)	S	40.6 ± 4.4	56.6 ± 10.2[a]	56.9 ± 13.8[a]
	C	40.5 ± 5.9	52.6 ± 12.1[a]	61.8 ± 6.7[a,b]
BMI (kg·m^{-2})	S	17.6 ± 1.5	19.9 ± 1.8[a]	19.8 ± 2.3[a]
	C	17.8 ± 1.6	19.8 ± 2.4[a]	20.2 ± 1.6[a]
Body fat (%)	S	12.8 ± 5.1	12.3 ± 6.6	11.9 ± 3.8
	C	15.5 ± 5.0[c]	12.9 ± 6.5	9.5 ± 4.0[a,b]
Fat mass (kg)	S	5.1 ± 2.1	6.3 ± 3.8	5.9 ± 1.9
	C	7.1 ± 5.4[c]	7.0 ± 3.9	5.5 ± 2.6
Fat-free mass (kg)	S	33.0 ± 3.6	49.6 ± 12.1[a]	47.8 ± 11.7[a]
	C	29.1 ± 8.7[c]	38.4 ± 14.1[a,c]	51.8 ± 7.5[a,b]
$\dot{V}O_{2peak}$ (L·min^{-1})	S	2.62 ± 0.52	2.73 ± 0.47	3.00 ± 0.87
	C	1.38 ± 0.42[c]	2.46 ± 0.75[a]	3.02 ± 0.52[a,b]

[a]Significant maturation effect compared with Group I; $p < 0.05$; [b]Significant maturation effect compared with Group II, $p < 0.05$; [c]Significant group effect compared with swimmers; $p < 0.05$; S = swimmers; C = controls.

Table 34.2 Blood biochemical values (mean $\pm$ SD) of the subject groups

		Group I (9 pairs)	Group II (11 pairs)	Group III (8 pairs)
Ghrelin (pg·mL^{-1})	S	1230.8 ± 386.0	1126.8 ± 406.0	1105.5 ± 337.5
	C	1272.7 ± 424.4	868.3 ± 411.2[a,c]	850.8 ± 306.0[a,c]
Leptin (ng·mL^{-1})	S	1.7 ± 0.7	1.4 ± 0.8[a]	1.1 ± 0.4[a,b]
	C	2.3 ± 1.1[c]	2.0 ± 0.6[a]	1.2 ± 0.9[a,b]
Testosterone (nmol·mL^{-1})	S	2.4 ± 1.2	6.4 ± 3.7[a]	13.2 ± 6.7[a,b]
	C	1.5 ± 1.3[c]	9.3 ± 6.9[a]	18.8 ± 3.3[a,b,c]
IGF-I (μg·mL^{-1})	S	275.9 ± 85.7	244.5 ± 141.2	306.9 ± 128.3[b]
	C	189.3 ± 68.4[c]	307.7 ± 176.9[a]	431.3 ± 90.7[a,b,c]
IGFBP-3 (mg·mL^{-1})	S	5.4 ± 0.7	4.7 ± 0.5	5.4 ± 1.0
	C	4.2 ± 0.7[c]	5.1 ± 0.6[a]	5.8 ± 0.7[a,b]

[a]Significant maturation effect compared with Group I; $p < 0.05$; [b]Significant maturation effect compared with Group II, $p < 0.05$; [c]Significant group effect compared with swimmers; $p < 0.05$; S = swimmers; C = controls.

according to pubertal development in all boys. However, the increases in testosterone and IGF-1 were lower in swimmers compared to the controls and swimmers had also significantly lower testosterone and IGF-1 levels in group III compared to the controls (Table 34.2).

Ghrelin was significantly correlated with $\dot{V}O_{2peak}$ in the control ($r = -0.530$; $p < 0.05$), but not in the swimmers group. In the control group, plasma ghrelin concentrations were significantly correlated with body mass, BMI, fat mass and fat free mass ($r =$ from -0.43 to -0.59). Grehlin was significantly related to testosterone, IGF-1 and IGFBP-3 ($r =$ from -0.49 to -0.65) in controls. No significant relationships were observed in the swimmers group between ghrelin and other biochemical parameters.

Discussion

Fasting plasma ghrelin concentrations were significantly decreased at the onset of puberty in physically inactive healthy boys, while no changes in fasting plasma ghrelin concentration were observed in physically active boys throughout puberty. This demonstrates that regular physical activity may have an influence on ghrelin concentration during puberty in boys.

A decrease in plasma ghrelin concentration during puberty has been previously reported (Haqq *et al.*, 2003; Whatmore *et al.*, 2003). However, Bellone *et al.* (2002) showed no relationship between ghrelin and pubertal status in boys. Ghrelin is known to stimulate appetite and it is well known that appetite and food intake are increased during puberty. However, this increased appetite and food intake in puberty is not associated with an increase, but with a decrease in plasma ghrelin levels in healthy, but physically inactive boys (Haqq *et al.*, 2003; Whatmore *et al.*, 2003). It is proposed that there could be an increased sensitivity for appetite stimulation by ghrelin over puberty (Whatmore *et al.*, 2003). Our study showed that regular physical activity is associated with higher plasma ghrelin levels, perhaps to stimulate appetite and food intake to cover the higher energy expenditure.

It was interesting to find that in the swimmers' group there were no significant correlations between ghrelin and anthropometric and metabolic parameters, except fat-free mass ($r = -0.51$). Therefore, physical activity may attenuate the ghrelin relationships to these selected parameters.

References

Bellone, S., Rapa, A., Vivenza, D., Castellino, N., Petri, A., Bellone, J., Me, E., Broglio, F., Prodam, F., Ghigo, E. and Bona, G., 2002, Circulating ghrelin levels as function of gender, pubertal status and adiposity in childhood. *Journal of Endocrinology Investigation*, **5**, pp. 13–15.

Haqq, A., Farooqi, I., O'Rahilly, S., Stadler, D., Rosenfeld, R., Pratt, K., LaFranchi, S. and Purnell, J., 2003, Serum ghrelin levels are inversely correlated with body mass index, age, and insulin concentrations in normal children and are markedly increased in Prader-Willi Syndrome. *Journal of Clinical Endocrinology and Metabolism*, **88**, pp. 174–178.

Kojima, M., Hosoda, H., Date, Y., Nakazato, M., Matsuo, H. and Kangawa, K., 1999, Ghrelin is a growth-hormone-releasing acylated peptide from stomach. *Nature*, **402**, pp. 656–660.

Whatmore, A., Hall, C., Jones, J., Westwood, M. and Clayton, P., 2003, Ghrelin concentrations in healthy children and adolescents. *Clinical Endocrinology*, **59**, pp. 649–654.

Yilmatz, D., Ersoy, B., Bilgin, E., Gümüser, G., Onur, E, and Pinar, E., 2005, Bone mineral density in girls and boys at different pubertal stages: Relation with gonadal steroids, bone formation markers, and growth parameters. *Journal of Bone Mineral Metabolism*, **23**, pp. 476–482.

35 The relationship between exercise-induced changes in stress hormones and immune responses

R.G. McMurray,[1] F. Zaldivar,[2] A. Eliakim,[2] D. Nemet[2] and D.M. Cooper[2]
[1]Department of Exercise and Sport Science, University of North Carolina, Chapel Hill, NC; [2]Pediatric Exercise Research Center, University of California, Irvine, CA, USA

Introduction

During strenuous exercise in adults several of the cytokines and inflammatory cells increase, with increases in leukocytes and IL-6 preceding the other cells (Ostrowski et al., 1999). These changes in immune cells are proposed to be related to increases in the catecholamines (Steensberg et al., 2001; Ortega et al., 2005). Also, the exercise-induced increase in IL-6 is hypothesized to cause elevations of cortisol and cortisol causes the elevations of circulating leukocytes (Steensberg et al., 2003). Strenuous exercise has consistently increased growth hormone (hGH) in both adults (Zaldivar et al., 2006) and children (Eliakim et al., 2006). Further, the increase in hGH has been linked to increases in neutrophils (Zaldivar et al., 2006). The exercise-induced increase of hGH appears to be related to the andrenergic response to exercise (Vettor et al., 1997; Eliakim et al., 2006). Thus, in adults there appear to be relationships between the exercise-induced inflammatory responses and the stress hormone responses (Kappell et al., 1991b; Gabriel et al., 1992; Pedersen et al., 1997). These relationships have not been examined systematically in youth; thus, the purpose of this study was to examine these relationships in youth.

Methods

Subjects were 38, 7–17 y; 19 of each sex. They were recruited from the community. Informed assent was obtained and consent was obtained from parents before participation. The study was approved by the University of California at Irvine Institutional Review Board. All trials were completed at the General Clinical Research Center at the University of California-Irvine Medical Center.

Each participant completed two exercise trials on separate days. During the first trial participants completed a progressive exercise test on a cycle ergometer to determine her/his peak oxygen uptake, peak power output, and anaerobic threshold (McMurray *et al.*, 2007). Breath-by-breath gas exchange was obtained from a Sensor Medics metabolic system. The anaerobic threshold was estimated from gas exchange.

During this second trial the participants completed ten, 2 min bouts of high-intensity exercise at 50 per cent above their anaerobic threshold, with 1 min rest between bouts. Pre-, immediate post-exercise, and 2 h post-exercise blood samples were obtained from an indwelling venous catheter. Two-hour post samples were used to evaluate the potential of a delayed response. During the 2 h recovery period the subjects remained in the laboratory and completed quiet activities. The blood samples were immediately cold-centrifuged and the serum decanted and frozen at −80°C for later analysis. Whole blood was analyzed for leukocytes and lymphocyte subsets using standard clinical haematological techniques (Zaldivar *et al.*, 2006). Catecholamine concentrations were measured using a radio-enzymatic technique (Kennedy and Ziegler, 1990), cortisol was determined by commercial RIA kit (Diagnostic Products, Los Angeles, CA), and hGH was determined by ELISA kit (Diagnostics System Laboratories, Webster, TX). The cytokines, IL-1B, IL-6, TNF-α were measured using commercially available ELISA kits (R&D Systems, Minneapolis, MN).

Results

The characteristics of the participants can be found in Table 35.1. The youth ranged from a BMI of 14.5 to 49.1 kg m^{-2} (6th to 99th percentile); with a mean of 25.14 ± 7.67. Mean peak aerobic power was low; somewhat related to their large sizes. All subjects completed the exercise protocol.

Exercise significantly increased the catecholamines and growth hormone ($p = 0.0001$), but not cortisol ($p > 0.582$). The increase in both the catecholamines and hGH returned to baseline 2 h post exercise. Exercise increased all leukocyte subsets ($p < 0.01$) except CD4 and CD8 cells. Two hours post exercise the neutrophil count remained elevated, while the majority of other leukocyte subsets had returned to baseline or were below baseline (CD4 and CD8 cells). Of the three cytokines, only IL-6 increased with exercise and remained elevated two hours post exercise ($p < 0.01$). Neither IL-1B nor TNF-α were significantly changed with exercise.

Table 35.1 Mean (±SD and ranges) characteristics of the 38 participants

Characteristic	Mean ± SD	Range
Age (y)	12.3 ± 2.6	7 – 17
Stature (cm)	155 ± 15	114 – 178
Body mass (kg)	62.2 ± 24.9	18.9 – 139.4
BMI	25.1 ± 7.7	14.5 – 49.1
BMI percentile	77.0 ± 28.7	6.1 – 99.8
$\dot{V}O_{2peak}$ (mL·kg^{-1}·min^{-1})	26.9 ± 7.8	14.2 – 41.1

Table 35.2 Resting, immediate post and 2-hour post concentrations of the leukocytes and cytokines

Marker	Baseline	Immediate post exercise	Two hour post exercise
Total WBC (cells·μL^{-1})	6963 ± 2069	9318 ± 2526*	8469 ± 2380*
Neutrophils (cells·μL^{-1})	3816 ± 1349	5003 ± 1698*	5132 ± 1677*
Monocyte (cells·μL^{-1})	425 ± 140	631 ± 236*	489 ± 202
Lymphocytes (cells·μL^{-1})	2483 ± 696	3459 ± 1437*	2592 ± 725
CD3 (cells·μL^{-1})	664 ± 479	2175 ± 860*	1804 ± 550
CD4 (cells·μL^{-1})	917 ± 284	728 ± 314*	720 ± 270*
CD8 (cells·μL^{-1})	613 ± 234	534 ± 282	460 ± 186*
CD19 (cells·μL^{-1})	426 ± 240	517 ± 276*	485 ± 229
CD1656 (cells·μL^{-1})	318 ± 154	653 ± 478*	226 ± 106
IL-1B (pg·mL^{-1})	0.17 ± 0.16	0.16 ± 0.14	0.16 ± 0.14
IL-6 (pg·mL^{-1})	2.80 ± 4.19	3.18 ± 4.36*	3.71 ± 4.03*
TNF-α (pg·mL^{-1})	2.19 ± 1.50	2.22 ± 1.39	2.07 ± 1.34
Norepinephrine (pg·mL^{-1})	287 ± 103	650 ± 373*	372 ± 237
Epinephrine (pg·mL^{-1})	28 ± 20	56 ± 40	25 ± 18
Dopamine (pg·mL^{-1})	18 ± 11	29 ± 19*	19 ± 13
Cortisol (μU·mL^{-1})	9.6 ± 5.1	10.0 ± 4.8	6.0 ± 2.7*
Growth hormone (ng·mL^{-1})	0.3 ± 0.6	6.2 ± 5.3*	0.1 ± 0.2

*$p < 0.05$ versus rest.

The exercise-induced increases in the catecholamines were moderately, but significantly ($p < 0.05$) associated with exercise-induced increases in monocytes, the majority of lymphocyte subsets, and IL-6 (Table 35.3). No significant correlations were found between the exercise-induced changes in hGH or cortisol and any of the leukocyte subsets or cytokine responses ($p > 0.31$). In addition, the exercise-induced changes in the stress hormones were not significantly associated with any two-hour post exercise changes in leukocytes or cytokines ($r \sim 0.26$ to -0.28).

Discussion

The results of this study suggest that the catecholamines may have a role in the exercise-induced responses of leukocytes and IL-6. However, the lack of significant relationships between the immune responses and either cortisol or hGH suggest that in youth, neither hormone has a significant impact on the immune responses to acute, high intensity exercise. Similar catecholamine responses to exercise have been reported in adults (Gabriel et al., 1992; Steensberg et al., 2001; Kohut et al., 2005; Ortega et al., 2005); thus, our results suggest that the exercise-induced immuno-reactance of adults is already present in children.

Cortisol did not significantly increase with the exercise; yet an immuno-reactance was evident; suggesting that cortisol is not needed to facilitate the

Table 35.3 Spearman correlations between the exercise-induced changes in stress hormones and the inflammatory markers immediate post exercise

Marker	Epinephrine	Norepinephrine	Dopamine	Cortisol	hGH
Total WBC	0.209	0.244	0.091	0.170	0.170
Neutrophil	0.075	0.163	0.077	0.307	0.189
Monocytes	0.421*	0.471*	0.143	0.162	0.220
Lymphocytes	0.470*	0.369*	0.321*	0.072	0.147
CD3	0.464*	0.332*	0.362*	0.060	0.147
CD4	0.269	0.256	0.333*	0.042	0.085
CD8	0.409*	0.474*	0.409*	0.044	0.024
CD19	0.366*	0.245	0.229	0.071	0.068
CD1656	0.479*	0.562*	0.388*	0.075	0.153
IL-1β	0.202	0.092	0.234	0.056	0.221
IL-6	0.274	0.321*	0.422*	0.121	0.166
TNF-α	0.219	0.313	0.174	0.288	0.116

*$p < 0.05$.

immune response to high intensity exercise in children. Kohut *et al.* (2005) has suggested that cortisol may be needed to sustain the immune response, but the catecholamines mediate the acute response. Our results agree. Steensberg *et al.* (2003) have suggested that the exercise-induced increase of IL-6 stimulates a rise in cortisol. An exercise-induced increase in IL-6 was evident in our subject, but no elevation in cortisol was noted. Further, IL-6 remained elevated 2 h post exercise; concomitantly, cortisol levels declined below baseline. These results suggest that, in youth, the exercise-induced cortisol response may be independent of IL-6.

Growth hormone has been linked to increases in neutrophils in adults (Kappel *et al.*, 1991a; Pedersen *et al.*, 1997; Zaldivar *et al.*, 2006). We found no such relationship in children. Although hGH increased with exercise and the majority of leukocyte subtypes increased, the magnitude of the increases were dissimilar: the mean hGH increase was 1900 per cent versus increases of 30–180 per cent for the leukocytes. Studies have suggested that hGH increases are associated with the catecholamines (Felsing *et al.*, 1992; Eliakim *et al.*, 2006). We found a significant relationship between the exercise-induced epinephrine and hGH response ($r = 0.348$); thus supporting these previous studies. However, no relationship between the magnitude of the hGH response and any measured immune response was evident. Thus the possibility exists that the catecholamines remain the initiator of the exercise-induced leukocytosis, while the hGH response is simply a simultaneous occurrence (Kappel *et al.*, 1991a).

Age influenced both the hormonal and immune responses to exercise. A posteriori, we correlated the age of the child with the magnitude of hormonal and immune responses and found significant and direct correlations ranging from $r = 0.26$ for neutrophils and IL-6 to $r = 0.631$ for CD1656 cells. Thus, young children appear to have less immune and hormonal responses to the exercise, which could potentially confound studies of exercise immunology.

Such relationships suggest that when evaluating exercise-induced hormonal and immune responses, a narrow age range of subjects should be obtained, or at least, the analyses adjusted for age. This is a limitation of the present study. Intriguingly, the correlations between age and exercise-induced change in hGH was not significant ($r = 0.039$); suggesting an independence of its action.

In conclusion, the results of this study suggest that in children the catecholamines may mediate the acute immune responses to high-intensity exercise. Further the magnitude of this effect appears to increase as the youth age. The results also suggest that in children cortisol does not have significant influence on the immediate post, or 2 h post exercise leukocytosis, as well as the responses of IL-1B, IL-6, and TNF-α. Furthermore, in children exercise-induced increases in IL-6 do not appear to cause a cortisol response. Although the hGH response to exercise was related to the catecholamines, the elevated hGH was not associated with the immune response to high-intensity exercise and, as such, may not have a major role in the immune response. Therefore the relationship between the stress hormones and the immune responses to exercise is not as apparent as in adults.

References

Eliakim, A., Nemet, D., Zaldivar, F., McMurray, R.G., Culler, F.L., Galissetti, P. and Cooper, D.M., 2006, Reduced exercise-associated response of the GH-IGF-1 axis and catecholamines in obese children and adolescents. *Journal of Applied Physiology*, **100**, pp. 1630–1637.

Felsing, N.E., Brasel, J. and Cooper, D.M., 1992, Effect of low- and high-intensity exercise on circulating growth hormone in men. *Journal of Clinical Endocrinology and Metabolism*, **15**, pp. 157–162.

Gabriel, H., Urhausen, A. and Kindermann, W., 1992, Mobilization of circulating leucocytes and lymphocyte subpopulations during and after short, anaerobic exercise. *European Journal of Applied Physiology*, **65**, pp. 164–170.

Kappel, M., Hansen, M.B., Diamant, M., Jorgensen, J.O., Gyhrs, A. and Pedersen, B.K., 1991a, Effects of an acute bolus growth hormone infusion of on the human immune system. *Hormone and Metabolism Research*, **25**, pp. 579–585.

Kappell, M., Tvede, N., Galbo, H., Haahr, P.M., Kjaer, M., Linstow, M., Klarlund, K. and Pedersen, P.K., 1991b, Evidence that the effect of physical exercise on NK cell activity is mediated by epinephrine. *Journal of Applied Physiology*, **70**, pp. 2530–2534.

Kennedy, B., and Ziegler, M.G., 1990, A more sensitive and specific radio-enzymatic assay for catecholamines. *Life Science*, **47**, pp. 2143–2153.

Kohut, M.L., Martin, A.E., Senchina, D.S. and Lee, W., 2005, Glucocorticoids produced during exercise may be necessary for optimal virus-induced IL-2 and cell proliferation wheras catecholamines and glucocorticoids may be required for adequate immune defense to viral inflection. *Brain Behavior and Immunology*, **19**, pp. 423–435.

McMurray, R.G., Zaldivar, F., Galassetti, P., Larson, J., Eliakim, A., Nemet, D. and Cooper, D.M., 2007, Cellular immunity and inflammatory mediator responses to intense exercise in overweight children and adolescents. *Journal of Investigative Medicine*, **55**, pp. 120–129.

Ortega, E., Marchena, J.M., Garcia, J.J., Barriga, C. and Rodriguez, A.B., 2005, Norepinephrine as mediator in the stimulation of phagocytosis induced by moderate exercise. *European Journal of Applied Physiology*. **93**, pp. 714–718.

Ostrowski, K., Rohde, T., Asp, S., Schjerling, P. and Pedersen, B.K., 1999, Pro- and anti-inflammatory cytokine balance during strenuous exercise in humans. *Journal of Physiology (London)*, **515**, pp. 287–291.

Pedersen, B.K., Bruunsgaard, H., Klokker, M., Kappel, M., Maclean, D.A., Nielsen, H.B., Rohde, T., Ullum, H. and Zacho, M., 1997, Exercise-induced immunomodulation – Possible roles of neuroendocrince and metabolic factors. *International Journal of Sports Medicine*, **18** (suppl 1), pp. 52–57.

Steensberg, A., Toft, A.D., Schjerling, P., Halkjaer-Kristensen, J. and Pedersen, B.K., 2001, Plasma interleukin-6 during strenuous exercise: Role of epinephrine. *American Journal of Physiology: Cell Physiology*, **281**, pp. C1001–C1004.

Steensberg, A., Fischer, C.P., Keller, C., Moller, K. and Pedersen, B.K., 2003, IL-6 enhances plasma IL-1ra, IL-10, and cortisol in humans. *American Journal of Physiology: Endocrinology and Metabolism*, **285**, pp. E433–E437.

Vettor, R., Macor, C., Rossi, E., Picmonte, G. and Federspil, G., 1997, Impaired counterregulatory hormonal and metabolic responses to exhaustive exercise. *Acta Diabetologica*, **34**, pp. 61–66.

Zaldivar, F., Wang-Rodrigeuz, J., Nemet, D., Schwindt, C., Galassetti, P., Mills, P.J., Wilson, L.D. and Cooper, D.M., 2006, Constitutive pro- and anti-inflammatory cytokine and growth factor response to exercise in leukocytes. *Journal of Applied Physiology*, **100**, pp. 1124–1133.

36 Insulin resistance and cytokines in adolescence

Are weight status and exercise possible moderators?

D.A. Rubin,[1,2] R.G. McMurray,[2] J.S. Harrell,[2] A.C. Hackney,[2] D.E. Thorpe[2] and A.M. Haqq[3]

[1]California State University Fullerton, Fullerton, CA, USA;
[2]University of North Carolina at Chapel Hill, Chapel Hill, NC, USA;
[3]Duke University Medical Center, Durham, NC, USA

Introduction

Increased adiposity has been strongly associated with insulin resistance in youth (Roemmich *et al.*, 2002). Cytokines released by the adipose tissue, such as adiponectin, resistin, interleukin-6 (IL-6), and tumor necrosis factor-α (TNF-α), appear to link adiposity with insulin resistance in adults (Fernandez-Real and Ricart, 2003). While adiponectin has a negative association with insulin resistance, resistin, TNF-α, and IL-6 appear to have a positive association (Esposito *et al.*, 2003; Fernandez-Real and Ricart, 2003; Silha *et al.*, 2003). Similar relationships may be expected in youth (Huang *et al.*, 2004). Moreover, these relationships may be exacerbated in overweight youth because of the excess of adiposity (Moon *et al.*, 2004). Since these cytokines appear to respond to chronic and acute exercise (Nemet *et al.*, 2002; Esposito *et al.*, 2003), physical activity or aerobic power might modify the association between these cytokines and insulin resistance. This study determined if cytokines (adiponectin, resistin, IL-6 and TNF-α) associated with adiposity are also correlated with insulin resistance in adolescence, and if these relationships are modified by weight status, vigorous physical activity (VPA), or aerobic power.

Methods

Sixty girls and 60 boys who participated in the Cardiovascular Health in Children Study were randomly selected from sub-groups of 437 adolescents. Half of the selected adolescents were overweight (body mass index >95th percentile), and half had a normal weight (BMI<75th percentile) according to the norms by the Center for Disease Control year 2000. Half of the adolescents also reported ≥ 180 min·week^{-1} of habitual VPA (High-VPA) while the others reported ≤ 120 min·week^{-1} of habitual VPA (Low-VPA).

Physical measures (height and weight), habitual physical activity, pubertal status, a fasting blood sample, and aerobic power were obtained in the school setting. Pubertal developmental stage (Tanner stages 1–5) was estimated using a self-administered validated survey. Habitual VPA was obtained from a validated physical activity survey containing 32 activities specific to youth in North Carolina, USA. Predicted maximal aerobic power was determined from a cycle-ergometer test. All these procedures have been described elsewhere (McMurray *et al.*, 2002). Plasma insulin concentrations were determined by Linco Laboratories (St. Charles, MO). Plasma adiponectin and resistin were assayed utilizing kits from Linco Research Inc. (St. Charles, MO). Plasma TNF-α and IL-6 concentrations were assayed utilizing kits from R & D Systems (Minneapolis, MN). Insulin resistance (IR) was determined using the Homeostatic Model Assessment (HOMA) for insulin resistance proposed by Turner *et al.* (1979).

Mean and standard deviation values were computed for all variables for all subjects in the study by sex and ethnic group. To determine if the cytokines were associated with insulin resistance, multiple regression models were computed for each cytokine controlling for gender using the enter method. The models included the cytokine and either weight status (normal weight vs overweight), levels of VPA (High vs Low) or aerobic power. Those parameters that were significant in preliminary models were used to test a final model. The cytokines and the HOMA were transformed logarithmically to conduct the regression analyses. Statistical significance was set at $p < 0.05$.

Results

Subjects' demographic, physical, and metabolic characteristics are presented in Table 36.1. Racial distribution was 57 per cent African-American, 37 per cent Caucasian, and 6 per cent other races. The pubertal status of the adolescents ranged from early (Tanner stage 2) to mid-late puberty (Tanner stages 3 and 4).

Adiponectin ($R^2 = 0.280, p < 0.001$), and TNF-α ($R^2 = 0.054, p = 0.016$) were associated with IR. In contrast, IL-6 was not related to IR ($R^2 = 0.055, p = 0.054$).

Table 36.1 Subject demographic, physical, and metabolic characteristics

	Girls	*Boys*
Age (years)	12.0 ± 1.0	12.0 ± 1.0
BMI (kg·m^{-2})	23.9 ± 7.4	23.2 ± 7.0
VPA (sessions·wk^{-1})	10.0 ± 8.0	12.0 ± 9.0
Aerobic power (mL·kg^{-1}·min^{-1})	33.6 ± 10.0	38.3 ± 11.5
Adiponectin (ng·mL^{-1})	10.47 ± 5.53	9.68 ± 4.17
Resistin (ng·mL^{-1})	10.76 ± 5.61	10.76 ± 4.63
TNF-α (pg·mL^{-1})	1.53 ± 1.2	1.71 ± 1.09
IL-6 (pg·mL^{-1})	1.74 ± 1.83	1.54 ± 1.84
HOMA	4.5 ± 3.5	3.5 ± 3.3

Resistin was associated with IR only in the boys ($R^2 = 0.069, p = 0.024$). Weight status interacted in the association between adiponectin and IR ($p < 0.05$ for interaction term of weight status and adiponectin) but did not interact with any other association. VPA interacted only in the association between IR and resistin ($p < 0.05$), but aerobic power did not interact with any associations between the cytokines and IR. Both TNF-α ($p > 0.05$) and resistin ($p > 0.05$) were not associated with IR if weight status was included in the regression models for these cytokines. VPA was independently related to IR in the regression model for resistin ($p < 0.05$), and aerobic power was independently related to IR in the regression models for adiponectin and TNF-α ($p < 0.05$).

Discussion

As others have previously shown (Huang *et al.*, 2004), higher adiponectin concentrations were associated with lower IR. This association was more evident in overweight than in normal weight adolescents. Perhaps in normal weight adolescents, since the concentrations of adiponectin and other cytokines associated with IR were normal, the protective role of adiponectin was minimal.

This was the first study to support a relationship between resistin and IR in youth. Although Gerber *et al.* (2005) failed to show this association, Silha *et al.* (2003) showed similar results in adults to our findings in youth. We suggest that IR is weakly associated with resistin in adolescents, maybe due to the association between body fat and resistin.

The present study also supports the positive association between TNF-α and IR found in adults (Fernandez-Real and Ricart, 2003) and in overweight youth (Moon *et al.*, 2004). Since when weight status was considered in the multiple regression models, TNF-α did not explain a significant variance in IR, our findings suggest that adiposity may also mediate this association. Because the IR variance explained by either resistin or TNF-α was small, it is possible that these associations become stronger as youth age and adiposity levels increase.

Unlike the other three cytokines, IL-6 concentrations were not associated with IR. Results by others suggest that IL-6 concentrations are associated with increased adiposity (Weiss *et al.*, 2004), but not with IR. Therefore, our findings further confirm this concept. In this study, low VPA and aerobic power were significant predictors of IR in youth as has been shown before (Rubin *et al.*, 2008). We hypothesized that both factors would modify the associations between the cytokines and IR based on positive changes induced in the cytokines by physical activity or exercise training observed in adults and youth (Balagopal *et al.*, 2005; Esposito *et al.*, 2003). Although VPA and aerobic power were associated with IR, the results do not support a role for VPA or aerobic power as moderators of the relationship between IR and the cytokines. Perhaps the changes observed in cytokines and IR due to exercise training or increased physical activity are independent from each other.

Main limitations of this study were the use of a survey to determine VPA and the use of HOMA to indicate IR. A more sensitive measure of IR might have strengthened the relationships between the cytokines and IR. In summary, in youth as in adults, select cytokines are associated with IR. Increased adiposity appears to link this association. Increased physical activity of vigorous intensity and cardiovascular fitness are associated with lower IR but do not moderate the associations between the cytokines and IR.

Acknowledgement

This study was supported by NINR R01837 (DAR, JSH) and NIH K23 RR021979 (AMH).

References

Balagopal, P., George, D., Patton, N., Yarandi, H., Roberts, W., Bayne, E. and Gidding, S., 2005, Lifestyle-only intervention attenuates the inflammatory state associated with obesity: A randomized controlled study in adolescents. *Journal of Pediatrics*, **146**, pp. 342–348.

Esposito, K., Pontillo, A., Di Palo, C., Giugliano, G., Masella, M., Marfella, R. and Giugliano, D., 2003, Effect of weight loss and lifestyle changes on vascular inflammatory markers in obese women. *Journal of the American Medical Association*, **289**, pp. 1799–1804.

Fernandez-Real, J. and Ricart, W., 2003, Insulin resistance and chronic cardiovascular inflammatory syndrome. *Endocrine Reviews*, **24**, pp. 278–301.

Gerber, M., Boettner, A., Seidel, B., Lammert, A., Bar, J., Schuster, E., Thiery, J., Kiess, W. and Kratzsch, J., 2005, Serum resistin levels of obese and lean children and adolescents: Biochemical analysis and clinical relevance. *Journal of Clinical Endocrinology and Metabolism*, **90**, pp. 4503–4509.

Huang, K., Lue, B., Yen, R., Shen, C., Ho, S., Tai, T. and Yang, W., 2004, Plasma adiponectin levels and metabolic factors in non-diabetic adolescents. *Obesity Research*, **12**, pp. 119–224.

McMurray, R.G., Harrell, J.S., Bangdiwala, S.I., Bradley, C.B., Deng, S. and Levine, A., 2002, A school-based intervention can reduce body fat and blood pressure in young adolescents. *Journal of Adolescent Health*, **31**, pp.125–132.

Moon, Y., Kim, D. and Song, D., 2004, Serum tumor necrosis factor-alpha levels and components of the metabolic syndrome in obese adolescents. *Metabolism*, **53**, pp. 863–867.

Nemet, D., Oh, Y., Kim, H., Hill, M. and Cooper, D., 2002, Effect of intense exercise on inflammatory cytokines and growth mediators in adolescent boys. *Pediatrics*, **110**, pp. 681–689.

Roemmich, J.N., Clark, P., Lusk, M. and Friel, A., 2002, Pubertal alterations in growth and body composition. Pubertal insulin resistance: relationship to adiposity, body fat distribution and hormone release. *International Journal of Obesity*, **26**, pp. 701–709.

Rubin, D.A., McMurray, R.G. and Harrell, J.S., 2008, Insulin resistance and weight status in adolescents: Independent effects of intensity of physical activity and peak aerobic power. *Pediatric Exercise Science*, **20**, pp. 29–39.

Silha, J., Krsek, M., Skrha, J.V., Sucharda, P., Nyomba, B. and Murphy, L., 2003, Plasma resistin, adiponectin and leptin levels in lean and obese subjects: Correlations with insulin resistance. *European Journal of Endocrinology*, **149**, pp. 331–335.

Turner, R., Holman, R., Matthews, D., Hockaday, T.D. and Peto, J., 1979, Insulin deficiency and insulin resistance interaction in diabetes: Estimation of their relative contribution by feedback analysis from basal insulin and glucose concentrations. *Metabolism*, **28**, pp. 1086–1096.

Weiss, R., Dziura, J., Burgert, T., Tamborlane, W., Taksali, S., Yeckel, C. and Allen K., 2004, Obesity and metabolic syndrome in children and adolescents. *New England Journal of Medicine*, **350**, pp. 2362–2374.

37 Serum leptin but not adiponectin changes during a 12-week community-based diet and exercise intervention programme

J. Slinger, E. van Breda, J. Brouns and H. Kuipers

Department of Movement Sciences, Maastricht University, Maastricht, The Netherlands.

Introduction

The prevalence of overweight and obesity in children and adolescents has been increasing worldwide (Kosti and Panagiotakos, 2008). It has been shown that overweight leads to an augmented risk of health problems such as insulin resistance, impaired aerobic capacity, and disturbed hormonal levels, such as leptin and adiponectin (Ebbeling *et al.*, 2002). These adipokines have been suggested to be intermediate factors between overweight and health problems (Hung *et al.*, 2006).

In order to counteract the detrimental health effects of the upcoming pandemic of obesity, numerous weight management programmes for overweight adults and adolescents have been developed (Summerbell *et al.*, 2003). In the present study a community based lifestyle programme (Realfit) was evaluated. Realfit is a 12-week programme designed for overweight adolescents. The programme focuses on weight loss and sports participation and aims to assist adolescents in developing a healthier lifestyle. Until now it is unknown whether such a programme can manipulate the overweight associated health problems and the suggested intermediate factors. Therefore, the aim of this study was to evaluate the effects of a community-based lifestyle intervention programme (Realfit) on body composition, insulin resistance and serum leptin and adiponectin concentrations.

Methods

Study population and design

Thirty-two overweight (BMI = 29.2 ± 4.1 kg·m^{-2}) adolescents (age 12–18 y) were included in the study. Before (T0), immediately after the 12 week intervention period (T1), and 20 weeks after ending the intervention (T2) body composition as well as serum leptin and adiponectin concentrations were measured. Realfit is a 12-week intervention programme, which aims to stimulate a healthy lifestyle. The programme consists of 12 varied sports lessons, seven individual consultations (one intake, five consultations, and one closing session) with a dietician, three group sessions with the dietician and three group sessions for parents with the dietician and a pedagogue.

All subjects were informed about the nature and risks of the study beforehand and gave their written informed consent to participate. The study was approved by the local medical ethical committee (Maastricht).

Anthropometry

To calculate the body mass index (BMI), height and body weight (BW) were determined bare footed in light clothes.

Aerobic capacity

Aerobic fitness was assessed using the Åstrand-Rhyming test. The maximal oxygen uptake was estimated from a nomogram (5) based on sex, workload, and mean steady-state heart rate during exercise. A correction factor for age was used, and maximum oxygen uptake was expressed in $mL \cdot kg^{-1} \cdot min^{-1}$.

Leptin and adiponectin concentration and insulin resistance

After an overnight fast, blood was collected from a forearm vein in serum tubes. Serum leptin and adiponectin concentrations were measured with a double-antibody, sandwich-type, enzyme-linked immunosorbent assay that used a monoclonal antibody specific for human leptin (DSL, Webster, TX, USA) or adiponectin (Mediagnost, Reutlingen, Germany), respectively. Fasted glucose and insulin levels has been used to calculate Insulin Resistance using the HOMA-index.

Statistical analysis

Results are shown as means ($\pm$SD). Differences between the three measurements (T0, T1, T2) were calculated with the General Linear Model (GLM) approach for repeated measures. GLM with a between subjects component was used to test differences in the changes in leptin and adiponectin between the subgroup who increased and the subgroup who decreased BMI during the programme. For all tests $p < 0.05$ was considered statistically significant.

Results

In the total group there were no significant changes in leptin or adiponectin concentration, HOMA-IR or $\dot{V}O_2$ max, whereas the BMI decreased significantly during the intervention (Table 37.1). Twenty-five of the participants decreased their BMI during Realfit whereas in seven of them the BMI increased.

Table 37.1 BMI, HOMA-IR, $\dot{V}O_2$max, leptin and adiponectin concentration in the total group

	T0 (n = 32)	T1 (n = 32)	T2 (n = 32)	p
BMI (kg·m^{-2})	29.2 (4.1)	28.3 (4.4)	28.9 (4.7)	0.016^{T0-T1}
HOMA insulin resistance	3.9 (1.5)	3.5 (1.9)	3.5 (1.9)	0.321
$\dot{V}O_2$max (mL·kg^{-1}·min^{-1})	30.8 (8.3)	33.7 (8.7)	32.4 (10.7)	0.055
Leptin (µg·L^{-1})	89.0 (44.2)	83.2 (49.1)	83.3 (53.3)	0.590
Adiponectin (mg·L^{-1})	8.5 (3.3)	9.3 (3.5)	8.6 (3.6)	0.256

Table 37.2 HOMA-IR, $\dot{V}O_2$max, leptin and adiponectin concentration in BMI(+) and BMI(−) group

	BMI	T0	T1	T2	p-value for interaction
HOMA insulin	+	32.1 (4.5)	32.4 (4.5)	33.4 (3.9)	0.081
resistance	−	28.4 (3.7)	27.2 (3.8)	27.6 (4.0)	
HOMA insulin	+	4.2 (2.0)	4.8 (2.0)	3.7 (1.2)	0.032^{T0-T1}
resistance	−	3.7 (1.2)	2.9 (1.2)	3.4 (1.9)	
$\dot{V}O_2$max	+	2.3 (0.6)	2.5 (1.2)	2.1 (0.8)	0.129
(mL·kg^{-1}·min^{-1})	−	2.6 (0.8)	2.7 (0.9)	2.7 (0.8)	
Leptin (µg·L^{-1})	+	121.2 (45.4)	137.4 (36.8)	134.7 (45.4)	0.013$^{T0-T1\&T1-T2}$
	−	75.8 (37.4)	62.2 (36.3)	64.3 (43.1)	
Adiponectin	+	7.8 (1.4)	8.0 (1.3)	8.0 (2.0)	0.605
(mg·L^{-1})	−	8.8 (3.8)	9.8 (4.1)	8.9 (4.2)	

In 25 successful (subjects BMI declined during the intervention period), leptin concentration ($p = 0.013$) and HOMA-IR ($p = 0.032$) decreased significantly compared to the unsuccessful subjects ($N = 7$) between T0 and T1. There was no significant difference in the development of $\dot{V}O_2$ max ($p = 0.129$) and adiponectin concentration ($p = 0.605$) (T0–T1). Between T1 and T2 the difference in leptin and BMI changes in both groups was reversed (Table 37.2).

Discussion

The current study showed that in the total group of participants of a 12-week community-based diet and exercise intervention programme, significant decreases in BMI, but not leptin and adiponectin, could be shown. The overall results of the Realfit programme are in line with the results of other short-term weight management programmes. For instance, Eliakim *et al.* (2002) reported similar decreases in BMI and body weight using a slightly different 12-week programme.

It has to be mentioned that the succesful group started with a lower body weight and fat percentage, and subsequently a lower leptin concentration. In this successful group it was shown that in the short-term their leptin concentration decreased significantly in comparison to the unsuccessful group. Although adiponectin is another hormone that is produced by the fat mass, no significant changes were observed. As leptin is considered to be an intermediate factor for obesity related health problems, a decrease in leptin concentration may decrease changes in insulin resistance. This is supported by the significant decrease in HOMA-IR in the group of successful participants. Five months after the end of the programme BMI, leptin concentration and HOMA-IR reversed towards baseline values. Such a regain in weight after an intervention is not uncommon and is referred to as weight cycling. It emphasizes the importance of long-term follow-up supervision.

The current data showed that a population based programme like Realfit was able to decrease leptin concentration and insulin resistance of the successful participants in the short term. These findings suggest a possible association between leptin and insulin resistance in overweight individuals. Although the short-term improvements in insulin resistance and leptin concentration in successful participants were promising, in the future more emphasis should be placed on the long-term results of intervention programmes.

References

Åstrand, P.O. and Rodahl, K., 2003, *Textbook of Work Physiology*, 4th edn. Champaign, IL: Human Kinetics.

Ebbeling, C.B., Pawlak, D.B. and Ludwig, D.S., 2002, Childhood obesity: Public-health crisis, common sense cure. *Lancet*, **360**, pp. 473–482.

Eliakim, A., Kaven, G., Berger, I., Friedland, O., Wolach, B. and Nemet, D., 2002, The effect of a combined intervention on body mass index and fitness in obese children and adolescents – A clinical experience. *European Journal of Pediatrics*, **161**, pp. 449–454.

Hung, Y.J., Chu, N.F., Wang, S.C., Hsieh, C.H., He, C.T., Lee, C.H. and Fan, S.C., 2006, Correlation of plasma leptin and adiponectin with insulin sensitivity and beta-cell function in children – The Taipei Children Heart Study. *International Journal Clinical Practice*, **60**, pp. 1582–1587.

Kosti, R.I. and Panagiotakos, D.B., 2006, The epidemic of obesity in children and adolescents in the world. *Central European Journal Public Health*, **14**, pp. 151–159.

Summerbell, C.D., Ashton, V., Campbell, K.J., Edmunds, L., Kelly, S. and Waters, E., 2003, Interventions for treating obesity in children. *Cochrane Database Systematic Reviews*, CD001872.

Part V
Elite young athletes

38 Physical training in children with osteogenesis imperfecta

A randomized clinical trial

M. *van Brussel*,[1] T. *Takken*,[1] C.S.P.M. *Uiterwaal*,[2] H.J. *Pruijs*,[3] J. *van der Net*,[1] P.J.M. *Helders*[1] *and* R.H.H. *Engelbert*[1]

[1]Department of Pediatric Physical Therapy and Exercise Physiology; [2]Julius Centre for Health Sciences and Primary Care; [3]Department of Orthopedics Surgery, Wilhelmina Children's Hospital, University Medical Center Utrecht, Utrecht, The Netherlands.

Introduction

Osteogenesis Imperfecta (OI) is a congenital connective tissue disorder characterized by increased bone fragility and osteopenia. The biochemical basis in most cases involves a quantitative abnormality, qualitative abnormality, or both in the biosynthesis of type I collagen, the principal organic component of the skeleton (Sillence, 1994). Severity varies in a wide range, reaching from intrauterine fractures and perinatal lethality to very mild forms with incidental fractures (Plotkin *et al.*, 2003). Children with mild and moderate forms of OI are in general walkers, varying from household to community walkers (Engelbert *et al.*, 2000). Among these children, fatigue, diminished exercise capacity and exercise intolerance is a frequently reported limitation in their activities of daily living (Engelbert *et al.*, 2004). Takken *et al.* (2004) studied cardiopulmonary function in 17 children with OI type I. They found that heart and lung abnormalities in rest were absent. However, they also reported that exercise capacity and muscle force were significantly lower when compared to healthy peers. Complaints of fatigue were related to proximal muscle weakness and a reduced peak oxygen uptake ($\dot{V}O_{2peak}$). It was unclear whether the reduced $\dot{V}O_{2peak}$ and muscle force were a consequence of a hypoactive lifestyle or a specific consequence of the impaired muscle collagen synthesis. Takken *et al.* (2004) suggested that a physical intervention study in patients with OI might improve exercise capacity and muscle force. To our knowledge, no physical intervention studies have been performed in children with OI. Exercise might have no effect on the disease itself, but possibly may improve the performance level of activities of daily living, self-esteem, and fitness in many of these children. Therefore, we designed a randomized controlled trial to study the effects of a physical training programme on exercise capacity, muscle force, and subjective fatigue in patients with the mild to moderate forms of OI.

Methods

In this study 34 children with OI type I or IV were randomly assigned to either a 12-week graded exercise programme or care as usual. Exercise capacity and muscle force were measured as primary outcome measures; subjective fatigue, perceived competence, and health-related quality of life were secondary outcomes. Exercise capacity was determined by maximal exercise tests using an electronically broked cycle ergometer and a calibrated respiratory gas analysis system (Cortex Metamax B^3). Muscle force was measured with a hand-held dynamometer (Citec) in four muscle groups. Fatigue was measured with the subscale subjective fatigue of the self-report questionnaire Checklist Individual Strength-20 (CIS-20). The perceived competence and health-related quality of life were measured by the Self-perception Profile for Children (CBSK) and the child health questionnaire Parent-Form 50 (CHQ), respectively. The effects of the intervention were analyzed by using linear regression statistics with a group indicator as independent variable and the outcome variables as dependent separate variables. All outcomes were measured at baseline ($T = 0$), after intervention ($T = 1$), and after six and nine months ($T = 2$ and $T = 3$, respectively).

Results

Table 38.1 shows that after intervention ($T = 1$), $\dot{V}O_{2peak}$, relative $\dot{V}O_{2peak}$ ($\dot{V}O_{2peak/kg}$), peak working capacity (W_{peak}), and muscle force were significantly ($p < 0.05$) improved in the children of the intervention group (17, 18, 10 and 12 per cent, respectively) compared with the children of the control group. Subjective fatigue decreased also among the children of the intervention group ($p < 0.05$). Follow-up at $T = 2$ showed a significant ($p < 0.05$) decrease of the improvements measured at $T = 1$ of $\dot{V}O_{2peak}$, but $\dot{V}O_{2peak/kg}$, W_{max}, and subjective fatigue showed no significant difference between the two groups. At $T=3$, we found a further decrease of the gained improvements.

Discussion

In this study, a significant improvement in peak oxygen uptake and muscle force was found after three months of training in children with OI. However, the effects decreased with time after the intervention was stopped. The same pattern was also found for subjective fatigue. This clinically relevant improvement in $\dot{V}O_{2peak}$ is greater than reported in healthy children, who after a comparable training period (Payne *et al.*, 1993) in general improved approximately eight per cent in $\dot{V}O_{2peak/kg}$. These large improvements can be explained by the lower initial levels of $\dot{V}O_{2peak}$ of children with OI (Takken *et al.*, 2004). Although the intervention consisted only of low-resistance strength training, there was a 12 per cent improvement in muscle force in the children in the intervention group during the training period. Comparable studies have shown improvements in muscle force between five and 40 per cent (Faigenbaum *et al.*, 1999).

Table 38.1 $\dot{V}O_{2peak}$, $\dot{V}O_{2peak}/kg$, muscle strength during the intervention and follow-up regression coefficients are presented in bold when p-value is lower than 0.05

		Intervention group Mean (SD)	Control group Mean (SD)	Mean group difference (95% confidence interval)	Mean group difference (95% confidence interval) adjusted for baseline (T = 0) value
$\dot{V}O_{2peak}$ (L·min⁻¹)	T = 0	1.25 (0.4)	1.50 (0.6)	0.25 (−0.1; 0.6)	
	T = 1	1.49 (0.4)	1.54 (0.6)	0.05 (−0.3; 0.4)	**−0.19 (−0.3; −0.1)**
	T = 2	1.41 (0.4)	1.59 (0.6)	0.18 (−0.2; 0.5)	−0.06 (−0.2; 0.1)
	T = 3	1.42 (0.4)	1.64 (0.7)	0.21 (−0.2; 0.6)	−0.05 (−0.2; 0.1)
$\dot{V}O_{2peak}/kg$ (mL·kg⁻¹·min⁻¹)	T = 0	30.9 (5.8)	35.6 (10.4)	4.7 (−1.3; 10.7)	
	T = 1	36.4 (6.4)	35.5 (10.2)	−0.9 (−7.0; 5.3)	**−5.1 (−8.0; −2.2)**
	T = 2	33.8 (6.8)	36.3 (11.1)	2.5 (−4.2; 9.1)	−1.6 (−6.0; 2.9)
	T = 3	33.7 (9.3)	37.1 (12.0)	3.4 (−4.2; 11.0)	−1.5 (−6.1; 3.2)
W_{peak}	T = 0	107.3 (39.0)	128.6 (61.0)	21.3 (−15.3; 57.9)	
	T = 1	122.7 (42.1)	134.0 (63.0)	11.3 (−27.0; 49.6)	**−10.3 (−20.0; −0.5)**
	T = 2	117.6 (39.4)	135.3 (63.4)	17.7 (−20.1; 55.4)	−3.6 (−13.0; 5.8)
	T = 3	114.9 (45.1)	135.6 (73.0)	20.7 (−22.7; 64.1)	−2.5 (20.2; 15.1)
Muscle force (Newton)	T = 0	537.8 (183.7)	589.3 (187.7)	51.5 (−80.3; 183.4)	
	T = 1	602.7 (182.6)	590.5 (184.5)	−12.2 (−142.6; 118.2)	**−61.4 (−96.7; −26.2)**
	T = 2	616.2 (169.8)	657.9 (196.6)	36.3 (−94.5; 167.1)	−5.2 (−53.0; 42.5)
	T = 3	621.3 (202.0)	680.1 (205.0)	58.8 (−85.8; 203.4)	6.5 (−49.7; 62.8)

Differences between our study results and other studies might be explained by the use of very low resistance. However, we think that the improvement in muscle force is clinically relevant for patients with OI since muscle force and the strength of bones are strongly associated (Schoenau, 2006). In our study, the children were not able to maintain the gained training effects three and six months (T = 2 and T = 3, respectively) after the completion of the intervention programme. Elucidating the effects of detraining (reversibility) on children is confounded by the child's continued growth and development during the detraining period. As in adults, it seems that adaptations to training are transient and will steadily decay once training has stopped (Lee, 1993). This decay is also seen in this study. A long-term benefit might depend on the continuation of training sessions into adult life (Lee, 1993). Many of the included patients were not involved in regular exercise with sufficient intensity. Patients might avoid these exercises because of the risk of fractures or environmental concerns such as neighbourhood safety (Weir *et al.*, 2006). This study indicates that children with mild to moderate OI can participate safely and benefit from a supervised and individual tailored training programme. Future studies should focus on the perceived barriers of these children to participate in physical exercise in their own neighbourhood or in school, on children with OI type IV and III who are wheelchair-bound, and when unsupervised training can be as safe and effective as the current training regimen. To maintain the improvement in exercise capacity and muscle force, the exercise regimen needs to be continued. For some of our secondary outcome measures, we did not find any improvements during training or follow-up (CHQ, CBSK). In conclusion, individual supervised training can be advised as a safe and beneficial addition to current treatment methods in the short term. The long-term efficacy of this intervention requires further evaluation.

References

Engelbert, R.H., Uiterwaal, C.S., Gerver, W.J., van der Net, J.J., Pruijs, H.E. and Helders, P.J., 2004, Osteogenesis imperfecta in childhood: Impairment and disability. A prospective study with 4-year follow-up. *Archives of Physical Medicine and Rehabilitation*, **85**, pp. 772–778.

Engelbert, R.H., Uiterwaal, C.S., Gulmans, V.A., Pruijs, H. and Helders, P.J., 2000, Osteogenesis imperfecta in childhood: Prognosis for walking. *Journal of Pediatrics*, **137**, pp. 397–402.

Faigenbaum, A.D., Westcott, W.L., Loud, R.L. and Long, C., 1999, The effects of different resistance training protocols on muscular strength and endurance development in children. *Pediatrics*, **104**, p. e5.

Lee, M., 1993. *Coaching Children in Sport; Principles and Practice*. Cambridge: F&N Spon.

Payne, V.G. and Morrow, J.R. Jr., 1993, Exercise and VO_2 max in children: A meta-analysis. *Research Quarterly of Exercise and Sport*, **64**, pp. 305–313.

Plotkin, H., Primorac, D. and Rowe, D., 2003, Osteogenesis imperfecta. In: *Pediatric Bone*, edited by Glorieux, F.H., Pettifor, J., Jeuppner, H. San Diego: Academic Press, pp. 443–471.

Schoenau, E., 2006. Bone mass increase in puberty: What makes it happen? *Hormones Research*, **65** (Suppl 2), pp. 2–10.

Sillence, D.O., 1994, Craniocervical abnormalities in osteogenesis imperfecta: Genetic and molecular correlation. *Pediatric Radiology*, **24**, pp. 427–430.

Takken, T., Terlingen, H.C., Helders, P.J., Pruijs, H., Van der Ent, C.K. and Engelbert, R.H., 2004. Cardiopulmonary fitness and muscle strength in patients with osteogenesis imperfecta type I. *Journal of Pediatrics*, **145**, pp. 813–818.

Weir, L.A., Etelson, D. and Brand, D.A., 2006, Parents' perceptions of neighborhood safety and children's physical activity. *Preventive Medicine*, **43**, pp. 212–217.

39 Multidimensional analysis of drop-out in youth basketball

Two-year follow-up among Portuguese initiates

C.E. Gonçalves, A. Figueiredo and M.J. Coelho e Silva
University of Coimbra, Portugal

Introduction

Drop-out is a major concern in youth sports. Classical studies (Gould *et al.*, 1981; Ewing and Seefeldt, 1995) adopted empirical inventories of reasons to explain drop-out. Previous studies also estimated an incidence ranging from 17–39 per cent among youth Portuguese male basketball players. Most studies approach drop-out issues from a point of view extrinsic to the training process. The understanding of a complex behaviour such as discontinuing from sport, requires a biocultural approach and a follow-up design. Practices and competitions represent the sport experience for children and adolescents and a field of social comparison. Motor competence is easily assessed by adults and peers, both in practices and in games. The accuracy of this assessment, that needs to be translated as relevant information to the young player, depends upon the specific knowledge and the communication skills of significant others.

In the age range 12–14 y, the coach is the main provider of information and he can be seen by the athlete as a source of support or of pressure and stress. It is also the period when the pubertal process begins and leaves its mark in the bodies and the minds of the youngsters. At the same time, it is the start of the sport specialization phase when, in basketball, the transition from the child-type games to the adult-like competitions occurs. Hence, the players want to show competent motor skills and are expected to perform at a higher level. In the core of the maturity process, many coaches do not pay the necessary attention to the athlete's sources of stress and are not able to manage the complex issues of their needs for satisfaction, skill level, maturity status, and the possibility of drop-out.

Therefore, reliable information is needed for youth sport coaches in order to improve the global quality of training and to prevent the occurence of drop-out. The study of the variables that can lead to drop-out is complex and it has to be approached from the point of view of different sciences, in order to reveal the critical factors that can influence the decision to discontinue the sport. Although many studies have been carried out on this theme, few of them have a design that integrates the contributions of various disciplines such as anthropometry, physiology or psychology.

The purpose of this 2 y longitudinal study is to describe the variables that can predict drop-out during the transition from initiates (12–13 y) to juveniles (14–15 y) among Portuguese basketball players.

Methods

The sample consisted of 84 male competitive basketball players with a chronological age of 13.0 ± 0.6 y, measured in 2003. In 2005 32 (38 per cent) of the original sample discontinued basketball participation, according to Basketball Association data.

Somatic characteristics included body weight, stature and sum of four skinfolds. Functional capacities were assessed through the counter movement vertical jump, squat-jump, 60 s sit-ups, hand grip strength, 2 kg ball throw, and 20 m shuttle run. Four basketball specific skills (shooting, dribbling, passing and defensive slide) were also considered, according to Kirkendall *et al.* (1987). In addition, athletes completed the *Portuguese Version of Task and Ego in Sport Questionnaire –TEOSQp* (Fonseca, 1999). After comparing players who continued participating for at least two seasons (2004 and 2005) with those who dropped out, discriminant function analysis was used to predict group membership.

Results

Players who continued their sport careers were heavier ($p \le 0.05$), fatter ($p \le 0.05$), attained poorer performances in the counter movement jump ($p \le 0.05$) and reached better scores in all manipulative skills (shooting, $p \le 0.01$; passing, $p \le 0.01$; dribbing, $p \le 0.05$), as shown in Table 39.1. Height, hand grip strength, 20 m shuttle run, 2 kg ball throw or defensive slalom did not reveal significant differences between the two groups.

The correlations between variables and standardized canonical discriminant function (Table 39.2) present shooting, counter movement jump, sum of skinfolds and weight as the variables with greater magnitude.

Discussion

Based on shooting, counter movement, sit-ups and body mass, it was possible to accurately predict 73 per cent of subjects according to their sport status [rc = 0.50, Wilks' lambda = 0.753, chi-squared (4) = 22.094, $p \le 0.01$]. The superior performance of drop-outs in countermovement jump suggests that jump power can be determined by other factors than anthropometric characteristics.

Canonical coefficients are relevant over 0.30 (Tabachnik and Fidell, 2001). It was not expected that muscle power (jumps) contributes to predict drop-out occurence, as shown by the counter movement jump negative coefficient (Table 39.2). As expected, manipulative skills show a significant difference

Table 39.1 Baseline mean values and comparisons between subjects who still participate in organized basketball and those who dropped out

Variables	Units	Players (n = 52)	Drop-outs (n = 32)	t	p
Height	cm	160.9	158.7	1.022	0.31
Weight	kg	54.8	48.8	2.090	0.04
Sum of 4 skinfolds	mm	101	80	2.117	0.04
Vertical jump [SJ]	cm	25.2	26.4	−1.067	0.29
Counter movement jump [CMJ]	cm	29.0	31.8	−2.405	0.02
Sit-ups	—	41.2	38.7	1.756	0.08
Hand grip strength	kg	30.4	30.0	0.298	0.72
2 kg ball throw	m	5.23	5.11	0.447	0.66
20 m shuttle run	m	53.7	52.9	0.195	0.85
Shooting	—	26.9	22.8	2.775	0.01
Passing	—	87.5	81.0	2.759	0.01
Dribbling	seconds	17.54	18.48	−2.318	0.02
Defensive slalom	seconds	21.08	21.73	−1.407	0.16
Task orientation	—	4.32	4.29	0.253	0.80
Ego orientation	—	0.56	1.54	0.175	0.86

Table 39.2 Correlations between variables and standardized canonical discriminant function

Variables	Structure matrix
Shooting	0.54
Counter movement jump	−0.46
Sum of skinfolds	0.43
Weight	0.40
Passing	0.38
Sit-ups	0.34
Squat-jump	−0.29
Dribbling	0.28
2 kg ball throw	0.24
Stature	0.18
20 m shuttle run	−0.15
Hand grip strength	0.12
Defensive slalom	0.06
Ego orientatiom	−0.05
Task orientation	0.04

between groups, but not the defensive slalom that does not require special coordinative abilities. At a level when for young athletes it is very important to exhibit motor competence, the poorer results in basketball fundamentals can explain an avoidance of performance by drop-outs. Surprisingly, height does not differentiate the groups. In a sport where stature is considered vital for better performances, it could be expected that those who continue to participate in sport would be taller than the drop-outs. This finding suggests that at this stage of competition, better performance does not correlate with bigger stature, with specific skills still playing a decisive role.

The variables weight and sum of skinfolds, as well as sit-ups, suggest that in a sport where physical contact in movements with and without the ball is a key factor for gaining ball possesion, the heavier players have a clear advantage. The maturity status represents probably the main reason for success at these ages, those advanced being the most physically ready for competition.

In summary, drop-out in basketball appears to be reasonably predicted by a small set of variables, including weight, strength and skill level. These findings contrast with sport selection that is based on stature (Coelho e Silva, 2002). It seems that sport organizations are not sophisticated in the selection of talented athletes, and that continuity or drop-out are complex processes. These findings have a clear importance for youth coaches and youth sport organizers, at all levels of competition, in order to promote a more balanced participation of youngsters, which includes satisfaction, well-being, prevention of injuries, and continuity in sport and more accurate sport selection. It is also of interest to note that achievement goal orientations failed to explain sport continuity, suggesting the need for new multidimensional approaches.

References

Coelho e Silva, M.J., 2002, Selecção desportiva: Análise prospectiva e retrospectiva. [Sport selection: Prospective and retrospective analysis]. In: *Tendências Actuais da Investigação em Basquetebol*, edited by Tavares, F., Janeira, M., Graça, A., Pinto, D. and Brandão, E. Porto: University of Porto, pp. 60–74.

Ewing, M.E. and Seefeldt, V., 1995, Patterns of participation and attrition in American agency-sponsored youth programs. In: *Children and Youth in Sport: A Biopsychosocial Perspective*, edited by Smoll, F. and Smith, R. Dubuque, IO: Brown & Benchmark, pp. 31–46.

Fonseca, A., 1999, Atribuições em contexto de actividade física ou desportiva – Perspectivas, relações e implicações. [Attributions in physical activity or sport context: Perspectives, relations, and implications]. PhD dissertation. University of Porto.

Gould, D., Feltz, D. and Weiss, M., 1981, Reasons for attrition in competitive youth swimming. *Journal of Sport Behavior*, **5,** pp. 155–165.

Kirkendal, D.R., Gruber, J.J. and Johnson, R.E., 1987, *Measurement and Evaluation for Physical Educators*. Champaign, IL: Human Kinetics.

Tabachnik, B. and Fidell, L., 2001, *Using Multivariate Statistics*. Needham Heights, MA: Allyn & Bacon.

40 Understanding participation among adolescent rugby union players

T.B. Hartwig,[1] *G. Naughton*[1] *and J. Carlson*[2]

[1]Australian Catholic University, School of Exercise Science, Centre of Physical Activity Across the Lifespan, Sydney, Australia; [2]Victoria University, Melbourne, Australia

Introduction

To facilitate optimal participation and performance in adolescent sport, coaches and sport scientists need to ensure appropriate load management. The training and game demands of some sports for adolescents are becoming increasingly more adult-like (Hollander, 1995). With a 'more is better' approach in some training programmes, detrimental effects on health, performance and participation are possible outcomes for adolescents (Polman and Houlahan, 2004). Consequently, there is a need to monitor young players' participation in sports to determine the most appropriate work loads. The overriding need is to ensure future participation and performance are not compromised (Smith, 2003).

Adolescents often participate in multiple team and individual sports simultaneously and incur intensive physical demands. The demands associated with participation in high-contact, high-intensity sports such as rugby union are currently poorly documented. There is a paucity of evidence-based strategies to monitor and determine appropriate participation loads.

Quantifying volume and intensity in team sports such as rugby union is challenging. However, advances in notational analysis technology such as global positioning satellite systems (GPS) and video analysis software systems permit an acceptable assessment of previously relatively imprecise estimates of training and game speeds, distances and intermittent movement intensities. Therefore, the purpose of this study was to use notational analyses and self-reporting to define the current level of physical demands during a typical rugby season, including training, competitive games and all other sport and physical activities in adolescent male rugby union players. An additional purpose was to define the variation in activity patterns for varying levels of participation.

Methods

Participants and research design

Seventy-five male rugby union players aged 14 to 18 years were recruited for the study. In addition to parental consent, players had to be free of injury and actively engaged in rugby training at the time of recruitment. Players were recruited from rugby teams representing three levels of rugby participation, (1) school boy, (2) national representative, and (3) a selective sports school's high-performance talent squad. Measures of volume and intensity of participation in rugby, as well as participation in other sport and physical activity, were estimated using Global positioning satellite (GPS) technology and heart rate monitoring, as well as subjective data on amounts and ratings of perceived exertion in training was recorded in weekly training diaries. Measures were taken twice a week for 12 weeks representing a full schoolboy competitive rugby season, for six weeks leading into the end of the representative rugby season, and for 10 weeks leading into the end of the selective high-performance squad rugby season.

Statistical treatment

One-way ANOVA analyses were used to compare differences among the three groups and, where appropriate, unadjusted Bonferroni post hoc analyses were used to locate and assess the magnitude of group differences. Significance was accepted at an alpha level of $p < 0.05$ for analyses.

Results

Rugby training

Schoolboy players covered (mean ± SD) 3511 ± 836 m per training session, representative squad players covered 3576 ± 956 m, and talent squad players covered 2208 ± 637 m. One-way ANOVA results showed differences between groups in average distance covered per session [F $(2, 158) = 43.96, p < 0.001$]. Unadjusted Bonferroni post hoc analysis showed the mean distance covered in talent squad sessions was less than the representative squad sessions ($p < 0.001$) and schoolboy sessions ($p < 0.001$). Mean distance covered during sessions was not different between the representative squad and schoolboy players ($p = 1.000$).

Weekly training

Weekly duration of sports and other physical activities in minutes per week and a breakdown of specific activities that comprise the weekly duration for each of the three groups are presented in Figure 40.1. Results of the one-way ANOVA analyses identified group differences [F $(2, 392) = 21.02, p < 0.001$] with the representative squad recording the highest weekly duration (515 ± 222 min $\cdot$ wk^{-1}) followed by

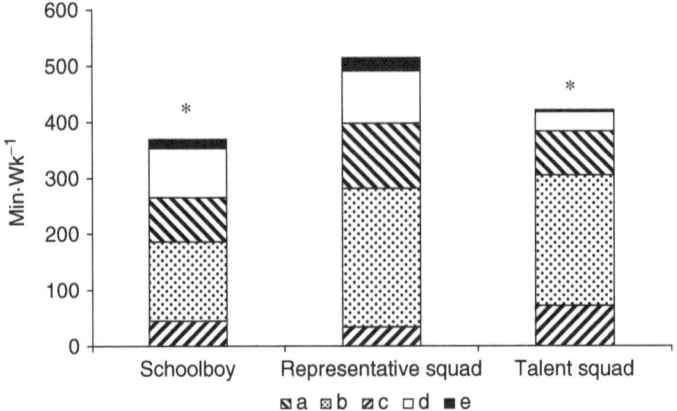

Figure 40.1 Mean total weekly duration and a breakdown of weekly activities in min wk^{-1} reported in training diaries. (*Significantly different from representative squad, $p < 0.001$. [a]Rugby game, [b]rugby training, [c]rugby related, [d]school/other organised, [e]recreational.)

the talent squad (421 ± 211 min·wk^{-1}) and schoolboy group (370 ± 135 min·wk^{-1}). Unadjusted Bonferroni post hoc analysis found that the weekly duration of activity of representative squad players' differed significantly from the talent squad players' ($p = 0.001$) and the schoolboy group ($p < 0.001$).

Diaries from individual players identified as group outliers for high training and game volumes showed participation in as many as three games and up to 11 training sessions per week. Profiles of selected 'highest load' players from each group revealed considerable weekly loading, with one player recording a weekly duration of 13.5 ± 5.5 hours comprising of three rugby games or as many as 11 rugby training sessions a week.

Discussion

Descriptions of the physical demands placed on adolescent rugby union players are lacking. Major findings on training profiles showed the discrepancies in distances travelled do not necessarily increase with the talent rating of players. Mean training distance of the talent squad was less than the other two teams but could have been more efficient in intensity demands. Profiles of weekly training found that mean weekly duration varied considerably among groups. Group means of weekly training duration provide potentially useful information, but can mask high-effort individual outliers.

Despite a lack of comparative data, the game and training demands of adolescent rugby union participation appear high. A major finding of this research is the notable differences within the same group of players, suggesting a strong need to monitor individuals to ensure training loads and activity types are appropriately managed. Defining optimum participation levels for adolescent rugby players remains a challenge. Maximizing athlete potential is often a major goal of participation in sports and physical activities. Links exist between voluminous training hours during the younger years and athletic success among elite netball, basketball and field hockey players (Baker *et al.*, 2003). Indeed, theories such as deliberate practice purport a direct relationship between hours engaged in deliberate practice, effortful, sport specific training, (Ericsson *et al.*, 1993) and the level of performance achieved (Helsen *et al.*, 1998). Despite purported benefits of such training approaches, there may be associated risks. Injury rates are reported as being relatively high among rugby union players (Bathgate *et al.*, 2002). Players with increased weekly training and game loads or periods of intensified participation are therefore at greater risk of injury. The possible outcomes of high volume, high intensity training is not confined to injury and could include potentially harmful consequences such as overtraining syndrome, sports burnout, increased susceptibility to illness, psychological disturbances, and performance decrements (Brenner, 2007).

The question of how ideal participation should be structured is yet to be answered. A better understanding of successful training loads is required to implement systematic planning of training prescription for adolescent athletes. A more informed approach will ideally maximize performance outcomes and minimize adverse effects such as fatigue, injury and overtraining.

Acknowledgements

We wish to acknowledge the support of the Australian Rugby Union and the New South Wales Sporting Injuries Committee.

References

Baker, J., Cote, J. and Abernethy, B., 2003, Sport-specific practice and the development of expert decision-making in team ball sports. *Journal of Applied Sport Psychology*, **15**, pp. 12–25.

Bathgate, A., Best, J.P., Craig, G., Jamieson, M. and Wiley, J.P., 2002, A prospective study of injuries to elite Australian rugby union players. *British Journal of Sports Medicine*, **36**, pp. 265–269.

Brenner, J.S., 2007, Overuse injuries, overtraining and burnout in child and adolescent athletes. (Clinical Report) *American Academy of Pediatrics*, www.pediatrics.org/cgi/doi/10.1542/peds.2007-0887

Ericsson, K.A., Krampe, R.T. and Tesch-Romer, C., 1993, The role of deliberate practice in the acquisition of expert performance. *Physiological Reviews*, **100**, pp. 363–406.

Helsen, W.F., Starkes, J.L. and Hodges, N.J., 1998, Team sports and the theory of deliberate practice. *Journal of Sport and Exercise Psychology*, **20**, pp. 12–34.

Hollander, D.B., Meyers, M.C. and LeUnes, A., 1995, Psychological factors associated with overtraining: Implications for youth sport coaches. *Journal of Sport Behavior*, **18**, pp. 3–20.

Polman, R. and Houlahan, K., 2004, A cumulative stress and training continuum model: A multidisciplinary approach to unexplained underperformance syndrome. *Research in Sports Medicine*, **12**, pp. 301–316.

Smith, D.J., 2003, A framework for understanding the training process leading to elite performance. *Sport Medicine*, **33**, pp. 1103–1126.

41 Intervertebral disc height, spinal curvature and low back pain in young rhythmic gymnasts

T. Kums,[1] *M. Pääsuke,*[1] *M. Leht*[2] *and A. Nurmiste*[3]
[1]Institute of Exercise Biology and Physiotherapy; [2]Department of Radiology, Tartu University Clinic, Estonia; [3]Tallinn Diagnostic Centre, Estonia

Introduction

Rhythmic gymnastics requires high hypermobility of the lumbar spine. Training in particular involves great concern about extreme positions and repetitive lumbar hyperextensions. Repetitive loading causes mostly an abnormality in the posterior elements of the spine. Low back pain is an extremely common complaint in competitive gymnasts and these athletes are at risk for multiple potential structural injuries to the spine. The true significance of early degenerative findings of the lumbar disc is not known (Harrison *et al.*, 2005). The purpose of the present study was to evaluate the effect of trunk posture on the disc height in thoracal and lumbar spine in gymnasts with and without low back pain (LBP), because the relationship between trunk posture and stresses acting on the intervertebral disc is not well understood.

Material and methods

Subjects

The subjects were 12 young rhythmic gymnasts aged 13–14 years. Gymnasts had been training for 5–6 years, 12–15 hours per week. Seven female rhythmic gymnasts with idiopathic LBP (with mean Oswestry index 19.8 per cent and mean ($\pm$SD) age of 13.3 ± 1.0 years, body mass of 37.02 ± 7.13 kg, height of 152.90 ± 8.15 cm, and body mass index (BMI) of 15.13 ± 2.35 kg·m^{-2}) were compared with five asymptomatic gymnasts (mean ($\pm$SD) age of 13.7 ± 0.6 years, body mass of 40.60 ± 6.75 kg, height of 158.60 ± 8.12 cm, BMI of 15.96 ± 1.73 kg·m^{-2}). The study was approved by the University of Tartu Ethics Committee.

Questionnaire

Idiopathic back pain score was determined in the subjects in accordance with the score of the Oswestry questionnaire. The Oswestry index covers 10 different areas of activities of daily living. These include pain intensity, personal care, lifting, walking, sitting, sleeping, social life, traveling and changing degree of pain (Cole *et al.*, 1994).

Spine curvature determination in the sagittal plane

Measurements were made from the lateral radiographs of 12 subjects clinically and radiographically. The technique used for the radiographs was to stand the subject in a relaxed position with the knees extended. The technique of using a digital level has already proven to be accurate and reproducible by Jackson *et al.* (1998). Cobb measurements of the thoracic kyphosis (TK) (T1–T12), the angle measured between the tangent lines along the vertebral body superior end plates of T1 and T12. The total segmental lumbar lordosis (LL) (L1–S1), the angle measured between the tangent lines along the vertebral body superior end plates of L1 and S1 (Gardocki *et al.*, 2002).

Anthropometric measurement

Body height of the subjects in standing and supine positions was measured using a Martin metal anthropometer with accuracy of ±0.5 mm. The difference in height in supine and standing positions (L, mm) was determined. The mean of three trials was calculated. This parameter characterizes indirectly the scope of deformation of the vertebral column in the sagittal profile and consequently is resilient. A higher value of L indicates better tolerance of impacts including stress on the musculoskeletal system (Vain and Kums, 2002).

Magnetic Resonance Imaging

All 12 girls were included in magnetic resonance imaging (MRI) studies. Each subject received a T1- and T2-weighted MRI scan of the spine. MRIs of the spine were acquired using a 1.5 T Siemens Symphony magnet (Siemens Medical Solutions, Erlangen, Germany). Sagittal T1- and T2-weighted images of the spine were obtained. Imaging parameters for the T1-weighted spin-echo sequence were: repetition time 500–600 ms, echo time 15 ms. The corresponding parameters for the T2-weighted turbo spin-echo sequence were 5000/122. MRI were analyzed by two experienced radiologists.

Measurements

The disc height was determined according to Frobin *et al.* (1997).

Statistics

Data are means and standard deviation (±SD). One-way analysis of variance (ANOVA) followed by Tukey post hoc comparisons were used to test for differences between groups. Pearson's correlation coefficients between measured parameters were also calculated. A level of $p < 0.05$ was selected to indicate statistical significance.

Results

There were no significant differences in age, height, body mass and BMI between measured groups. The spine angles of TK and LL were significantly lower ($p < 0.001$) in gymnasts with LBP in comparison with the asymptomatic gymnasts. In gymnasts with LBP, disc height in thoracal and lumbar spine was significantly lower ($p < 0.001$) than in the asymptomatic gymnasts. The difference in height in supine and standing position (L) was lower ($p < 0.05$) in LBP gymnasts than in the asymptomatic group. Oswestry questionnaire score form 19.8 per cent and this correlated significantly ($p < 0.05$) negatively with TK, LL and mean disc height in L1–S1 part ($r = -0.87, -0.86, -0.89$, respectively). A high positive correlation between mean lumbar L1–S1 disc height and L was observed in LBP gymnasts ($r = 0.96, p < 0.002, n = 7$).

Discussion

Clinically accepted radiographic values of thoracic kyphosis in growing children range from 20° to 40°, and lumbar lordosis from 20° to 45° (Willner and Johnson, 1983). The current study has shown that gymnasts with LBP had a more flattened spine in the thoracal and lumbar part. On the whole in asymptomatic gymnasts sport activity elicits the development of normal curves. These results are consistent with those of Tsai and Wredmark (1993), which showed that elite gymnasts had a flattened thoracic kyphosis. The majority of investigators, reported an association between larger degrees of kyphosis and lordosis and incidence of LBP (Ohlen *et al.*, 1989). In the present study it appeared that gymnasts with LBP have reduced disc height in the thoracic and lumbar spine in comparison with asymptomatic gymnasts. Oswestry questionnaire scores were high and negatively correlated with disc height in the lumbar spine ($r = -0.89, p < 0.017$) and with the angle of

Table 41.1 Mean (±SD) spinal curvature, disc height and anthropometric measurements in gymnasts with and without LBP

Parameter	Gymnasts with LBP (n = 7)	Gymnasts without LBP (n = 5)
TK(°)	17.7±3.1	33.5±7.9***
LL (°)	19.7±5.3	34.2±4.2***
T7–T12 (mm)	4.1±0.2	7.6±1.2***
L1–S1 (mm)	7.0±0.9	9.0±1.7***
L (mm)	4.0±1.7	16.7±6.6*

TK – thoracal kyphosis; LL – lumbar lordosis; T7–T12 – intervertebral disc morphology in thoracal and L1–S1 – lumbar part of the spine; L – the difference in height in supine and standing position. $p < 0.001$***, $p < 0.05$* compared to asymptomatic gymnasts.

the thoracic kyphosis, and lumbar lordosis ($r = -0.87$, $p < 0.024$; $r = -0.86$, $p < 0.028$, respectively). This indicates that gymnasts with more presented LBP have flattened spinal curvature in the thoracal and lumbar part and more reduced disc height in the lumbar part. These data suggest that the flattened posture decreases the elasticity of the vertebral column, and that the spine is stiff and prone to injuries, because only the normal lumbar spine is best suited to withstand compressive loads. Smaller height differences in the supine and standing position in gymnasts with LBP in comparison with asymptomatic gymnasts showed this in the present study. These height differences were positively correlated with lumbar disc height in gymnasts with LBP ($r = 0.96$, $p < 0.002$). Hypolordotic spine is smaller still. Flatback syndrome, a product of loss of lumbar lordosis, causes decreased spinal range of motion and loss of sagittal spinal balance, which places the erector spinae muscle group in a mechanically disadvantageous position (Gardocki *et al.*, 2002). In flat-back patients, the sagittal balance is generally displaced, well anterior to normal. Harrison *et al.* (2005) have indicated that anterior trunk translation (maintaining sagittal alignment of T1–T12 anterior to S1) in a standing subject increases extensor muscle activity and increases loads and stresses on the intervertebral disc in the lower thoracic and lumbar region. We presume that this causes disc height in the thoracal and particularly in the lumbar part of the spine to be much lower in gymnasts with LBP in our study. Most studies show that disc height and signal intensity have been used as indicators for disc degeneration (Luoma *et al.*, 2001). In our study T2-weighted signal intensity of the nucleus pulposus of disc in thoracal T7–T12 and lumbar L1–S1 part were measured. All gymnasts with idiopathic LBP showed the lowest disc height in the thoracal and lumbar part, but had highest signal intensity which did not differ from asymptomatic gymnasts. We conclude that disc degeneration was not presented in the T7–T12 region or in the lumbar spine in all investigated gymnasts. Disc height reduction in our study is not related to early degeneration, but is a result of functional overloading of the spine in gymnasts with LBP.

References

Cole, B., Finch, E., Gowland, C. and Mayo, N., 1994, Oswestry low back pain disability questionnaire. In: *Physical Rehabilitation Outcome Measures*, edited by Basmajian, J. Toronto, Canada Communication Group Publ., p. 90.

Frobin, W., Brinckmann, P., Biggemann., M., Tillotson, M. and Burton, K., 1997, Precision measurement of disc height, vertebral height and sagittal plane displacement from lateral radiographic views of the lumbar spine. *Clinical Biomechanics*, **12**, pp. S1–S64.

Gardocki, R.J., Watkins, R.G. and Williams, L.A., 2002, Measurements of lumbopelvic lordosis using the pelvic radius tehnique as it correlates with sagittal spinal balance and sacral translation. *Spine Journal*, **2**, pp. 421–429.

Harrison, D.E., Colloca, C.J., Harrison, D.D., Janik, T.J., Haas, J.W. and Keller, T.S., 2005, Anterior thoracic posture increases thoracolumbar disc loading. *Eur Spine Journal*, **14**, pp. 234–242.

Jackson, R.P., Peterson, M.D., McManus, A. and Hales, C., 1998, Compensatory spinopelvic balance over the hip axis and better reliability in measuring lordosis to the pelvic radius on standing lateral radiographs of adult volunteers and patients. *Spine*, **23**, pp. 1750–1767.

Luoma, K., Vehmas, T., Riihimaki, H. and Raininko, R., 2001, Disc height and signal intensity of the nucleus pulposus on magnetic resonance imaging as indicators of lumbar disc degeneration. *Spine*, **26**, pp. 680–686.

Ohlen, G., Wredmark, T. and Spangfort, E., 1989, Spinal sagittal configuration and mobility related to low-back pain in the female gymnast. *Spine*, **14**, pp. 847–850.

Tsai, L. and Wredmark, T., 1993, Spinal posture, sagittal mobility, and subjective rating of back probleme in former female elite gymnasts. *Spine*, **18**, pp. 872–875.

Vain, A. and Kums, T., 2002, Criteria for preventing overtraining of the musculoskeletal system of gymnasts. *Biology of Sport*, **19**, pp. 329–345.

Willner, S. and Johnson, B., 1983, Thoracic kyphosis and lumbar lordosis during the growth period in children. *Acta Paediatrica Scandinavica*, **72**, pp. 873–878.

42 Biomechanics and bioenergetics of front crawl swimming in young female swimmers

E. Lätt,[1] J. Jürimäe,[1] K. Haljaste,[1] A. Cicchella,[2] P. Purge[1] and T. Jürimäe[1]

[1]Institute of Sport Pedagogy and Coaching Sciences, Centre of Behavioural and Health Sciences, University of Tartu, Tartu, Estonia; [2]Faculty of Exercise and Sport Science, University of Bologna, Bologna, Italy

Introduction

Performance in swimming is related to different biomechanical, bioenergetical and anthropometrical parameters (Poujade et al., 2002; Zamparo et al., 2005). Different biomechanical studies have assessed the relationship of swimming performance with stroke rate and stroke length in swimmers (Poujade et al., 2002). However, Costill et al. (1985) chose stroke index (SI) as an indicator of swimming economy since it describes the ability of a swimmer to move at a given velocity with the fewest number of strokes. In any event, maximal performance in swimming is dependent on a number of factors, including body size, stroke efficiency and also on the amount of metabolic energy (Cs) spent in transporting the body mass of the athlete over the unit of swimming distance (Zamparo et al., 2005). However, very few investigations have studied the importance of different biomechanical, bioenergetical and anthropometrical characteristics to determine swimming performance in children (Poujade et al., 2002; Jürimäe et al., 2007). It is important to consider that changes from prepuberty to puberty are important and include different biomechanical, bioenergetical and anthropometrical characteristics that all determine swimming performance in children (Poujade et al., 2002). The purpose of this study was to examine the influence of energy cost of swimming, anthropometrical and technical parameters on swimming performance in prepubertal and pubertal female swimmers.

Methods

Twenty-six young swimmers, 14 prepubertal (11.1 ± 0.7 y; Tanner stages 1–2) and 12 pubertal (14.7 ± 1.6 y; Tanner stages 3–4) girls participated in the study. All swimmers had a training background of 3.5 ± 1.6 years and had trained for an average of 6.1 ± 1.8 hours/week for the last two years. The study was approved by the Medical Ethics Committee of the University of Tartu.

Initially, main anthropometric parameters, biological age, and $\dot{V}O_{2peak}$ on the bicycle ergometer were measured. Height (Martin metal anthropometer) and body mass (A&D Instruments, UK) of the participants were measured and body mass index (BMI) was calculated. Arm span was also measured (Jürimäe *et al.*, 2007). $\dot{V}O_{2peak}$ was measured on a bicycle ergometer (Tunturi T8, Finland) using portable open circuit system (MedGraphics $\dot{V}O_{200}$, St. Paul, MN, USA) (Jürimäe *et al.*, 2007). The second measurement session consisted of maximal 400 m front crawl swimming test in the 25 m pool, where the energy cost of swimming and stroking parameters were assessed (Jürimäe *et al.*, 2007). The backward extrapolation technique was used to evaluate $\dot{V}O_{2peak}$ during the test (Costill *et al.*, 1985). In addition, capillary blood samples were analysed enzymatically for blood lactate levels (Dr. Lange, Berlin, Germany) at the recovery time to find the net increase of blood lactate (ΔLa) (Zamparo *et al.*, 2005). The energy cost of swimming (Cs; kJ·m^{-1}) was calculated from the obtained $\dot{V}O_2$ and ΔLa values (Zamparo *et al.*, 2005). To exclude the influence of turning, the effective swimming speed (v; m·s^{-1}) maintained by each swimmer during the trial was measured over 15 m distance within two points from each end of the pool by a video camera (Sony DCR-TRV 130E, Japan). The video recording covered at least five stroke cycles for each trial. Average stroke rate (SR; cycles·min^{-1}) and the distance per stroke (SL; m·cycle^{-1}) were obtained (Jürimäe *et al.*, 2007). In addition, a stroke index (SI; m^{2}s^{-1}·cycles^{-1}) was calculated to gauge the economy of a swimmer's technique (Costill *et al.*, 1985). During the third measurement session, body composition parameters were measured by dual-energy X-ray absorptiometry using the DPX-IQ densitometer (Lunar Corp., Madison, USA) and analysed for fat (FM) and fat free (FFM) mass.

Statistical analysis was performed with SPSS 11.0 for Windows (Chicago, IL, USA). Means ($\pm$SD) were calculated. An unpaired, two-tailed t-test was used to assess differences between groups. Pearson product moment correlations were used to determine the degree of associations among selected variables. Regression analyses were used to evaluate the potential associations among selected variables. Significance was set at $p < 0.05$.

Results

Pubertal swimmers had significantly higher values ($p < 0.05$) for height, body mass, BMI, body fat percentage, FM, FFM and arm span than did prepubertal swimmers (Table 42.1). No differences ($p > 0.05$) were observed in body fat percentage values. Absolute $\dot{V}O_{2peak}$ measured on a bicycle ergometer was significantly higher in pubertal swimmers (3.26 ± 0.55 L min^{-1}) than in prepubertal swimmers (2.64 ± 0.60 L min^{-1}), but relative $\dot{V}O_{2peak}$ values were not different between groups (prepubertal: 60.3 ± 9.34 mL·kg^{-1}·min^{-1}; pubertal: 56.3 ± 7.38 mL·kg^{-1}·min^{-1}). Performance time, v, SL, SR, SI, Cs and ΔLa values were not different between the two groups, while $\dot{V}O_{2peak}$ values were higher in pubertal swimmers compared to prepubertal swimmers (Table 42.2). The results of

Table 42.1 Mean (±SD) anthropometrical and body composition parameters in prepubertal and pubertal female swimmers

Variable	Prepubertal (n = 14)	Pubertal (n = 12)	Total (n = 26)
Age (y)	11.1 ± 0.7	14.7 ± 1.6*	12.7 ± 2.2
Height (cm)	155.2 ± 8.1	167.6 ± 5.5*	160.9 ± 9.3
Body mass (kg)	43.0 ± 5.0	58.9 ± 4.0*	50.3 ± 9.2
BMI (kg·m^{-2})	17.9 ± 2.3	21.4 ± 2.3*	19.5 ± 2.9
Body fat%	19.3 ± 6.5	22.3 ± 4.3	20.7 ± 5.7
FM (kg)	8.0 ± 3.4	12.3 ± 2.9*	10.0 ± 3.8
FFM (kg)	32.8 ± 3.5	42.4 ± 3.4*	37.2 ± 6.0
Arm span (cm)	157.2 ± 4.8	171.8 ± 6.8*	163.9 ± 9.4
Tanner stage	1–2	3–4	2.3 ± 0.8

*Significantly different from prepubertal girls; $p < 0.05$.

Table 42.2 Mean (±SD) biomechanic and bioenergetic values obtained from the maximal 400 metre front crawl swim in prepubertal and pubertal female swimmers

Variable	Prepubertal (n = 14)	Pubertal (n = 12)	Total (n = 26)
Time (s)	385.6 ± 28.8	360.1 ± 46.2	373.9 ± 39.2
v (m·s^{-1})	1.02 ± 0.07	1.08 ± 0.13	1.05 ± 0.10
SL (m·cycle^{-1})	0.89 ± 0.08	0.98 ± 0.15	0.94 ± 0.12
SR (cycle·min^{-1})	68.8 ± 5.3	66.6 ± 5.2	67.8 ± 5.3
SI (m^2·s^{-1}·cycles^{-1})	0.92 ± 0.13	1.08 ± 0.27	0.99 ± 0.22
Cs (kJ·m^{-1})	1.38 ± 0.36	1.72 ± 0.51	1.55 ± 0.46
$\dot{V}O_2$ (L·min^{-1})	2.34 ± 0.41	2.93 ± 0.50*	2.61 ± 0.54
ΔLa (mmol·L^{-1})	3.5 ± 1.4	4.8 ± 2.4	4.2 ± 2.0

*Significantly different from prepubertal girls; $p < 0.05$.

the indirect measurement of $\dot{V}O_{2peak}$ in the whole group of studied swimmers were related to the $\dot{V}O_{2peak}$ results obtained on a cycle ergometer test in the laboratory ($R^2 = 0.679$; $p < 0.05$). Correlation analysis indicated that biological age, height, FFM and arm span values were related to stroking parameters (v, SL, SI) in young swimmers ($r > 0.44$; $p < 0.05$). Stroke rate was only related to arm span ($r = -0.41$; $p < 0.05$) from the measured anthropometric and body composition parameters. No relationships were observed between Cs, $\dot{V}O_{2peak}$ and ΔLa values for the maximal swimming test with the measured anthropometric and body composition values. In addition, Cs were not related to the studied stroking parameters. Stepwise regression analysis revealed that SI ($R^2 = 0.713$; $p < 0.05$), $\dot{V}O_{2peak}$ ($R^2 = 0.319$; $p < 0.05$) and FFM ($R^2 = 0.352$; $p < 0.05$) were the best predictors of swimming performance from measured stroking, bioenergetic and body composition parameters in studied young swimmers.

Discussion

Swimmers usually start with heavy training before the onset of puberty and achieve international competitive level at a relatively early age. This makes it necessary to study different parameters that may affect swimming performance in complex, taking into account various anthropometric/body composition, bioenergetical and biomechanical aspects of swimming already before puberty (Jürimäe *et al.*, 2007). Our previous study with prepubertal and pubertal boys demonstrated that biomechanical factors (i.e. SI) contributed most to swimming performance, followed by anthropometric/body composition (i.e. arm span) and bioenergetic (i.e. in-water measurement of $\dot{V}O_{2peak}$) factors (Jürimäe *et al.*, 2007). The same pattern was observed also in this study with prepubertal and pubertal female swimmers, where biomechanical factors (i.e. SI) characterized best 400 m front crawl swimming performance, followed by anthropometric/body composition (i.e. FFM) and bioenergetic (i.e. in-water measurement of $\dot{V}O_{2peak}$) values. These results demonstrate that it is very important to consider specific stroke technique parameters when predicting success of young swimmers already in the prepubertal years.

The backward extrapolation method of $\dot{V}O_{2peak}$ values recorded immediately after the 400 m maximal trial appeared to be a valid method and allowed the calculation of Cs in young female swimmers. It should be noted that the evaluation of Cs in young swimmers allows the estimation of energy expenditure during swimming training and could be used to evaluate the training load in young female swimmers (Poujade *et al.*, 2002).

In conclusion, the backward extrapolation method could be used to assess $\dot{V}O_{2peak}$ in young swimmers in sport specific conditions. Stroke index, FFM and $\dot{V}O_{2peak}$ are the major determinants of front crawl swimming performance in young female prepubertal and pubertal swimmers.

References

Costill, D.L., Kovaleski, J., Porter, D., Kirwan, J., Fielding, R. and King, D., 1985, Energy expenditure during front crawl swimming: Predicting success in middle-distance events. *International Journal of Sports Medicine*, **6**, pp. 266–270.

Jürimäe, J., Haljaste, K., Cicchella, A., Lätt, E., Purge, P., Leppik, A. and Jürimäe, T., 2007, Analysis of swimming performance from physical, physiological, and biomechanical parameters in young swimmers. *Pediatric Exercise Science*, **19**, pp. 70–82.

Poujade, B., Hautier, C.A. and Rouard, A., 2002, Determinants of the energy cost of front-crawl swimming in children. *European Journal of Applied Physiology*, **87**, pp. 1–6.

Zamparo, P., Bonifazi, M., Faina, M., Milan, A., Sardella, F., Schena, F. and Capelli, C., 2005, Energy cost of swimming of elite long-distance swimmers. *European Journal of Applied Physiology*, **94**, pp. 697–704.

Part VI

Aerobic and anaerobic fitness

43 Effect of training intensity on heart rate variability in prepubescent children

F.-X. Gamelin,[1] *G. Baquet,*[1] *S. Berthoin,*[1]
D. Thevenet,[2] *C. Nourry,*[1] *S. Nottin*[3] *and*
L. Bosquet[4]

[1]University of Lille 2; [2]University of Nantes; [3]University of Avignon;
[4]University of Montreal

Introduction

The measurement of heart rate variability (HRV) is a useful tool to quantify the activity of the autonomic nervous system on cardiovascular function in adults as well as in children (Task Force, 1996; Mandigout *et al.*, 2002). Low heart rate variability is considered as a general risk marker of several diseases in children (Massin and von Bernuth, 1998; Gutin *et al.*, 2000; Javorka *et al.*, 2005).

It is well established that endurance training is the main non-pharmacological means of increasing HRV in adults (Aubert *et al.*, 2003). Nevertheless, the literature on HRV in prepubescent children is poor and leads to inconsistent conclusions (Mandigout *et al.*, 2002; Triposkiadis *et al.*, 2002; Franks and Boutcher, 2003; Nagai *et al.*, 2004; Vinet *et al.*, 2005). Training intensity plays a major role in autonomic nervous adaptations and could be the explanation for the discrepancies in these studies.

Thus, the aim of this study was to compare the effects of seven weeks of either submaximal or supramaximal exercise training on autonomic cardiovascular control in prepubescent children, as measured by HRV.

Methods

Experimental design

Children (age: 9.3 ± 1.0 years) were randomly assigned to one of the three following groups: submaximal training (CT, $n = 18$) supramaximal training (IT, $n = 22$), and control (CON, $n = 16$). They performed an autonomic test to determine HRV and a graded running test to determine maximal aerobic velocity (MAV, the minimal velocity to attain maximal oxygen consumption) before and after a seven-week training period with three 30-minute sessions each week.

Training design

For seven weeks, children in CT and IT groups followed three 30 min running sessions per week. The training intensity was determined for each individual based his own MAV. The CT group trained at velocities ranging from 80–85 per cent of the MAV during exercise/recovery sequences lasting 4×6 min, 3×8 min, 2×10 min, 2×12 min, 1×15 min, 1×18 min, 1×20 min with 5 min of recovery between sets. Whereas, intermittent training consisted of short intermittent runs with exercise/recovery sequences lasting 5/15s, 10/10s, 15/10s, 20/20s and 30/30s. Intensities were set from 100–190 per cent of MAV.

Heart rate variability

They rested comfortably for 10 min in a supine position before a 5 min supine recording. No attempt was made to control breathing frequency or tidal volume. Intervals R–R (period between two consecutive beats) were measured continuously using a heart rate monitor (S810, Polar Electo Oy, Kempele, Finland).

HRV was performed on short-term recording in the time and frequency domains to determine the standard deviation of all NN intervals (SDNN), root mean square of differences of successive NN intervals (RMSSD), the power spectral density of the low frequency (LF; 0.04 to 0.15 Hz) and the high frequency (HF; 0.15 to 0.40 Hz) bands.

Statistical analysis

Standard statistical methods were used for the calculation of means and standard deviations. A logarithmic transformation was performed before the analysis when data were skewed or exhibited heteroscedasticity. A two-way analysis of variance (group by time) was used to evaluate the effect of training modality on HRV and other relevant parameters. Multiple comparisons were made with the Bonferroni post hoc test.

Results

MAV increased significantly in the CT and IT group (from 10.8 ± 1.1 to 11.8 ± 1.1 km·h^{-1} and from 11.3 ± 0.7 to 12.1 ± 0.7 km·h^{-1} respectively; $p < 0.05$).

Results are shown in Table 43.1.

Discussion

The aim of this study was to compare the effect of seven weeks of either supramaximal or submaximal training on the autonomic cardiovascular control of prepubescent children, as measured by HRV. The increase in MAV was not accompanied by significant autonomic gains.

Table 43.1 HRV spectral parameters (Mean RR: mean interval R–R; Standard deviation: SD; Root means square of successive differences; LF: low-frequency; HF: high-frequency) before and after seven weeks of submaximal (CT), supramaximal (IT) training and in the control group (CON). Values are mean ± SD

	CT		IT		CON	
	Before	After	Before	After	Before	After
Time domain						
Mean RR (ms)	801.7 ± 117.3	766.0 ± 102.4	753.3 ± 86.8	765.3 ± 76.5	756.3 ± 68.1	740.4 ± 80.7
SD (ms)	79.6 ± 35.1	92.3 ± 42.3	58.1 ± 20.4	58.4 ± 20.0	70.2 ± 33.9	61.9 ± 28.7
RMSSD (ms)	79.4 ± 37.4	101.3 ± 55.1	53.5 ± 26.3	54.2 ± 25.8	67.4 ± 32.8	61.5 ± 38.3
Frequency domain						
ln (LF+HF) (ms^2)	6.9 ± 0.9	7.1 ± 1.1	6.3 ± 0.8	6.2 ± 0.9	6.6 ± 0.9	6.3 ± 0.9
ln LF (ms^2)	6.2 ± 0.8	6.3 ± 1.0	5.5 ± 0.8	5.5 ± 0.7	5.7 ± 1.1	5.5 ± 0.8
ln HF (ms^2)	6.1 ± 1.0	6.4 ± 1.4	5.6 ± 1.1	5.4 ± 1.3	6.1 ± 0.8	5.7 ± 1.1

An explanation of this absence of results could be attributed to the training duration. In fact, in our study training duration was shorter than the study that showed a beneficial effect of training on HRV (Mandigout *et al.*, 2002).

Nevertheless, it seems that nervous autonomic control in prepubescent children is less sensitive to physical training than in adults, at least in relation to oxygen consumption adaptations (Baquet *et al.*, 2003).

Additional data with a longer training period are needed to study the effect of intensity on HRV.

References

Aubert, A.E., Seps, B. and Beckers, F., 2003, Heart rate variability in athletes. *Sports Medicine*, **33**, pp. 889–919.

Baquet, G., van Praagh, E. and Berthoin, S., 2003, Endurance training and aerobic fitness in young people. *Sports Medicine*, **33**, pp. 1127–1143.

Franks, P.W. and Boutcher, S.H., 2003, Cardiovascular response of trained preadolescent boys to mental challenge. *Medicine and Science in Sports and Exercise*, **35**, pp. 1429–1435.

Gutin, B., Barbeau, P., Litaker, M.S., Ferguson, M. and Owens, S., 2000, Heart rate variability in obese children: Relations to total body and visceral adiposity, and changes with physical training and detraining. *Obesity Research*, **8**, pp. 12–19.

Javorka, M., Javorkova, J., Tonhajzerova, I., Calkovska, A. and Javorka, K., 2005, Heart rate variability in young patients with diabetes mellitus and healthy subjects explored by Poincare and sequence plots. *Clinical and Physiological Function Imaging*, **25**, pp. 119–127.

Mandigout, S., Melin, A., Fauchier, L., N'Guyen, L.D., Courteix, D. and Obert, P., 2002, Physical training increases heart rate variability in healthy prepubertal children. *European Journal of Clinical Investigation*, **32**, pp. 479–487.

Massin, M. and von Bernuth, G., 1998, Clinical and haemodynamic correlates of heart rate variability in children with congenital heart disease. *European Journal of Pediatrics*, **157**, pp. 967–971.

Nagai, N., Hamada, T., Kimura, T. and Moritani, T., 2004, Moderate physical exercise increases cardiac autonomic nervous system activity in children with low heart rate variability. *Childs Nervous System*, **20**, pp. 209–214; discussion p. 215.

Task Force, 1996, Heart rate variability: Standards of measurement, physiological interpretation and clinical use. *Circulation*, **93**, pp. 1043–1065.

Triposkiadis, F., Ghiokas, S., Skoularigis, I., Kotsakis, A., Giannakoulis, I. and Thanopoulos, V., 2002, Cardiac adaptation to intensive training in prepubertal swimmers. *European Journal of Clinical Investigation*, **32**, pp. 16–23.

Vinet, A., Beck, L., Nottin, S. and Obert, P., 2005, Effect of intensive training on heart rate variability in prepubertal swimmers. *European Journal of Clinical Investigation*, **35**, pp. 610–614.

44 Reliability of physical activity and heart rate measures in children during steady rate and intermittent treadmill exercise

The A-CLASS project

L. Graves

Liverpool John Moores University, Liverpool, UK

Introduction

To help clarify the dose-response relationship between physical activity (PA) and health outcomes, a PA measurement tool must be valid and demonstrate adequate reliability (Wareham and Rennie, 1998). To date only one reported study has assessed the test-retest reliability of field-based PA monitors with participants (Rowlands *et al.*, 2007). In trained runners undergoing identical treadmill trials, ActiGraph accelerometer (GT1M, Fort Walton Beach, FL) reliability was high between 4–20 kph but RT3 triaxial accelerometer (Stayhealthy, Inc., Monrovia, CA) reliability was poor at midrange and high speeds (Rowlands *et al.*, 2007).

However, no information is currently available on the reliability of field-based monitors in children who may be less motor efficient, or between ecologically valid trials that attempt to simulate the intermittent, free-living activity patterns of children (Baquet *et al.*, 2007). The aim of this study was to assess the test-retest reliability of the Actiheart combined heart rate (HR) and movement sensor (Cambridge Neurotechnology, Cambridge, UK) and the GT1M ActiGraph accelerometer, in children during steady rate and intermittent exercise in controlled laboratory conditions.

Methods

Participants and settings

Three boys and seven girls (10.8 ± 0.2 years) from a primary school in a large urban city in North West England returned signed parental informed consent to participate in the present study. The school was located in a geographical area of high social and economic deprivation. Ethical approval was obtained from the university Ethics Committee.

Procedure

During a treadmill and monitor familiarisation session the maximum speed all children could run at for 30 s was established (10 km·h^{-1}) and informed the intensity of experimental trials. Over one night between familiarisation and the first experimental trial resting HR was assessed. Participants completed four non-randomly allocated experimental trials, each at least 48 hours apart. On visits one and two an intermittent trial was completed, which consisted of four repeated 30 s bouts of exercise interspersed with 15 s periods of rest, completed at four increasing intensities (4 km·h^{-1} 1 per cent incline, 4 km·h^{-1} 5 per cent incline, 7 km·h^{-1} 1 per cent incline, 10 km·h^{-1} 1 per cent incline). On visits three and four participants completed a continuous steady rate trial of 2.5 min exercise bouts at four increasing intensities (3.2 km·h^{-1} 1 per cent incline, 3.2 km·h^{-1} 5 per cent incline, 5.6 km·h^{-1} 1 per cent incline, 8 km·h^{-1} 1 per cent incline) followed by 4 min of standing rest. The procedures allowed for the same total work to be performed in both protocols. All participants completed all trials.

Instrumentation

Actiheart measured HR (beats·min^{-1}) and movement (counts per epoch (cpe)) and a GT1M measured activity (cpe) over 15 s epochs during trials. Monitors at test and retest were not intentionally matched. The Actiheart medial electrode attached to the base of the sternum and the lateral electrode horizontally to the left side. Participants wore the GT1M on the midaxillary line of the right hip.

Statistical analysis

Descriptive data are mean ± SD. Test-retest reliability for activity and PAHR was assessed for total trials and all speeds separately. Only exercise data were used for steady rate analysis. Data were analysed using customised macros in Microsoft Excel, and transferred into SPSS v.14 (SPSS Inc, Chicago, IL, USA) for statistical analysis. Statistical significance was set at $p \leq 0.05$.

Systematic error for PAHR was examined via paired t-tests and by comparing the mean difference between tests (± 95% CI) with an a priori defined acceptable level of agreement (Atkinson and Nevill, 2007) of ± 6 beats·min^{-1}. Systematic error for activity data was examined via paired t-tests and effect sizes (Cohen, 1969). Random error was scrutinised through coefficient of variation (CV) statistics. From repeatability CV statistics the sample size required to detect a 5 per cent change due to some hypothetical intervention in a simple pre-post design experiment was estimated using a novel nomogram (Batterham and Atkinson, 2005). This method assesses whether the test-retest variability of the outcome variable is so high that the required sample size becomes impractical (Batterham and Atkinson, 2005).

Results

Actiheart HR sensor

There were no significant test-retest differences at all speeds or for total trials ($p \geq 0.145$). Systematic bias was lower for the total intermittent (1.9 beats·min^{-1}) compared to steady rate trial (4.2 beats·min^{-1}). Mean differences fell within the acceptable region of ± 6 beats·min^{-1}, except 8 km·h^{-1} steady rate running. All upper 95 per cent CI exceeded the acceptable limit of ± 6 beats·min^{-1}.

The HR sensor, which had a repeatability CV of 6.8 per cent (95 per cent CI = 3.7–12.6) for total intermittent PAHR and 10.5 per cent (95 per cent CI = 5.4–20.3) for total steady rate PAHR would allow detection of a 5 per cent change in a pre-post design experiment and with sample sizes of approximately 40 and 80 participants, respectively. Reliability improved with intensity during intermittent trials but had no such linear relationship during steady rate.

Actiheart movement sensor

Sensors differed significantly across trials for 7 km·h^{-1} intermittent running and the total intermittent trial ($p \leq 0.046$). The movement sensor, which had a repeatability CV of 6.3 per cent (95 per cent CI = 3.4–11.7) for total intermittent activity and 8.4 per cent (95 per cent CI = 4.5–15.6) for total steady rate activity would allow detection of a 5 per cent change and with sample sizes of approximately 40 and 60 participants, respectively. Reliability improved at faster intermittent speeds but fluctuated with intensity across the steady rate trial.

GT1M actigraph

There were no significant test-retest differences for total steady rate or intermittent activity ($p \geq 0.132$). Bias was greatest at the fastest intermittent and steady rate speed. The GT1M, which had a repeatability CV of 9.1 per cent (95 per cent CI = 5.2–16.1) for total intermittent activity and 8.7 per cent (95 per cent CI = 4.7–16.2) for total steady rate activity, would allow detection of a 5 per cent change and with a sample size of approximately 70. Reliability improved with intensity in both exercise types.

Discussion

Test-retest reliability of the Actiheart sensors was greater across intermittent compared to steady rate treadmill trials in young children. The GT1M demonstrated similar reliability regardless of exercise type. Unlike the Actiheart movement sensor, the Actiheart HR sensor and GT1M appeared adequately reliable for assessing respective variables across intermittent treadmill trials. Estimated sample sizes appear feasible for simple pre-post design experiments, based on subject recruitment in previous studies (Corder *et al.*, 2005; Haerens *et al.*, 2007). Given the intermittent trial more closely recreated a child's habitual activity patterns, our results are encouraging for the reliable assessment of HR and activity, using the Actiheart HR sensor and GT1M, in children during free living.

Sample sizes estimated from Actiheart error statistics question its appropriateness in more complex design experiments, due to its invasiveness, cost and the availability of more convenient HR monitors and uniaxial accelerometers, such as the GT1M. Though it is appreciated that the Actiheart is primarily a tool for assessing energy expenditure, and not HR or activity in isolation, at present the monitor seems of best use as a validation tool in larger or more complex studies.

Biological and technical sources of variation that may have contributed to measurement error include within-participant variability, the use of different monitors at test and retest, and the consistency of monitor placement. Future research may investigate the extent to which such sources of variation influence monitor reliability, informing researchers how more reliable measures of activity and HR in children can be attained across repeated lab or field-based experiments.

References

Atkinson, G. and Nevill, A.M., 2007, Method agreement and measurement error in the physiology of exercise. In: *Sport and Exercise Physiology Testing: Guidelines: The British Association of Sport and Exercise Sciences Guide*, Vol.1, 1st edn, edited by Winter, E.M., Jones, A.M., Davison, R.R.C., Bromley, P.D. and Mercer, T.H. Oxford: Routledge, pp. 41–48.

Batterham, A.M. and Atkinson, G., 2005, How big does my sample size need to be? A primer on the murky world of sample size estimation. *Physical Therapy in Sport*, **6**, pp. 153–163.

Baquet, G., Stratton, G., Van Praagh, E. and Berthoin, S., 2007, Improving physical activity assessment in prepubertal children with high-frequency accelerometry monitoring: A methodological issue. *Preventive Medicine*, **44**, pp. 143–147.

Cohen, J., 1969, *Statistical Power Analysis for the Behavioural Sciences* (2nd edn). New York: Academic Press.

Corder, K., Brage, S., Wareham, N.J. and Ekelund, U., 2005, Comparison of PAEE from combined and separate heart rate and movement models in children. *Medicine and Science in Sports and Exercise*, **37**, pp. 1761–1767.

Haerens, L., De Bourdeaudhuij, I., Maes, L., Cardon, G. and Deforche, B., 2007, School-based randomized controlled trial of a physical activity intervention among adolescents. *Journal of Adolescent Health*, **40**, pp. 258–265.

Rowlands, A.V., Stone, M.R. and Eston, R.G., 2007, Influence of speed and step frequency during walking and running on motion sensor output. *Medicine and Science in Sports and Exercise*, **39**, pp. 716–727.

Wareham, N.J. and Rennie, K.L., 1998, The assessment of physical activity in individuals and populations: Why try to be more precise about how physical activity is assessed? *International Journal of Obesity and Related Metabolic Disorders*, **22**, pp. 30–38.

45 Comparison of training loads between two participation levels, apparatus and training phases of female gymnasts

L.A. Burt, G.A. Naughton, R. Landeo and D.G. Higham

Australian Catholic University, School of Exercise Science, Centre of Physical Activity Across the Lifespan, Sydney, Australia

Introduction

Previous studies of young gymnasts frequently separate growth, maturation, injury, training load and biomechanical analyses (Baxter-Jones *et al.*, 2003; Caine *et al.*, 2003; Davidson *et al.*, 2005; Seeley and Bressel, 2005). Research recognising the potential synergy among factors affecting young gymnasts is required to assist in peak performance and injury prevention. To this end, a recent initiative of Gymnastics Australia has been the recommendation of periodised training programmes. The primary aim of this study was to determine the effects of participation level (international and national levels), apparatus (beam and floor) and training phase (pre-competition and competition) on estimates of training load among female artistic gymnasts aged seven to 13 years. In particular, the gymnastic-specific dependent variables involved observations of the frequency of wrist and ankle impacts, landings, balance-related skills and rotations. The study also quantified the non-gymnastic-specific movement components of accelerations and total steps per apparatus.

Methods

Twenty-five gymnasts from an international [$n = 12$; (mean $\pm$ standard deviation) aged 9.25 ± 1.86 y, height 1.30 ± 0.10 m, mass 27.66 ± 4.83 kg] and national ($n = 13$; aged 9.77 ± 1.24 y, height 1.35 ± 0.08 m, mass 30.46 ± 5.23 kg) levels programme were assessed during two training sessions in both pre-competition and competition phases of the training year on the balance beam and floor apparatus. This apparatus was selected because of links to high injury prevalence (Caine *et al.*, 2003; Kirialanis *et al.*, 2002). Two 50 Hz digital video cameras (GR-DVL820EA, JVC, Japan) were used to determine the frequency of observed gymnastic-specific movements, including estimates of ankle and wrist impacts (contact with the apparatus for less than one second), landings (contact with the apparatus for greater than one second), balance-related skills (any pose or hold maintained for greater than three seconds), and rotations (circular movements around any of the three body axes). Additional movement measurement for vertical accelerations and total steps was provided by an accelerometer (GT1M, Actigraph, LLC, model 5032, Fort Walton Beach, FL.) placed on the gymnasts' right iliac crest. To further estimate training load, 16 gymnasts performed additional skills, common to both groups, on a portable force platform (Quattro Jump 9290AD, Kistler Instruments Corp., Amherst, NY.). Statistical analysis following tests for normality consisted of two-sample t-tests for differences between participation level, apparatus, training phase and baseline descriptive data using SPSS 12.0.1 for Windows (SPSS Inc., Chicago, IL.). The effects of participation level, apparatus and phase on gymnastics movements were then explored using three-way ANOVA and linear regression. Significance was set at $p \leq 0.05$ for all analyses.

Results

Regression analyses showed participation level, apparatus and training phase only partially explained skill-specific variance (from 34 per cent to 51 per cent) in gymnastics-specific movements. Therefore, other factors in addition to participation level, apparatus and training phase must have influenced the dependent variables. Three-way interactions were observed for ankle impacts [$F(1, 180) = 18.925$, $p < 0.0001$] and landings [$F(1, 173) = 4.831$, $p = 0.006$]. Two-way interactions were strongest for participation level by phase as significance was achieved for all dependent variables with the exception of accelerations. Participation level was the strongest main effect variable as it was statistically significant for all dependent variables.

Figure 45.1 shows the three-way interaction effect for participation level by apparatus by phase for landing observations. Overall, more landings occurred in both groups during the competition than pre-competition phase. However, international level gymnasts had higher mean landing observations than national level gymnasts for both apparatus and training phases, with the exception of the floor during the competition phase. During the competition phase, national level gymnasts performed more landings on the floor than beam, with similar landing observations on both apparatus during pre-competition. National level gymnasts performed more landings on floor than beam during the competition training phase. In agreement with results for international level gymnasts, pre-competition landing observations of national level gymnasts were similar on the beam and floor.

Two-sample t-tests revealed no significant differences for international and national level gymnasts' peak vertical ground reaction forces (PGRF) for both ankle and wrist impacts for any of the selected skills performed on the force platform. However, the floor apparatus consistently exposed gymnasts to greater forces relative to bodyweight than the beam. Similarly, the lower extremity was exposed to greater PGRF than the upper extremity, on both apparatus.

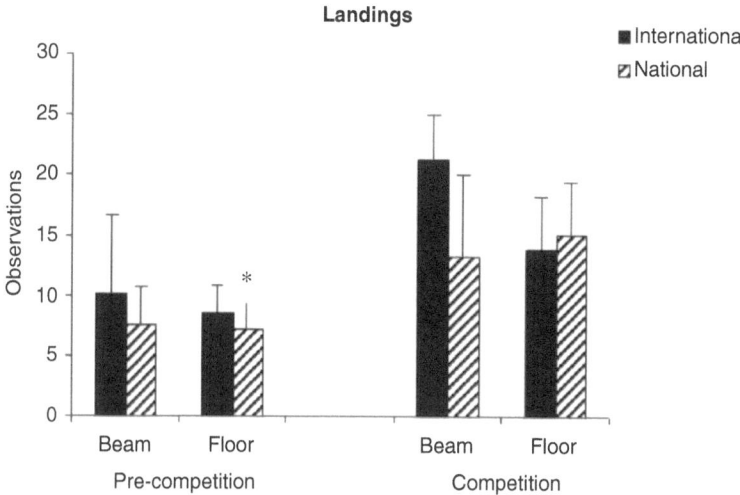

Figure 45.1 Three-way participation level × apparatus × training phase interaction effect for landing observations. (*Denotes significant three-way interaction).

Conclusion

This study showed differences exist in estimates of training load for the two groups of gymnasts performing on floor and beam apparatus and in the pre-competition and competition phases of the periodised year. International level gymnasts were exposed to a higher frequency of impacts than national level gymnasts across both apparatus throughout the periodised program. This effect is even more pronounced with the greater hours of exposure to 'loading' opportunities in the higher skilled group. Coaches must be aware that as the frequency and magnitude of impacts increases, there is a greater need for injury prevention measures. The high mechanical loading of the lower body regions must be closely monitored to ensure the longevity of athletes and minimise the risk of injury.

In the present study, the international level gymnasts followed a more refined periodised training programme. Markers of a quality periodised programme, such as greater variation in training load (intensity and volume) between phases, maximise the opportunity for peak performance during the competition phase and concurrently minimise the potential for overtraining or under recovery.

References

Baxter-Jones, A., Maffulli, N. and Mirwald, R., 2003, Does elite competition inhibit growth and delay maturation in some gymnasts? Probably not. *Pediatric Exercise Science*, **15**, pp. 373–382.

Caine, D., Knutzen, K., Howe, W., Keeler, L., Sheppard, L. and Henrichs, D., 2003, A three-year epidemiological study of injuries affecting young female gymnasts. *Physical Therapy in Sport*, **4**, pp. 10–23.

Davidson, P.L., Mahar, B., Chalmers, D.J. and Wilson, B.D., 2005, Impact modeling of gymnastic back-handsprings and dive-rolls in children. *Journal of Applied Biomechanics*, **21**, pp. 115–128.

Kirialanis, P., Malliou, P., Beneka, A., Gourgoulis, V., Giofstidou, A. and Godolias, G., 2002, Injuries in artistic gymnastic elite adolescent male and female athletes. *Journal of Back and Musculoskeletal Rehabilitation*, **16**, pp. 145–151.

Seeley, M. K. and Bressel, E., 2005, A comparison of upper-extremity reaction forces between the yurchenko vault and floor exercise. *Journal of Sports Science and Medicine*, **4**, pp. 85–94.

46 Comparison of peak oxygen uptake in boys exercising on treadmill and cycle ergometers

A. Mamen,[1] G.K. Resaland,[1] D.A. Mo[2] and L.B. Andersen[2,3]

[1]Sogn og Fjordane University College, Faculty of Teacher Education and Sport, Sogndal, Norway; [2]Norwegian School of Sport Sciences, Section for Sport Medicine, Oslo, Norway; [3]Institute of Exercise and Sport Sciences, University of Southern Denmark, Odense, Denmark

Introduction

Measurement of $\dot{V}O_{2peak}$ is the gold standard of aerobic fitness assessment, and the assessments are usually conducted on either a treadmill or a cycle ergometer. Each test form has advantages and shortcomings but measures are not identical. Use of a smaller muscle mass in cycling may explain the lower values usually found for that type of exercise. Most studies of the difference between running and cycling results have been carried out on adults (LeMura et al., 2001) and the volume of research investigating children is much less (Boileau et al., 1977). The aim of the present study was to compare the $\dot{V}O_{2peak}$ values in nine-year-old boys measured on the treadmill and during cycling to enable comparison between populations tested with different exercise modes.

Methods

Subjects

Subjects were 20 Caucasian boys aged 9.1 ± 0.3 y (mean $\pm$ SD). The height was 1.38 ± 0.6 m, body mass 30.9 ± 4.8 kg, and BMI was 16.3 ± 1.6 kg m^{-2}. Each boy received written consent from their parents/guardians, and they knew they participated voluntarily and could leave the testing at any time without giving a reason for doing so.

Metabolic cart

A MetaMax CBS metabolic cart (Cortex Biophysik, Leipzig, Germany) analysed expiration gasses using the MetaSoft 1.11.05 software without any curve smoothing. The metabolic cart has been investigated for reliability by Medbø et al. (2002), and found reliable. The cart was thoroughly calibrated before each test.

Test procedure

All tests were done within a week. The treadmill and cycle protocols differed. The protocol for running was custom made to our needs. When the subject demonstrated adequate technique, the maximal test started. Load was increased every minute by raising the speed 1 $km \cdot h^{-1}$, or if a maximal speed of 10 $km \cdot h^{-1}$ was reached, by raising the inclination by 1.5 per cent. This ensured that the test was not prematurely ended due to difficulties with keeping the pace of the treadmill. In the cycling test, cadence was kept at 70 $rev \cdot min^{-1}$ and the load increased by 20 or 25 W every third minute until exhaustion, as described by Hansen et al. (1989). This test protocol was used in another project that recorded Norwegian children's fitness; choosing this protocol allows us to compare cycling fitness data for our children with other Norwegian children (Mo, 2007). We applied strong verbal encouragement at the end of each test to make sure the boys made their best effort.

A Polar heart rate monitor (Polar OY, Kempele, Finland) measured the heart rate continuously.

Criteria for a maximal test

A test was considered maximal if end heart rate was 95 per cent of age adjusted maximal HR, or showed a RER > 0.95, or the test person was unable to continue despite strong verbal encouragement. All children fulfilled at least one of these criteria.

Statistics

Means were compared with paired t-tests. Correlation analysis was done with Pearson's r. (SigmaPlot v.10.0/SigmaStat v.3.5, Systat Software GmbH, Erkrath, Germany).

Results

The absolute $\dot{V}O_{2peak}$ was 1.71 ± 0.21 $L \cdot min^{-1}$ when running and 1.63 ± 0.17 $L \cdot min^{-1}$ in the cycling test. This difference of 0.08 $L \cdot min^{-1}$ (4.7 per cent) was highly significant ($p < 0.01$). Relative $\dot{V}O_{2peak}$ was 56.0 ± 6.0 and 53.5 ± 6.2 $mL \cdot kg^{-1} \cdot min^{-1}$ respectively ($p < 0.01$). The correlation between the two test modalities for oxygen uptake was high ($r = 0.81$, SEE 0.1 $L \cdot min^{-1}$ (absolute) and 3.7 $mL \cdot kg^{-1} \cdot min^{-1}$ (relative), $p < 0.01$). For five of the children, the best $\dot{V}O_{2peak}$ result was obtained during cycling. HR_{max} was higher in the running mode, 203 ± 6 vs 195 ± 5 $beats \cdot min^{-1}$, $p < 0.01$. The percentage differences between running and cycling for several variables are shown in Fig 46.1.

Discussion

We found that in children 9.1 years old the $\dot{V}O_{2peak}$ was about 5 per cent lower during cycling compared with running. This difference is less than most others

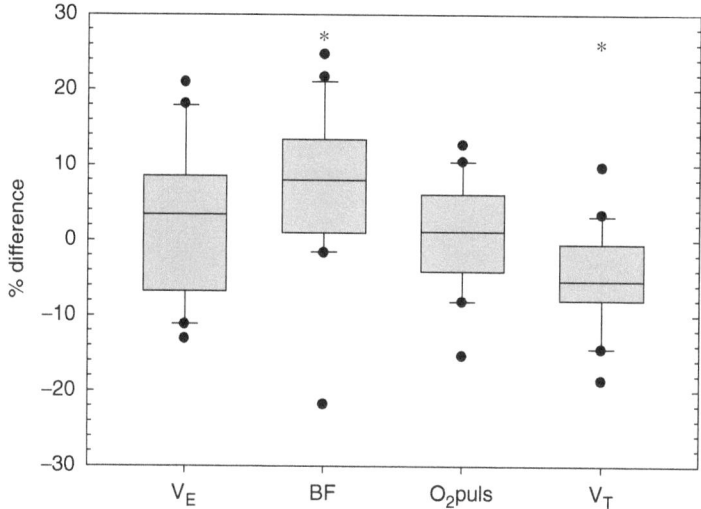

Figure 46.1 Percentage difference between running and cycling for pulmonary ventilation (V_E), breathing frequency (BF), O_{2puls} and tidal volume (V_T). Positive difference indicates higher values from running. (* = $p < 0.01$. Boxes are 25th and 75th percentiles, whiskers are 10th and 90th percentiles, dots are outliers, the horizontal lines show median values.)

have found for children (Ikai and Kitagawa, 1972; Macek *et al.*, 1976; Boileau *et al.*, 1977; LeMura *et al.*, 2001) who all report values of about 8 per cent. Because we had five children who performed better during the cycling test, our average result is lower than expected. The majority of children who performed best during running, showed, on average, a difference of 8.1 per cent between running and cycling.

HR_{max} was significantly lower during the cycle test, 8 beats·min^{-1} (3.9 per cent), $p < 0.01$. This agrees with most other findings in adults (Hermansen *et al.*, 1970), and in children (Boileau *et al.*, 1977). Use of a smaller muscle mass can explain this difference, as local muscular fatigue might be more pronounced during cycling and so give less metabolic stress. Another factor might be reduced venous return; this we did not measure, but the oxygen pulse, which is indicative of stroke volume, did not show a statistical difference (Running 8.47 ± 1.09 vs Cycling 8.37 ± 0.91, $p = 0.77$).

The only variable to be lower while running was V_T; 0.93 ± 0.03 vs 0.97 ± 0.03 L. Cycling reduced the breathing frequency more than the V_E, leading to a significant ($p < 0.01$) increase in cycling V_T. In rhythmic exercise, the breathing pattern tends to be influenced by the rhythm of the movement (Bechbache and Duffin, 1977).

In this experiment, we did not randomise the order of testing for practical reasons. When the children had done their treadmill testing, they were asked to do the cycling tests to compare results with another study. A possibility exists therefore for an order effect that can mask the real difference between the two testing methods; it might be either a learning effect, a training effect, a developed negative feeling for such maximal testing or apparatus variations.

In conclusion, we have found both test modalities feasible for children, but if comparison of group data between the two forms is to be made, the cycling value should be adjusted up about 5 per cent relative to running values.

References

Bechbache, R.R. and Duffin, J., 1977, The entrainment of breathing frequency by exercise rhythm. *Journal of Physiology* (London), **272**, pp. 553–561.

Boileau, R.A., Bonen, A., Heyward, V.H. and Massey, B.H., 1977, Maximal aerobic capacity on the treadmill and bicycle ergometer of boys 11–14 years of age. *Journal of Sports Medicine*, **17**, pp. 153–162.

Hansen, H.S., Froberg, K., Nielsen, J.R. and Hyldebrandt, N., 1989, A new approach to assessing maximal aerobic power in children: The Odense School Child Study. *European Journal of Applied Physiology*, **58**, pp. 618–624.

Hermansen, L., Ekblom, B. and Saltin, B., 1970, Cardiac output during submaximal and maximal treadmill and bicycle exercise. *Journal of Applied Phyiology*, **29**, pp. 82–86.

Ikai, M. and Kitagawa, K., 1972, Maximum oxygen uptake of Japanese related to gender and age. *Medicine and Science in Sports and Exercise*, **4**, pp. 127–131.

LeMura, L.M., von Duvillard, S.P., Cohen, S.L., Root, C.J., Chelland, S.A., Andreacci, J., Hoover, J. and Weatherford, J., 2001, Treadmill and cycle ergometry testing in 5- to 6-year-old children. *European Journal of Applied Physiology*, **85**, pp. 472–478.

Macek, M., Vavra, J. and Novosada J., 1976, Prolonged exercise in prepubertal boys. *European Journal of Applied Physiology*, **35**, pp. 208–213.

Medbø, J.I., Mamen, A., Welde, B., von Heimburg, E. and Stokke, R., 2002, Examination of the Metamax 1 and II oxygen analysers during exercise studies in the laboratory. *Scandinavian Journal of Clinical and Laboratory Investigations*, **62**, pp. 585–598.

Mo, D.A. 2007, $\dot{V}O_2$ peak hos rurale og urbane barn, og en validering av maksimalt arbeid på ergometersykkel og tredemølle [VO_2 peak in rural and urban children, and a validation of maximal work on the cycle ergometer and treadmill. [In Norwegian]. Master thesis, Norwegian School of Sport Science, Oslo.

47 Effects of age on skeletal muscle oxidative capacity

A^{31}P-MRS study

S. Ratel,[1] *A. Tonson,*[2] *Y. Le Fur,*[2] *P. Cozzone*[2] *and D. Bendahan*[2]

[1]Laboratory of Exercise Biology, University of Blaise Pascal, UFR STAPS, Aubière, France; [2]CRMBM, UMR CNRS 6612, University of Méditerranée, Faculty of Medicine, Marseille, France

Introduction

Although it has been previously described that children display a greater resistance to fatigue as compared to adults during repeated bouts of high-intensity exercise (Ratel *et al.*, 2002), the exact causative factors have not been clearly discriminated. Several hypotheses related to metabolic changes during or between exercise bouts could be put forth. In that respect, the greater resistance to fatigue in children could be linked to a higher skeletal muscle oxidative capacity allowing a faster phosphocreatine (PCr) resynthesis and a faster restoration of short-term muscle power following each exercise bout (Bogdanis *et al.*, 1996). Oxidative capacity can be estimated non-invasively from the rate of post-exercise PCr resynthesis using 31-phosphorus magnetic resonance spectroscopy (^{31}P-MRS). However, using this method, conflicting results have been reported between children and adults (Kuno *et al.*, 1995; Taylor *et al.*, 1997) which could lead to misinterpretations. For instance, confounding factors such as end-of-exercise pH and PCr concentration have not been systematically taken into account (Roussel *et al.*, 2000).

The aim of the present study was to compare skeletal muscle oxidative capacity between children and adults taking into account confounding factors.

Methods

Seven young boys (11.7 ± 0.6 y) and ten men (35.6 ± 7.8 y) volunteered to be included in the study. They were involved in different recreational physical activities, such as athletics, water-polo and tennis. Written informed consent was signed by each subject or his parents. The experimental protocol was approved by the Ethics Timone Hospital Committee (Marseille, France).

The subjects sat on a chair close to the magnet and inserted their forearm horizontally into the magnet bore over the 50 mm diameter surface coil.

The forearm was placed approximately at the same height as the shoulder to ensure a good venous return. After a 3 min resting period, the subjects performed finger flexions at 1.5 s intervals for 3 min, followed by a 15 min recovery period. Exercise consisted of lifting a weight adjusted to 15 per cent of the MVC in a 50/50 duty cycle (0.75 s contraction, 0.75 s relaxation). Exercise frequency was imposed by a metronome. The sliding amplitude of the weight and the frequency of the corresponding signal were recorded using a displacement transducer connected to a personal computer running ATS software (SYSMA-FRANCE). Calculated power output was averaged over each 15 s of exercise. Magnetic resonance spectra from forearm flexor muscles were obtained at 4.7T (Bruker 47/30 Biospec).

Intracellular pH was calculated from the chemical shift difference between the inorganic phosphate (Pi) and PCr signals. Muscle oxidative capacity was measured from the rate constant of PCr recovery (kPCr) calculated from the fitting of the raw data to a single exponential curve. In addition, the half-time of PCr recovery ($t_{1/2 \; PCr}$) was calculated as follows: $t_{1/2 \; PCr}$ (min) $= \ln (2)/(k_{PCr})$. Also, the theoretical maximum rate of oxidative phosphorylation (V_{max}) was calculated according to the model of Michaëlis-Menten, as previously reported (Roussel et al., 2000).

Values are reported as mean $\pm$ SD. Unpaired Student t-tests were used in order to analyze the effects of age on the different metabolic variables. The limit for statistical significance was set at $p < 0.05$. Statistical procedures were performed using the StatView software (StatView SE+ Graphics®, Abacus Concepts, Inc.).

Results

End-of-exercise pH values were not significantly different between children and adults (6.6 ± 0.2 vs 6.5 ± 0.2, respectively). PCr consumption measured at the end of exercise was significantly lower in children than in adults (45.1 ± 4.8 vs 64.8 ± 16.1 per cent of the resting level, $p < 0.05$). The rate constants of PCr recovery (k_{PCr}) and V_{max} were significantly higher in boys as compared to men (Table 47.1). In addition, the half-time of PCr recovery ($t_{1/2 \; PCr}$) was about twofold lower in young boys (33.0 ± 14.4 s) than in men (62.4 ± 19.7 s).

PCr changes during the standardized rest-exercise-recovery protocol in children and adults are shown in Figure 47.1.

Table 47.1 Metabolic variables measured throughout the post-exercise-recovery period

	Boys	p	Men
k_{PCr} (min^{-1})	1.7 ± 1.2	< 0.05	0.7 ± 0.2
$t_{1/2 PCr}$ (s)	33.0 ± 14.4	< 0.01	62.4 ± 19.7
V_{max} (mM $\cdot$ min^{-1})	49.7 ± 24.6	< 0.05	29.4 ± 7.9

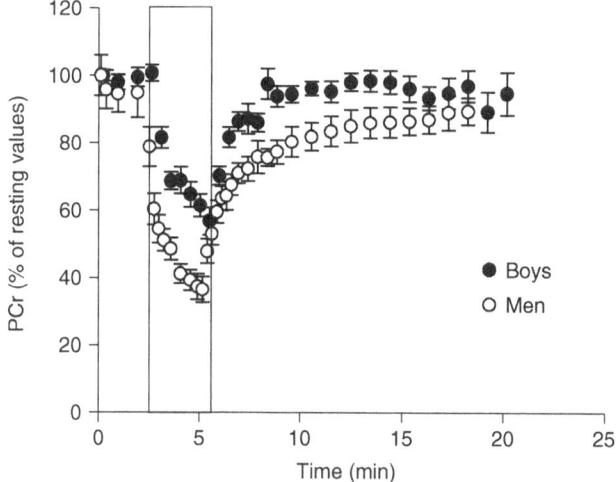

Figure 47.1 PCr changes during the standardized rest-exercise-recovery protocol in boys
(●) and men (O).

Discussion

The main finding of the present study is that the skeletal muscle oxidative capacity
is larger in young boys as compared to men, as indicated by the higher k_{PCr} and
V_{max} values.

It has been demonstrated that k_{PCr} was inversely related to the extent of
intracellular acidosis, whereas V_{max} would be insensitive to end-of-exercise
conditions (Roussel *et al.*, 2000). Therefore, k_{PCr} can be used on its own in order
to compare different subjects as long as end-of-exercise metabolic conditions are
similar. In the present study, end-of-exercise pH values were similar in the two
age groups so that oxidative capacity can be compared between the two groups
from k_{PCr} values. V_{max} could also be used as an additional index.

The present results are in line with those of Taylor *et al.* (1997) who reported
that, after a graded exercise protocol, $t_{1/2\ PCr}$ was approximately twofold lower
in children aged 6–12 y as compared to adults aged 20–29 y (12 ± 4 vs 27 ± 8 s,
respectively) while V_{max} was also larger in children as compared to adults (91 ± 46
vs $54 \pm 17\ mM\ min^{-1}$). In contrast, these child-adult differences are not consistent
with the results from Kuno *et al.* (1995) showing similar k_{PCr} values between 12-
year-old children and 25-year-old adults following a graded exercise protocol.
However, in this latter study, V_{max} values were not reported. In addition, given
that end-of-exercise metabolic conditions were different between the two groups
(i.e. lower post-exercise pH values in adults), these results should be interpreted
with caution.

The higher oxidative capacity measured in children could be due to a higher
relative content of type I fibers (Lexell *et al.*, 1992). During exercise protocols

involving repeated bouts of high-intensity exercise and recovery periods, the ability to recover quickly to the pre-exercise level plays an important role in limiting fatigue. Currently, it is accepted in adults that the restoration of short-term muscle power following exercise is dependent on PCr resynthesis, a purely oxidative process (Bogdanis *et al.*, 1996). Considering that the fatigue phenomenon commonly reported during repeated bouts of high-intensity exercise would be due to a shortfall in aerobic ATP synthesis (Bogdanis *et al.*, 1996), one can reasonably hypothesize that individuals with a high oxidative capacity can recover their initial PCr stores faster thereby limiting the fatigue phenomenon. On the basis of the present results, the greater fatigue resistance of children during intermittent type fatigue protocols could be explained by their higher muscle oxidative activity allowing them a faster PCr recovery between exercise bouts.

In conclusion, post-exercise recovery measurements illustrate a greater mitochondrial oxidative capacity in children. This faster aerobic ATP generation could partially explain their greater resistance to fatigue during high-intensity intermittent exercise.

Acknowledgement

This work was supported by the French association against myopathy (AFM).

References

Bogdanis, G.C., Nevill, M.E., Boobis, L.H. and Lakomy, H.K., 1996, Contribution of phosphocreatine and aerobic metabolism to energy supply during repeated sprint exercise. *Journal of Applied Physiology*, **80**, pp. 876–884.

Kuno, S., Takahashi, H., Fujimoto, K., Akima, H., Miyamaru, M., Nemoto, I., Itai, Y. and Katsuta, S., 1995, Muscle metabolism during exercise using phosphorus-31 nuclear magnetic resonance spectroscopy in adolescents. *European Journal of Applied Physiology*, **70**, pp. 301–304.

Lexell, J., Sjostrom, M., Nordlund, A.S. and Taylor, C.C., 1992, Growth and development of human muscle: A quantitative morphological study of whole vastus lateralis from childhood to adult age. *Muscle Nerve*, **15**, pp. 404–409.

Ratel, S., Duché, P., Hennegrave, A., Van Praagh, E. and Bedu, M., 2002, Acid-base balance during repeated cycling sprints in boys and men. *Journal of Applied Physiology*, **92**, pp. 479–485.

Roussel, M., Bendahan, D., Mattei, J.P., Le Fur, Y. and Cozzone, P.J., 2000, ^{31}P magnetic resonance spectroscopy study of phosphocreatine recovery kinetics in skeletal muscle: The issue of intersubject variability. *Biochimica et Biophysica Acta*, **1457**, pp. 18–26.

Taylor, D.J., Kemp, G.J., Thompson, C.H. and Radda, G.K., 1997, Ageing: Effects on oxidative function of skeletal musclee in vivo. *Molecular and Cellular Biochemistry*, **174**, pp. 321–324.

48 Physical performance characteristics of Finnish boys aged 10 and 14 years

T. Vänttinen, M. Blomqvist and S. Vänttinen
KIHU – Research Institute for Olympic Sports, Finland

Introduction

Hormonal changes, e.g. rapidly increasing testosterone after age 12 y (Winter, 1978), leads to peak height and weight velocity during growth in boys at the age of around 14 y (Tanner *et al.*, 1966). During the adolescent spurt, marked development in anthropometrical stature (Malina, 1991) and various performance tests (Mero, 1990) can also be observed. The purpose of this study was to examine the physical characteristics of 10-and 14-year-old Finnish males with reference to anthropometrics, hormonal levels and oxygen transport capacity of the blood cells.

Methods

The subjects of this study were 10- ($n = 26$) and 14- ($n = 23$) year-old Finnish males. The anthropometrics were determined with height, weight, percentage of fat, total muscle mass, average lean mass of arms and legs and total lean mass of trunk measured using conventional methods and with the InBody720 body composition analyzer. Erythrocytes, haemoglobin, haematocrit, cortisol, growth hormone and testosterone were analyzed from a basal venous blood sample (between 7.30 and 8.30 a.m. after 12 h fasting). The subjects' physical performance was measured in speed (30 m sprint), strength (107° isometric leg press and grip) and endurance ($\dot{V}O_2$ on a 1° grade treadmill starting at a speed of 7 $km \cdot h^{-1}$ with a 1 $km \cdot h^{-1}$ increase each minute until exhaustion and a YoYo shuttle run). A *t*-test was applied to detect differences between the age groups. The relationships between physical performance and other measured variables were examined using Pearson's correlation coefficient.

Results

Means and SDs of subjects' anthropometrical measurements for both age groups are presented in Table 48.1. The weight, muscle mass and lean body mass of different body parts in the 10-year-old group was between 50–60 per cent of that found in the 14-year-old group. All other measured variables increased with age

Table 48.1 Anthropometrics of 10- and 14-year-old Finnish males

	Height (m)	Weight (kg)	Muscle (kg)	Arms (kg)	Trunk (kg)	Legs (kg)	Fat %
10 y	1.45	36.0	16.5	2.5	14.1	9.4	13.1
	(5.5)	(5.7)	(1.9)	(0.4)	(1.4)	(1.2)	(6.5)
14 y	1.72	61.0	30.4	4.5	24.0	17.8	10.6
	(8.1)	(10.9)	(4.4)	(1.0)	(3.2)	(2.5)	(6.6)
Sig.	***	***	***	***	***	***	ns.

Table 48.2 Blood and hormonal variables of 10- and 14-year-old Finnish males.

	RBC ($E12\,L^{-1}$)	HB ($g\,L^{-1}$)	HCT (%)	COR ($nmol\;L^{-1}$)	GH ($mU\,L^{-1}$)	T ($nmol\,L^{-1}$)
10 y	4.85	139	40	472	3.79	0.5
	(0.27)	(8)	(2)	(143)	(5.61)	(0.8)
14 y	5.13	149	43	484	2.35	18.0
	(0.31)	(10)	(2)	(174)	(4.11)	(4.7)
Sig.	**	***	***	ns	ns	***

except percentage of body fat which was lower (ns) in the 14-year-olds than in the 10-year-old group.

The hormonal stature and variables related to oxygen transport capacity of the blood are presented in Table 48.2. The red blood cell quantities in the 10-year-old group were around 90 per cent of those found in 14-year-olds. The most significant difference was found in the concentration of testosterone which increased from 0.5–18 mmol·L^{-1} from age 10–14 years. It is important to notice that, as analyzed from one blood sample, the cortisol and especially the growth hormone values include more uncertainty due to diurnal variation and burst like expression.

The results of the physical performance test are presented in Table 48.3. In the 10-year-old group grip strength was around 51 per cent and leg strength 73 per cent of that found in the 14-year-olds. Oxygen uptake ($\dot{V}O_2$, L·min^{-1}) was almost twice as high in the group of 14-year-olds compared to the 10-year-old group but the difference diminished when oxygen uptake was adjusted to body weight (mL·kg^{-1}·min^{-1}). Even though no significant differences where found

Table 48.3 Physical performance characteristics of 10- and 14-year-old Finnish males

Age	Grip (N)	Legs (N)	30 m (s)	$\dot{V}O_2$ ($L\cdot min^{-1}$)	$\dot{V}O_{2max}$ ($mL\cdot kg^{-1}\cdot min^{-1}$)	Shuttle (m)
10 y	214	1491	5.52	1.69	44.7	1382
	(42)	(579)	(0.45)	(0.28)	(6.8)	(456)
14 y	421	2031	4.79	3.04	46.1	1813
	(73)	(795)	(0.39)	(0.47)	(7.2)	(676)
Sig.	***	***	***	***	ns.	*

in $\dot{V}O_{2max}$, the endurance performance (shuttle run) increased significantly with increasing age.

The correlation analysis revealed the following relationships:

10-year-olds

1 Lower percentage of body fat was related to better grip strength ($r = 0.41^*$), leg strength ($r = 0.67^{**}$), speed ($r = -0.48^*$), $\dot{V}O_{2max}$ ($r = 0.45^*$) and shuttle run ($r = 0.53^{**}$);
2 Lower skeletal muscle mass was related to better grip strength ($r = -0.44^*$) and $\dot{V}O_{2max}$ ($r = -0.50^{**}$); and
3 Higher level of cortisol was related to better speed ($r = -0.51^{**}$) and shuttle run performance ($r = 0.53^{**}$) (Figure 48.1).

14-year-olds

1 Lower percentage of body fat was related to better speed ($r = -0.54^{**}$), $\dot{V}O_{2max}$ ($r = 0.43^*$) and shuttle run ($r = 0.50^*$);
2 Lower lean body mass in legs was related to better leg strength ($r = -0.59^{**}$) and shuttle run ($r = -0.51^*$);
3 Lower skeletal muscle mass was related to better leg strength ($r = -0.58^{**}$), $\dot{V}O_{2max}$ ($r = -0.46^*$) and shuttle run performance ($r = -0.55^{**}$);
4 Higher skeletal muscle mass was related to better $\dot{V}O_2$ ($r = 0.54^{**}$);
5 Higher haemoglobin was related to better $\dot{V}O_2$ ($r = 0.45^*$);
6 Higher level of testosterone was related to better speed ($r = -0.49^*$);
7 Lower level of growth hormone was related to better shuttle run performance ($r = -0.45^*$); and

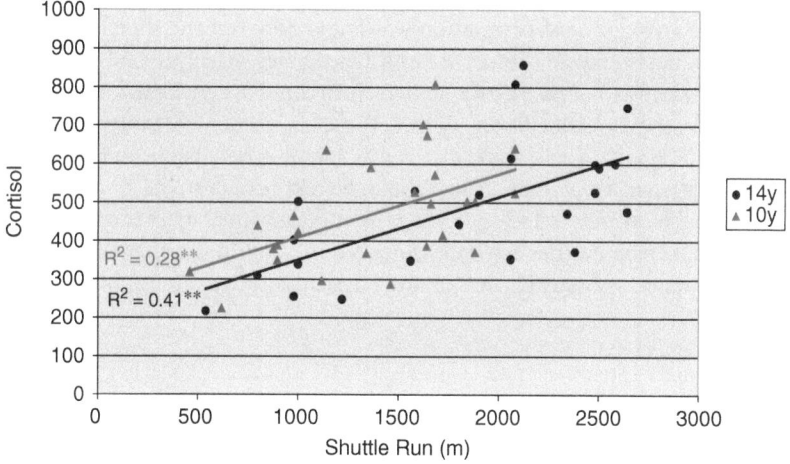

Figure 48.1 Relationships between basal cortisol level and endurance performance.

8   Higher level of cortisol was related to better grip strength ($r = 0.42^{**}$), leg strength ($r = 0.53^{**}$), speed ($r = -0.59^{**}$), $\dot{V}O_{2max}$ ($r = 0.48^{*}$) and shuttle run performance ($r = 0.64^{**}$) (Figure 48.1).

Conclusions

The results of this study suggest that the reason for rapid improvement in various performance tests from 10–14 years is maturation through hormonal changes and following an increase in muscle mass. The testosterone concentration of Finnish boys increased from practically zero at the age of 10 y to around 75 per cent of that typically found in adults at the age of 14 y. The anthropometrical analysis revealed that the total muscle mass was almost doubled during this stage of development. It was also observed that the lean body mass was increased relatively more in arms and legs compared to the trunk. The performance ability in the 10-year-old group when compared to the 14-year-old group was around 50 per cent in grip strength, 75 per cent in leg strength and shuttle run (endurance performance) and 85 per cent in speed. The difference in oxygen uptake per unit of body weight was minimal.

There have been concerns in western societies that more and more children are becoming overweight and as a consequence their physical fitness also decreases. Even though the children and youths in this study were normal weight, clear evidence was found that physical fitness is better when children/youths have less fat. At the age of 10 y, the leaner boys were better in speed and endurance performance but not in strength, as would be expected. In the 14-year-old group all performance variables were related to subjects' percentage of body fat. It seems that during the growth spurt the percentage of body fat slightly decreases in boys. This could be a convenient time to motivate inactive children to exercise, especially when other changes in the body (hormones and muscles) make progression in physical fitness easier.

In this study, a significant correlation was found between the shuttle run test and all other measured performance tests (speed, leg strength and $\dot{V}O_{2max}$) in both age groups. Therefore the shuttle run can be considered to be the best test to describe overall fitness within these experimental groups. In both age groups the result of the shuttle run was better when basal cortisol level was higher. Higher level of cortisol could be explained to be a metabolic adaptation to a more active life-style, exercise induced stress marker or plainly a methodological error. Further research is needed to confirm whether the level of cortisol really reflects physical fitness or/and physical activity among children and youths.

References

Malina, R.M., 1989, Models and methods for studying body composition. In: *Growth, Maturation and Physical Activity*, edited by Malina, R.M. and Bouchard, C. Champaign, IL: Human Kinetics, pp. 87–100.

Mero, A., 1990, Perusteet lasten ja nuorten harjoittelussa, In: *Lasten ja Nuorten Harjoittelu.* JKL: Gummerus Oy, pp. 49–190.

Tanner, J.M., Whitehouse, R.H. and Takaishi, M., 1966, Standards from British children for maturity for height, weight, height velocity and weight velocity: British Children, 1965–I. *Archives of Disease in Childhood*, **41**, pp. 454–471.

Winter, J.S.D., 1978, Prepubertal and pubertal endocrinology. In: *Human Growth*, Vol 2, edited by Falkner, F. and Tanner, J.M. New York: Plenum, pp. 183–213.

49 Sports participation in children and their parents is associated with higher aerobic fitness of children

L. Zahner,[1,2] M. Schmid,[1] B. Steffen,[1] J.J. Puder,[3]
T. Mühlbauer[1] and S. Kriemler[1]

[1]University of Basel; [2]Swiss Federal Office of Sports; [3]University of
Lausanne, Switzerland

Introduction

Increased fatness, decreased aerobic fitness and a low level of physical activity are thought to be relevant factors for decreased health in children (e.g. Armstrong, 1989; Thompson et al., 2002; Lobstein et al., 2004). However, regular sports club participation is associated with a lower fatness and higher aerobic fitness level (e.g. Washington et al., 2001; Jago and Baranowski, 2004). Previous studies have mainly focused on the association between sports club participation and fatness and/or fitness in adults and adolescents. In contrast, the role of sports club participation on children's fatness and fitness has not yet been addressed. Furthermore, parental support to perform physical activity, the performance of physical activity by parents and children together, and an environment which is promoting activity are PA enhancing factors (Sallis et al., 1992; Heitzler et al., 2006). Thus, the purpose of the present study was to assess the influence of sports club participation of children and their parents on fatness and aerobic fitness of the children.

Methods

Study sample and recruitment

Data were drawn from the baseline examination of the Children and Youth Sport Study (Kinder-Sportstudie, KISS), a randomized controlled trial (Zahner et al., 2006). Children ($n = 553$) from the first and fifth grade from two provinces of Switzerland were randomly selected and stratified for ethnicity and living area. Sports club participation (at least once a week) of the children (chi-yes: $n = 288$, chi-no: $n = 150$) and their parents (par-yes: $n = 143$, par-no: $n = 295$) were acquired by questionnaire. The main characteristics of the children for the two groups are presented in Table 49.1.

Table 49.1 Description of the study sample by sports club participation of the children

	Chi-yes	Chi-no
Age (years)	9.5 ± 2.1	8.9 ± 2.2
Height (cm)	137.0 ± 13.0	133.6 ± 13.5
Mass (kg)	33.1 ± 9.9	30.8 ± 9.3
BMI ($kg \cdot m^{-2}$)	17.3 ± 2.6	16.9 ± 2.7

Measurements

Body height, mass and four skinfold thicknesses (biceps, triceps, subscapular, suprailiacal) were measured. Body mass index (BMI) and the sum of the four skinfolds were calculated. Aerobic fitness was assessed with the 20 m shuttle run test.

Data analysis

Descriptive statistics (mean and standard deviation) were run on all data using SPSS version 13.0. All analyses were adjusted for gender and grade. To assess the influence of sports club participation on fatness and fitness a univariate analysis of variance using the General Linear Model procedure was conducted. The significance level was set at $p < 0.05$.

Results

For skinfold thickness (see Figure 49.1), no differences were found concerning children's and/or parental sports club participation (p-values were 0.21 and 0.07).

For aerobic fitness (see Figure 49.2), significantly higher values were obtained for children, who participated in a sports club ($p < 0.001$) and for children with parental sport club participation ($p = 0.033$).

Discussion

The aim of the present study was to examine the effect of sports club participation of children and their parents on fatness and aerobic fitness of the children. Children showed a higher aerobic fitness if they and their parents regular participate in a sports club. This result is in line with the findings of Ara *et al.* (2004), who also reported a significantly higher aerobic fitness of boys with regular sport participation compared with boys without. In contrast to Ara and colleagues, our study included not only boys but children of both sexes as well as children from two different grades (first and fifth grade).

For skinfold thickness, no differences were found according to sports club participation of the children as well as their parents. This result is in contrast to the findings of Ara *et al.* (2004), because they reported a significantly lower value for the boys who regular participated in a sports club. With regard to this

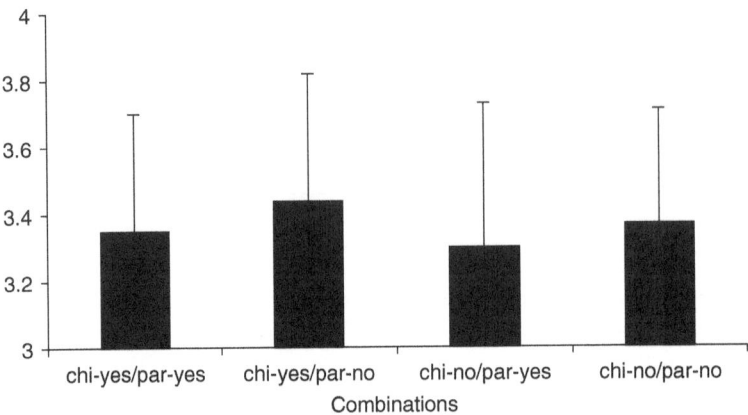

Figure 49.1 Sum of the four skinfolds (transformed to the natural logarithm) based on sports club participation of the children and their parents.

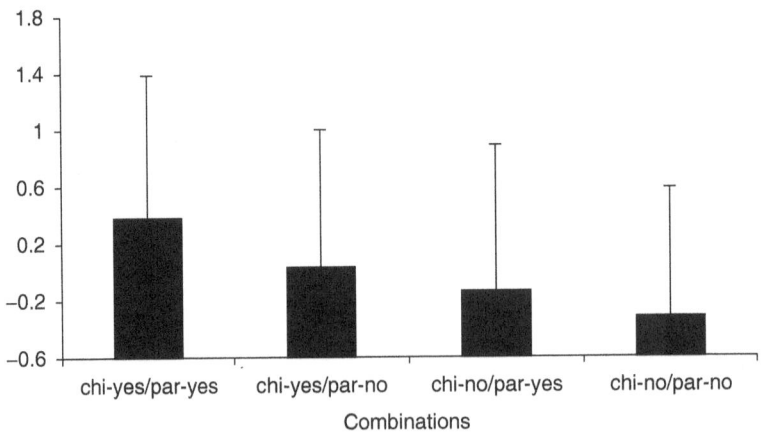

Figure 49.2 Performance of the 20 m shuttle run test (z-score) based on sports club participation of the children and their parents.

inconsistency between the data of Ara *et al.* (2004) and our own results, it is important to point out the different definition of regular sports participation. We considered regular sports participation of at least once a week, whereas Ara *et al.* (2004) thought of at least three hours a week. Hence, it is presumed that more differences will be discovered through a higher level of sports participation. This interpretation is supported by data that were already been reported (Steffen *et al.*, 2007).

The finding of a higher aerobic fitness in children, if they and their parents regularly participate in a sports club, suggests that children and their parents should be actively supported to participate in a sports club, since this is an easy tool to improve total physical activity and aerobic fitness.

Acknowledgement

This work was supported by a grant from the Swiss Federal Office of Sport (SW105-013 KISS).

References

Ara, I., Vincente-Rodriguezs, G., Jimenez-Ramirez, J., Dorado, C., Serrano-Sanchez, J.A., and Calbet, J.A.L., 2004, Regular participation in sports is associated with enhanced physical fitness and lower fat mass in prepubertal boys. *International Journal of Obesity and Related Metabolic Disorders*, **28**, pp. 1585–1593.

Armstrong, N., 1989, Children are fit but not active! *Education & Health*, **7**, pp. 28–32.

Heitzler, C.D., Martin, S.L., Duke, J., and Human, M., 2006, Correlates of physical activity in a national sample of children aged 9–13 years. *Preventive Medicine*, **42**, pp. 254–260.

Jago, R., and Baranowski, T., 2004, Non-curricular approaches for increasing physical activity. *Preventive Medicine*, **39**, pp. 157–163.

Lobstein, T., Baur, L. and Uauy, R., 2004, Obesity in children and young people: A crisis in public health. *Obesity Reviews*, **5**, pp. 4–104.

Sallis, J.F., Simons-Morton, B.G. and Stone, E.G., 1992, Determinants of physical activity and interventions in youth. *Medicine & Science in Sports & Exercise*, **24**, pp. 248–257.

Steffen, B., Zahner, L., Puder, J., Schmid, M.and Kriemler, S., 2007, Das aktive Mitmachen im Sportverein von Kindern und ihren Eltern ist positiv assoziiert mit dem Fitnessgrad von Schulkindern. *Schweizerische Zeitschrift für Sportmedizin und Sporttraumatologie*, **55**, pp. 69–76.

Thompson, A.M., Baxter-Jones, A.D.G., Mirwald, R.L. and Bailey, D.A., 2002, Secular trend in the development of fatness during childhood and adolescence. *American Journal of Human Biology*, **14**, pp. 669–679.

Washington, R.L., Bernhardt, D.T. and Gomez, J. 2001, Organized sports for children and preadolescents. *Pediatrics*, **107**, pp. 1459–1462.

Zahner, L., Puder, J.J., and Roth, R. 2006, A school-based physical activity program to improve health and fitness in children aged 6–13 years (Kinder-Sportstudie KISS): Study design of a randomized controlled trial. *BMC Public Health*, **6**, p. 147.

Part VII
Muscle physiology

50 The effect of the central and peripheral factors in adults' and children's fatigability

K. Hatzikotoulas, D. Patikas, E. Bassa, H. Kitsas, A. Giannakos and C. Kotzamanidis
Department of Physical Education and Sports Science, Aristotle University of Thessaloniki, Greece

Introduction

Fatigability in adults has been studied thoroughly. However, this phenomenon in children lacks extensive investigation. Comparisons between adults and children were performed during maximal efforts (Paraschos *et al.*, 2007; Ratel *et al.*, 2006). These studies showed that adults were more fatigued than children. This was attributed mainly to metabolic factors. However, there is no information to our knowledge concerning the fatigue topography differences between children and adults during maximal sustained contraction. Specifically, we do not know to what extent the neuronal and muscular factors contribute to fatigue in children and adults.

For this reason the purpose of this study was to examine to what extent central and peripheral mechanisms contribute to the fatigue differences between adults and prepubertal boys during a maximal sustained fatigue test.

Methods

Ten healthy boys (mean ± SD age: 10.9 ± 0.8 yrs, body mass: 43.1 ± 10.9 kg, height: 150.1 ± 7.7 cm) and men (age: 25.4 ± 1.9 yrs, body mass: 74.9 ± 7.8 kg, height: 180.4 ± 6.3 cm) volunteered to participate in this study. The subjects were informed for the purpose and the measurements of this study prior to the test. Written inform consent forms were completed by all subjects. As far as the boys were concerned, their parents were informed about the purpose of the experimental procedure prior to the test and parental written consent was given in all cases. The experimental procedure was performed according to the ethical rules of the Aristotle University of Thessaloniki.

A Cybex Norm dynamometer was employed to determine Maximal Isometric Voluntary Contraction (MIVC). EMG activity from medial gastrocnemius (MG) and tibialis anterior (TA) muscles was recorded using the BTS EMG device. Supramaximal electrical stimulation was applied to the Posterior Tibial nerve for Voluntary Muscle Activation (VMA) estimation, delivered by DSA7H Digitimer stimulator.

All tests were performed from a seated position (hip flexion angle of 170°) with the knee fully extended (0°) and the ankle at the anatomical zero (90°). The antagonist activity of TA was expressed as a percentage of the activity of the respective muscle when acting as agonist.

The MIVC, the agonist and antagonist EMG were evaluated prior, during and at the end of a maximal sustained plantar flexion fatigue test. The fatigue procedure was terminated when the torque output decreased to 50 per cent of the MIVC. Immediately following the fatigue task, one final MIVC was performed by the subjects.

All torque and EMG values during fatigue were expressed as a percentage of the maximal measurement prior to the fatigue protocol. All torque and EMG values were normalized relative to the first measurement during the fatigue protocol. The level of VMA was calculated as [(voluntary torque – torque with stimulation)/voluntary torque] × 100.

Results are presented as mean values and standard deviation of mean (SD). The analyzed independent variables were the age (adult-prepubertal) and trial (prior-after fatigue protocol). The analyzed dependent variables were the torque, the EMG of MG, the coactivation of TA and the VMA. The results were analyzed with a two factors ANOVA.

During the fatigue protocol, the analyzed independent variables were a age (adult-prepubertal) and fatigue time (percentage). The analyzed dependent variables were the torque, the EMG of MG and the coactivation of TA. A two-way analysis of variance (ANOVA) for repeated measurement was applied for each dependent variable. The Scheffè post hoc test for multiple comparisons was performed when the ANOVA indicated an interaction between the independent variables. The level of significance was set at $p < 0.05$ in all cases.

Results

The fatigue time to reach the 50 per cent of MIVC was 123 s and 98 s for boys and men, respectively. The MVC torque following the fatigue protocol declined significantly for both groups ($F_{(1,18)} = 2137.7$, $p \leq 0.001$; Figure 50.1). During the fatigue protocol there was a significant main effect of age ($F_{(1,18)} = 12.19$, $p \leq 0.01$). The interaction was also statistically significant ($F_{(9,162)} = 7.29$, $p \leq 0.01$). The post hoc test showed that for the men after the 30 per cent of fatigue time, values were significantly differentiated from the initial value. The respective percentage of the boys was the 50 per cent. Between 30 and 50 per cent of the fatigue time, the men showed a higher decline of the torque than boys ($p < 0.05$).

The EMG of MG in maximal isometric plantarflexion declined significantly after the fatigue protocol in both groups ($F_{(1,18)} = 642.95$, $p \leq 0.001$). As far as men are concerned, immediately after the fatigue session EMG values of MG were decreased relative to the pre-fatigue values by 42.39 ± 6.85 per cent. For the boys, the respective EMG values were 37.13 ± 6.86 per cent. Nonetheless, the post hoc test revealed no significant differences between men and

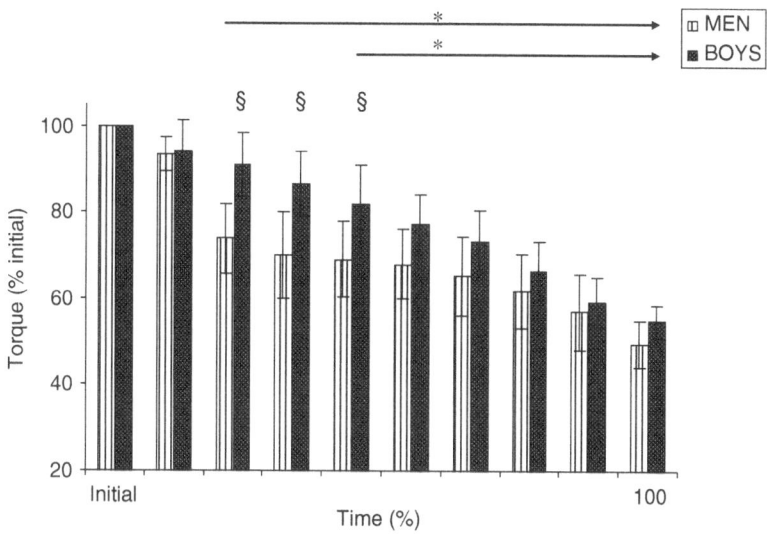

Figure 50.1 Torque decrease during fatigue test (*significant difference within group, § significant differences between groups).

boys ($p > 0.05$). However, during the fatigue protocol all subjects showed a decrease in the EMG amplitude of MG ($F_{(9,162)} = 154.36, p \leq 0.001$). There was also a significant main effect for age ($F_{(1,18)} = 8.15, p \leq 0.05$) and a statistically significant interaction MG ($F_{(9,162)} = 5.89, p \leq 0.01$). More specifically, the EMG of MG decreased by 41.97 ± 6.16 per cent and 42.82 ± 7.35 per cent for men and boys, respectively. Additionally, the EMG values were significantly differentiated from the initial ones after 30 per cent of fatigue protocol duration for the men and 60 per cent for the boys. Between 30–50 per cent of the fatigue time the men showed a higher decline of the MG EMG compared to boys ($p < 0.05$).

Similar to the agonist muscles activation was the coactivation of TA as well. The EMG values showed significant decrease after the fatigue session ($F_{(1,18)} = 26.12, p \leq 0.01$). More specifically, the values were 82.97 ± 9.25 per cent and 85.52 ± 7.90 per cent of pre-fatigue ones in men and boys, respectively ($p > 0.05$). Also in this case, the Scheffè post hoc test revealed no significant differences between genders. The coactivation of the TA decreased gradually, becoming significantly lower ($F_{(9,162)} = 80.54, p \leq 0.001$) from the initial value in the 60 per cent and 80 per cent of fatigue time for men and boys, respectively.

The VMA values also decreased statistically after the fatigue session ($F_{(1,18)} = 144.45, p \leq 0.001$). Also in this case, the Scheffè post hoc test revealed no significant differences between age groups ($p > 0.05$).

Discussion

The present study showed that, during a maximal sustained contraction test, fatigue was higher in adults. The agonist activity decreased to a higher extent in adults. Antagonist activity was decreased in both groups without significant differences between them. No differences were found in the decrease of voluntary activation while the maximal evoked torque decreased more in adults.

The higher fatigability in adults after a maximal sustained contraction was also shown in a previous study (Halin *et al.*, 2003) and it was attributed mainly to a higher inhibition of the agonist activity which is also shown in the present study and especially with fast motor units.

The coactivation decrease could be explained by the torque decrease. It is well known that antagonist activity contributes to joint stabilization (Solomonow *et al.*, 1987) opposing agonist joint torque. Consequently, when the agonist torque decreases then the strain in the joint decreases as well and thus there is no specific reason for the antagonist activity to remain constant. Therefore, it is normal consequence to decrease.

The maximal voluntary activation decreased to the same extent in both of the two groups. This finding is supported by previous studies as well (Kent-Braun, 1999) and indicates that contribution of the central neuronal mechanism to fatigue is equal between the selected groups.

The findings of this study indicate that the higher fatigue occurrence in adults compared to boys was not caused by the central nervous system or by the agonist activity. Hence, this difference could be attributed to muscular factors.

References

Halin, R., Germain, P., Bercier, S., Kapitaniak, B. and Buttelli, O., 2003, Neuromuscular response of young boys versus men during sustained maximal contraction. *Medicine and Science in Sports and Exercise*, **35**, pp. 1042–1048.

Kent-Braun, J., 1999, Central and contributions to muscle fatigue in humans during sustained maximal effort. *European Journal of Applied Physiology*, **80**, pp. 57–63.

Paraschos, I., Hasani, A., Hatzikotoulas, K., Patikas, D. and Kotzamanidis, C., 2007, Differences in neuromuscular activation between adults and prepubertal males during maximal isokinetic knee extension fatigue test. *International Journal of Sports Medicine*, **28**, pp. 958–963.

Ratel, S., Duche, P. and Williams, C., 2006, Muscle fatigue during high-intensity exercise in children. *Sports Medicine*, **36**, pp. 1031–1065.

Solomonow, M.R., Baratta, R.V., Zhou, B.H., Shoji, H., Bose, W., Beck, C. and D'Ambrosia, R., 1987, The synergistic action of the ACL and thigh muscles in maintaining joint stability. *American Journal of Sports Medicine*, **15**, pp. 207–213.

51 Differences in voluntary activation between adult and prepubertal males

K. Hatzikotoulas, D. Patikas, E. Bassa, I. Paraschos and C. Kotzamanidis

Department of Physical Education and Sports Science, Aristotle University of Thessaloniki, Greece

Introduction

The strength increase during developmental ages is affected by various factors such as neuronal, hormonal and biomechanical and these factors cause the appropriate structural and functional adaptations for the strength gain (Blimkie, 1989).

Relevant studies have shown that absolute strength is higher in adults compared to children but this is not the case for the relative torque where in other cases it was higher in adults and in others equal between them (Fukunaga *et al.*, 1995). The activation issue during maximal voluntary conctraction (MVC) has not been analyzed extensively in children. Specifically, the agonist activity has been investigated (Grosset *et al.*, 2006) with no differences observed between children and adults. Regarding the activity of the antagonist muscles, the coactivation was analyzed during isokinetic (Bassa *et al.*, 2005) and isometric contraction (Grosset *et al.*, 2006) giving conflicting results. Specifically, in the first case no differences were observed between groups, while in the second one children presented higher coactivation.

Furthermore, only a few studies have investigated the differences in voluntary activation in children. To our knowledge only Belanger and McComas (1989) investigated the differences between children and pubertal boys. According to this study, boys activated their motor units to a lesser extent compared with adults. However, in their study they chose children with no homogenous age and specifically from 6–13 years old and it is well accepted that there are big differences in the exerted torque among the mentioned ages, which possibly contaminates the reported results.

For this reason the purpose of this study was to re-examine the differences in the relative torque, agonist, antagonist activity and voluntary activation between children and adults.

Methods

Ten untrained, healthy boys (mean ± SD age: 10.9 ± 0.8 y, body mass: 43.1 ± 10.9 kg, height: 150.1 ± 7.7 cm) and men (age: 25.4 ± 1.9 y, body mass: 74.9 ± 7.8 kg, height: 180.4 ± 6.3 cm) volunteered to participate in this study. The subjects were informed of the purpose and measurements of this study prior to the test. Written informed consent forms were completed by all subjects. As far as boys were concerned, their parents were informed about the purpose of the experimental procedure prior to the test and parental written consent was given in all cases. The experimental procedure was performed according to the ethical rules of the Aristotle University of Thessaloniki.

A Cybex Norm dynamometer (Cybex division of Lumex, Ronkonkoma, NY) was employed to determine maximal isometric voluntary contraction (MIVC). EMG activity from soleus (Sol), medial gastrocnemius (MG) and tibialis anterior (TA) muscles was recorded using the device teleEMG of BTS (Bioengineering Milano, Italy).

Supramaximal electrical stimulation was applied to the posterior tibial nerve for voluntary muscle activation (VMA) estimation, delivered by DSA7H, Digitimer stimulator. The maximal amplitude of the M-wave was used as a criterion for determining the supramaximal intensity of the stimulus and normalization of EMG signals.

All tests were performed from a seated position (hip flexion angle of $170°$) with the knee fully extended ($0°$) and the ankle at the anatomical zero ($90°$). Concerning EMG activity, Sol, MG and TA were selected as representative plantar flexor and dorsal flexor muscles, respectively. On the testing day each participant performed five minutes warm-up on a cycle-ergometer and stretching exercises for the lower limbs muscles. At the beginning of each session, a single stimulus was given at rest for M-wave estimation. The voltage was increased until the M-wave took the maximal amplitude. Then, 3–5 MVC were performed for the plantar flexors and 3–5 for the dorsal flexors on the anatomical zero of the ankle joint. For VMA measurements the Interpolated Twitch Technique (ITT) was used. The level of VMA was calculated as [(voluntary torque − torque with stimulation)/voluntary torque] × 100. Visual feedback of the torque output and verbal encouragement was provided during the whole experimental session.

Statistical analysis

Results are presented as mean values and standard deviation of mean (SD). The analyzed independent variable was the age (adult-prepubertal). The analyzed dependent variables were the torque, the normalized torque (peak torque/body mass), the EMG of MG and Sol, the coactivation of TA and the level of activation (VMA). Analysis of t-tests for independent samples was used for the statistical data analysis. The level of significance was set at $p < 0.05$.

Results

The t-test showed that men (187.20 ± 27.06 Nm) had higher peak torque output ($t = 8.89$, $p < 0.001$) than boys (95.30 ± 18.32 Nm). The main effect for age

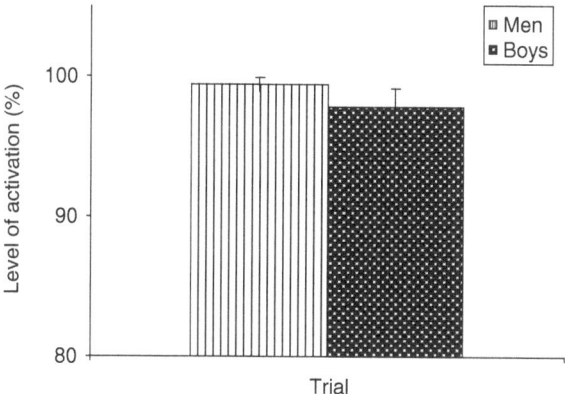

Figure 51.1 Differences between men and boys during maximal voluntary activation.

was also statistically significant ($t = 7.19$, $p < 0.01$) concerning torque/body mass ratio, with adults (2.47 ± 0.29 Nm·kg^{-1}) having a higher ratio than prepubertal (1.73 ± 0.15 Nm·kg^{-1}).

No significant differences in agonist EMG were found among the groups ($p > 0.05$). In contrast, the antagonistic EMG activity of the TA was significantly affected by age ($t = 2.84$, $p < 0.05$). More specifically, the coactivation was 0.13 ± 0.05 mV and 0.25 ± 0.01 mV for men and boys, respectively.

As far as VMA concerns (Figure 51.1) the results showed that did not differ significantly ($p > 0.05$) between men (99.4 ± 1.5 per cent) and boys (97.8 ± 1.3 per cent).

Discussion

The main findings of this study were that children exerted lower absolute and relative torque, higher coactivation but equal VMA. The higher absolute torque in adults is well documented by previous studies and it was attributed both in neuronal and morphological factors (Blimkie, 1989). The difference in relative torque between children and adults is a conflicting issue, showing higher values for adults (Fukunaga *et al.*, 1995) or equal to children (Pääsuke *et al.*, 2000). It seems that the estimation of relative torque is affected by many factors, such as the applied methodology, the joint angle, the muscle group and the gender (Fukunaga *et al.*, 1995). The obtained results are in agreement with previous studies which examined the relative torque in the same gender, joint angle, muscle group and muscle action (Fukunaga *et al.*, 1995).

The antagonist activity is controlled mainly by spinal and supraspinal mechanisms (Lévénez *et al.*, 2005). However, it has not been investigated until now to what extent the coactivation was involved in the obtained results of the present study. There are not many studies which have investigated this issue during maximal isometric voluntary contraction in children. In a previous study, related with maximal isokinetic contraction, it was found that coactivation was equal between prepubertal children and adults (Bassa *et al.*, 2005). However, during maximal isometric contraction the coactivation was higher in children (Grosset *et al.*, 2006), a fact which indirectly supports our data. Nonetheless, for this issue further investigation is required.

The voluntary activation was examined until now only by Belanger and McComas (1989). In this study the voluntary activation of children aged from 6–13 years old was found to be lower than pubertal boys. Nevertheless, selecting boys of similar age (9–12 y) as in the present study, it was found that five out of six children were able fully to activate their motor units and the other one only by 85 per cent. This indicates that, for the plantar flexor muscles, prepubertal children and adults are able to activate their motor units to the same extent as do adults. The basic explanation for that could be the findings from previous studies that the corticospinal track has been matured since early childhood (Fietzek *et al.*, 2000).

The present finding indicates that voluntary activation is equal for children and adults at least concerning the plantar flexor muscles. However, this case has not been well studied and needs further research, especially for other joint muscles.

References

Bassa, H., Patikas, D. and Kotzamanidis, C., 2004, Activation of antagonist knee muscles during isokinetic efforts in prepubertal and adult males. *Pediatric Exercise Science*, **17**, pp. 65–75.

Belanger, A. and McComas, A., 1989, Contractile properties of human skeletal muscle in childhood and adolescence. *European Journal of Applied Physiology*, **58**, pp. 563–567.

Grosset, J., Mora, I., Lambertz, D. and Perot, C., 2008, Voluntary activation of the triceps surae in prepubertal children. *Journal of Electromyography and Kinesiology*, **18**, pp. 455–465.

Fietzek, U., Heinen, F., Berweck, S., Maute, S., Hufschmidt, A., Schulte-Monting, J., Lucking, C. and Korinthenberg, R., 2000, Development of the corticospinal system and hand motor function: Central times and motor performance tests. *Developmental Medicine and Child Neurology*, **42**, pp. 220–227.

Kanehisa, H., Yata, S., Ikegawa, S. and Fukunaga, T., 1995, A cross-sectional study of the size and strength of the lower leg muscles during growth. *European Journal of Applied Physiology*, **72**, pp. 150–156.

Lévénez, M., Kotzamanidis, C., Carpentier, A. and Duchateau, J., 2005, Spinal reflexes and coactivation of ankle muscles during a submaximal fatiguing contraction. *Journal of Applied Physiology*, **99**, pp. 1182–1188.

Pääsuke, M., Ereline, J. and Gapeyeva, H., 2000, Twitch contraction properties of plantar flexor muscles in pre- and post-pubertal boys and men. *European Journal of Applied Physiology*, **82**, pp. 459–464.

52 Perceived and measured fatigue of lumbar muscles in young competitive swimmers, fin swimmers and master swimmers

A. Cicchella[1,2] *and A.M. Bassi*[1]

[1]Faculty of Exercise and Sport Sciences; [2]Department of Psychology, University of Bologna, Italy

Introduction

One outcome of the high physical demands of sport training is joint pathologies, and among these back pain (Johnson, 1993). Training hours in young swimmers can be up to 30 hours per week during peak training periods, and this can lead to injuries.

A limited number of studies on the relation between back pain epidemiology and fatigue in swimming exist (Goldstein *et al.*, 1991). Our aim in the present study was to determine differences in lumbar muscle endurance and objective and perceived fatigue levels between different groups of aquatic sports athletes (competitive, masters and fin swimmers). In particular we hypothesized that the fin swimmers would show less fatigue and lower objective and subjective pain levels than competitive and master swimmers.

Methods

Competitive athletes ($n = 64$) performed a modified Biering-Sorensen Test consisting of holding the trunk suspended for one minute at hip level in the horizontal position laying supine on a bench with the leg secured (Latimer *et al.*, 1999). A total of 64 athletes were tested; 31 competitive swimmers, 16 female (mean age 14.9, range 13–19 y) and 15 male (mean age 16.8, range 14–24 y), 15 master swimmers, five female (mean age 32.4, range 27–36 y) and 10 male (mean age 25.6, range 21–43 y), and 18 fin swimmers, seven female (mean age 14.0, range 12–18 y) and 11 male (mean age 16.5, range 13–18 y).

Surface EMG (SEMG) was recorded from the erector spinae muscle with bipolar surface disc electrodes at L1–L2 level monolaterally, in accord with the international norms for SEMG studies. The raw EMG signal was detected with a sampling frequency of 1000 Hz. The system used was a ME3000P portable surface

EMG system (Mega Electronics, Finland) and stored in a computer for subsequent analysis (Elfving et al., 1999).

Median frequency of the power spectrum of surface EMG was extracted with progressive single spectrum Fast Fourier Transform algorhythm (FFT). Prior to FFT, a flat-topped window of 1024 points with 50 per cent overlap on the raw EMG signal was used (Hagg, 1992).

Regression analysis was made over one minute, and the intercept of the regression line at time zero was used as the initial median frequency. The slope ($Hz \cdot min^{-1}$) was normalized to percent per minute. All the calculations were performed using the software Megawin (v.2.14, Mega Electronics, Finland). Borg (1998) RPE (rate of perceived exertion) has been validated with EMG and used previously with swimmers (Wolff, 2000). We adopted the CR-10 version (Italian language). Immediately after the Sorensen test, the subjects were asked to rank the perceived exertion.

Measurement of S-EMG began immediately after the subjects reached the horizontal position. Statistical analysis was performed by means of t-test for independent samples with the SPSS v.14.0 Statistical Package (SPSS Inc., Chicago, IL.).

Results

EMG decline per minute is shown in Table 52.1.

A significant difference (Student $t = 4.651, p = 0.010$,[a]) in MF-SEMG decline percentage was found between female competitive swimmers and female master swimmers, the master swimmers having less fatigue. This result is consistent with findings in normal populations – a better lumbar muscle endurance was found in older females. A significant difference in MF-SEMG decline was found ($t = 2.904, p = 0.027$[b]) between female competitive swimmers and female fin swimmers, showing the female fin swimmers had a better endurance of lumbar muscles. For the Borg scale scoring (Table 52.2), significant differences ($t = 2.6, p = 0.048$[c]) were found between male fin swimmers and male master swimmers. The male fin swimmers thus seem to better tolerate fatigue localized at the lumbar muscles. Our results are in accordance with those of Dedering et al. (2000).

Table 52.1 Surface EMG median frequency decay (% per minute)

	Competitive swimmers (n = 31, 16♀15 ♂)	Master swimmers (n = 15, 5♀10 ♂)	Fin swimmers (n = 18, 7♀11 ♂)
Male	−20.5 (−5.8/30.0)	−22.4 (−8.4/−39.2)	−24.5 (−14.8/−37.8)
Female	−22.8 (−4.8/−40.1)	−17.1*[a] (−10.5/−28.3)	−10.0*[b] (−4.9/−19.1)

*[a] Significant difference ($p = 0.010$) between female competitive and master swimmers.
*[b] Significant difference ($p = 0.027$) between female competitive and fin smimmers.

Table 52.2 Borg CR-10 rating of perceived exertion

	Competitive swimmers (n = 31, 16♀15♂)	Master swimmers (n = 15, 5♀10♂)	Fin swimmers (n = 18, 7♀11♂)
Male	12.6 (8–17)	11.5 (8–15)	9.5 (8–11)*c
Female	11.7 (7–15)	11.0 (7–13)	12.0 (11–13)

*c Significant difference ($p = 0.048$) between male fin and master swimmers.

Discussion

Age seems to be a major determinant in the perception of local lumbar muscle fatigue in females, as shown by the comparison among the young female swimmers and female master swimmers.

Another finding of this study was that the male fin swimmers showed differences from the master swimmers in objective and perceived fatigue.

A possible hypothesis for the differences found in the Borg scale between male fin swimmers and male master swimmers is the specificity of movements performed by fin swimmers, with the lumbar muscles of these athletes better trained than other athletes as a consequence of the adaptation induced by the specific movement of fin swimming which involves massive lumbar muscle.

Conclusions

Swimmers often report lumbar pain (Goldstein, 1991). The relationship between measured (SEMG) and reported (Borg) effort of the lumbar muscles was presented. The age of the female swimmers is a major determinant of measured fatigue of lumbar muscles – young female fin swimmers show values similar to female master swimmers. Young male fin swimmers show less sensitivity to perceived lumbar fatigue, probably due to the adaptation induced by the lumbar motion of fin swimming.

References

Borg, G., 1998, *Borg's Perceived Exertion and Pain Scales*. Champaign IL: Human Kinetics.

Dedering, A., Ross, A.F., Hjelmsater, M., Elfving, B., Harms-Ringdahl, K. and Nemeth, G., 2000, Between-days reliability of subjective and objective assessment of back extensor muscle fatigue in subjects without lower-back pain. *Journal of Electromyography and Kinesiology*, **10**, pp. 151–158.

Elfving, B., Nemeth, G., Arvidsson, I. and Lamontagne, M., 1999, Reliability of EMG spectral parameters in repeated measurements of back muscle fatigue. *Journal of Electromyography and Kinesiology*, **17**, pp. 235–243.

Goldstein, J.D., Berger, P.E., Windler, G.E. and Jackson, D.W., 1991, Spine injuries in gymnasts and swimmers. An epidemiologic investigation. *American Journal of Sports Medicine*, **19**, pp. 463–468.

Hagg, G., 1992, Interpretation of EMG spectral alterations and alteration indexes at sustained contraction. *Journal of Applied Physiology*, **73**, pp. 1211–1217.

Johnson, R.J., 1993, Low back pain in sports. *The Physician and Sports Medicine*, **21**, pp. 53–59.

Latimer, J., Maher, C.G., Refshauge, K. and Colaco, I., 1999, The reliability and validity of the Biering-Sorensen test in asymptomatic subjects and subjects reporting current or previous non-specific low back pain. *Spine*, **24**, pp. 2085–2089.

Wolff, G.M., 2000, The relationship of the Borg rate of perceived exertion (RPE) scale and Borg category-ratio scale (CR-10) to mechanical and physiological intensity of untethered freestyle swimming in trained swimmers. Thesis (MS Ed)-Northern Illinois University. Eugene: Microform Publications, University of Oregon.

53 Isometric contraction differentiation in 12–15-year-old boys and girls

G. *Knipshe*[1] *and L. Cupriks*[2]

[1]University of Latvia; [2]Latvian Academy of Sport Education, Riga, Latvia

Introduction

Human movements and their results depend on various factors. One of these is the work of muscles making a dynamic structure of movement act (Brown, 2000). The second one is the fact that isometric contraction is present in every movement or every physical action. A man is always aware of movement regulation with the help of the only directly regulating force – muscle dynamic force. However, muscle co-ordination mainly depends on muscle tension co-ordination, which occurs in separate muscle group tension and action duration control, which leads to the most optimal execution of movement. The aim of this research was to investigate the differentiation of isometric contraction – how the ability to evaluate muscle tension at the load of 25 per cent, 50 per cent and 75 per cent of the maximal training load changes in different movements (flexion and extension) in 12–15-year-old boys and girls. Separate muscle groups (upper arm and forearm, trunk, thigh, calf flexors and extensors) were analysed.

Methods

Forty-five boys and 40 girls aged 12–15 years attending state schools took part in the research. The isokinetic dynamometer (REV 9000) in isometric measurement mode was used in the research. The test included: muscle stretching (5 min), warming-up free movements (8 min), and a special warm-up using the isokinetic device (3 min). The measurement of muscles' flexion – extension movements was done in the following conditions: for leg muscles the regime in knee joint was at an angle of 90°, in the hip joint at an angle of 70°; for trunk muscles at an angle of 70°; for arm muscles in the elbow joint at an angle of 50° (Orlovsky, 1972; Murray *et al.*, 1978; Brown, 2000).

Results and discussion

The results of the study are shown in Table 53.1 and Figures 53.1 and 53.2. As the analysis of the results shows the repetition accuracy at the load of 25 per cent of the maximal training load is higher with some muscle groups in 13-year-old

Table 53.1 Summary parameters of isometric contraction differentiation in
12–15-year-old boys and girls

Muscle groups		Summary mistakes (%)									
		Forearm		Upper arm		Trunk		Thigh		Calf	
Age	Sex	flex	ext	flex	ext	flex	ext	flex	ext	flex	ext
12 year	boys	40.4	36.1	34.5	40.5	43.1	35.0	41.9	33.3	47.2	36.0
	girls	40.0	35.2	35.6	40.0	41.3	35.2	40.9	33.0	45.9	36.1
13 year	boys	37.6	37.9	33.4	43.2	38.7	33.9	40.1	31.2	40.9	35.3
	girls	38.2	37.6	31.2	40.0	39.9	34.4	40.0	32.3	43.3	36.0
14 year	boys	32.5	35.0	32.0	34.6	33.7	28.9	38.5	28.5	38.2	28.5
	girls	35.3	36.0	32.6	36.2	36.2	30.2	39.3	30.0	40.7	34.0
15 year	boys	30.1	31.2	30.0	31.7	29.8	27.8	35.5	26.8	38.5	31.5
	girls	30.1	30.1	31.4	33.6	32.7	30.2	37.1	37.1	28.3	32.5

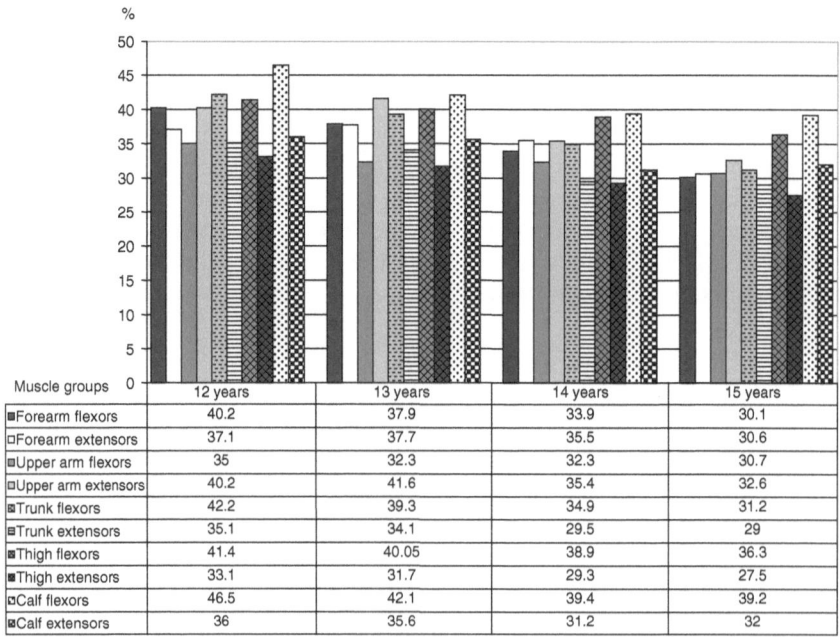

Figure 53.1 Isometric contraction differentiation in 12–15-year-old boys and girls (%).

boys in comparison with 12-year-old boys. For other muscle groups the accuracy
variations were not significant and did not exceed 2 per cent. The muscle tension
accuracy was improved significantly in the trunk, thigh and upper arm flexors and
thigh extensors in 15-year-old boys in comparison with 14-year-old boys. In the
girls starting from 12 years in all age groups, the repetition accuracy at a load

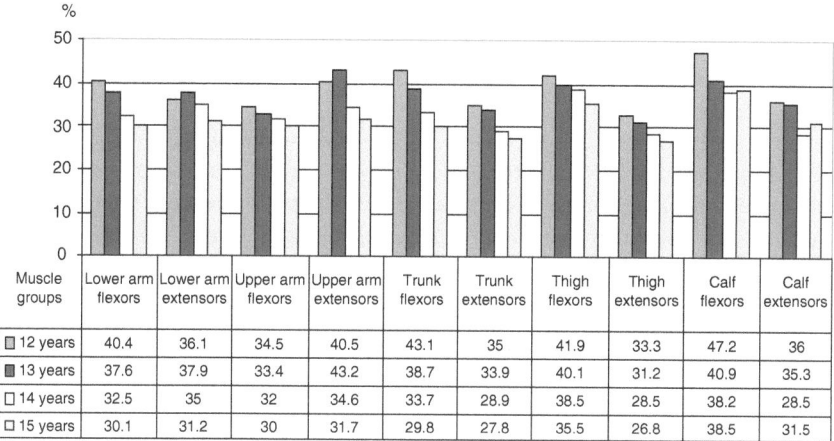

Muscle groups	Lower arm flexors	Lower arm extensors	Upper arm flexors	Upper arm extensors	Trunk flexors	Trunk extensors	Thigh flexors	Thigh extensors	Calf flexors	Calf extensors
☐ 12 years	40.4	36.1	34.5	40.5	43.1	35	41.9	33.3	47.2	36
■ 13 years	37.6	37.9	33.4	43.2	38.7	33.9	40.1	31.2	40.9	35.3
☐ 14 years	32.5	35	32	34.6	33.7	28.9	38.5	28.5	38.2	28.5
☐ 15 years	30.1	31.2	30	31.7	29.8	27.8	35.5	26.8	38.5	31.5

Figure 53.2 Changes of muscle isometric contraction in 12–15-year-old boys.

of 25 per cent of the maximal training load in all muscle groups (especially in upper arm flexors and trunk extensors) was higher than in the same aged boys, but starting with the 14-year-olds this difference between boys and girls disappeared. Thus, having analysed the accuracy results of the execution at 25 per cent load at different ages, we can conclude that some muscle groups (the forearm, upper arm, calf and trunk flexors) increase with age in both genders, but at the age of 13 years the indices of these muscle groups decrease, followed by a significant increase at the age of 14 years.

Having analysed the muscle tension differentiation results at 50 per cent of maximum training load, more precise evaluation of muscle tension was observed in 13-year-old boys in comparison with 12-year-old boys. The accuracy of muscle tension control of the forearm, upper arm, trunk flexors, and forearm and thigh extensors was improved significantly. For 14-year-olds in comparison with 13-year-old boys the accuracy of evaluation of muscle tension of the upper arm, thigh and calf extensors and calf flexors changed significantly. At the age of 15 years a significant improvement of muscle tension differentiation was observed in trunk flexors and extensors. For other muscle groups the changes were not significant.

The analysis of the results of muscle tension differentiation at 75 per cent of maximum training load showed that, as children become older, the accuracy increases, however for functionally different muscle groups the increase is not simultaneous. At the age of 12 years the muscle tension differentiation of the trunk, upper arm and thigh extensors improves significantly. In other muscle groups there is a very small increase and the indices are lower for 13-year-old boys in comparison with 12-year olds. At 75 per cent of maximum training load all the results, both for the flexors and extensors, are higher for 14-year-old boys. At the age of 15, in comparison with 14 years, the degree of muscle tension differentiation does not increase or there is a slight difference. Having analysed the data we can say that the ability to repeat exact muscle tension correctly is characterised by the summary index of the parameters' accuracy, which includes the sum of mistakes in muscle isometric contraction differentiation at loads of 25 per cent, 50 per cent and 75 per cent of the maximal load.

Comparing the 12-year-old boys with the 13-year-old ones, 13-year-old boys have lower indices of muscle tension differentiation only in two cases (forearm and upper arm extensors). The accuracy of load evaluation of other muscle groups increases alongside the age. Moreover, the best muscle tension control is noticed in the forearm and thigh flexors in both genders. At the age of 14 years the indices of all investigated muscle group tensions increase; at the age of 15 years the accuracy of load evaluation of upper arm, trunk and thigh flexor increases. In increases of the other muscle tension control differentiation is not significant at this age, but the parameters of separate muscle groups are lower even than at the age of 13–14 years (calf flexors and extensors).

Having analysed the changes of flexors differentiation summary indices, it should be said that the biggest accuracy of load evaluation was observed at the age of 14 for the boys and at the age of 12 for the girls. Thus, comparing the summary indices of the increase that characterise the tension differentiation accuracy of all investigated muscle groups, it should be stated that, at the age of 13 and 15 y, they are practically equal, but for whole research at muscle differentiation loads of 25 per cent, 50 per cent and 75 per cent of the maximum training load, we can conclude that alongside the age the isometric contraction differentiation accuracy increases.

References

Brown, L.E., 2000, *Isokinetics in Human Performance*. Champaign, IL: Human Kinetics, pp. 149–377.

Murray, M., Guten, G.N., Sepic, S.B., Gardner, G.M. and Baldwin, I.M., 1978, Function of the triceps surae during gait. Compensatory mechanisms for unilateral loss. *Journal of Bone Joint Surgery*, **60**, pp. 412–419.

Orlovsky, G.N., 1972, The effect of different descending systems on flexor and extensor activity during locomotion. *Brain Research*, **46**, pp. 156–166.

54 Contractile properties of plantarflexor muscles in pre- and post-pubertal girls

M. Pääsuke,[1,2] J. Ereline,[1,2] H. Gapeyeva[1,2] and T. Kums[1]

[1]Institute of Exercise Biology and Physiotherapy; [2]Estonian Centre of Behavioural and Health Sciences, University of Tartu, Tartu, Estonia

Introduction

Skeletal muscles undergo both structural and functional changes with puberty. The majority of related studies have focused on changes in the voluntary force generating capacity of different muscle groups. Fewer studies have assessed changes in electrically evoked twitch contractile properties of human muscles that occur during puberty. It has been indicated that twitch peak torque (Pt) in post-pubertal compared with pre-pubertal children is significantly greater (Belanger and McComas, 1989; Pääsuke et al., 2000). Belanger and McComas (1989) have reported higher post-activation potentiation (PAP) of twitch Pt in pre- compared with post-pubertal children in dorsiflexor muscles, whereas these authors and our previous study (Pääsuke et al., 2000) indicated no significant differences in PAP between these children in plantarflexor (PF) muscles. Davies (1985) reported that in 14-year-old boys the twitch contraction (CT) and half-relaxation (HRT) time of the PF muscles have been shown to be shorter compared with 11-year-old boys, whereas Belanger and McComas (1989) have reported a prolongation of twitch CT and HRT of the dorsiflexor muscles in post-pubertal compared with pre-pubertal boys. Our previous study indicated no differences in twitch CT and HRT in pre- and post-pubertal boys (Pääsuke et al., 2000). Thus, the question of changes in twitch contraction characteristics and PAP with puberty is not yet clear.

The aim of this study was to compare force generating and potentiation capacity, and time-course characteristics of the isometric twitch in pre- and post-pubertal girls. Recordings were made from the PF muscles that are involved in many everyday work and sporting activities.

Methods

Subjects

Sixteen pre-pubertal (9–10 years old) and 15 post-pubertal (16 years old) healthy girls participated in this study. Pubertal stages were determined according to the criteria of Tanner by a paediatrician of the same gender as the subjects. All 9–10-year-old girls were in Tanner stage 1 and all 16-year-old girls were in Tanner stage 5 and they were classified as pre-pubertal from the appearance of their breast development and pubic hair. All the subjects were informed of the procedures, informed parental consent was obtained prior to the pre-pubertal children's participation in the experiment, and the post-pubertal girls gave written informed consent. The study carried the approval of the University Ethics Commitee. The anthropometric parameters and isometric maximal voluntary contraction (MVC) torque characteristics of the subjects are presented in Table 54.1.

Apparatus

During the experiment the subjects were seated in a custom-made dynamometer with the dominant leg flexed 90° at the knee and ankle angles, and mounted inside a metal frame. The foot was strapped to an aluminium foot plate. The inclination of the foot could be altered by rotating the foot plate about an axis that corresponded to that of the ankle joint, i.e. the medial malleolus. Torques acting on the foot plate were sensed by a standard strain-gauge transducer (DST, Russia) connected with the foot plate. The point of application of force to the foot plate was located on articulation regions between the metatarsus and ossa digitorum pedis. The force signals were sampled at a frequency of 1 kHz and stored on a hard disk for further analysis.

Electrical stimulation

The posterior tibial nerve was stimulated through a pair of 2-mm-thick, self-adhesive surface electrodes (Medicompex SA, Ecublens, Switzerland). The cathode (5 × 5 cm) was placed over the tibial nerve in popliteal fossa and anode (5 × 10 cm) was placed 2–3 cm proximally to the patella. Supramaximal square wave pulses of 1ms duration were delivered from an isolated voltage stimulator Medicor MG-440 (Budapest, Hungary) and were controlled by M-wave amplitude of the soleus muscle. Three maximal isometric twitches of the PF muscles were

Table 54.1 Mean (±SE) anthropometric parameters and isometric maximal voluntary contraction (MVC) torque of the plantarflexor muscles of the subjects

Parameter	Pre-pubertal girls (n = 16)	Post-pubertal girls (n = 15)
Age (years)	10.3 ± 0.1	16.1 ± 0.1*
Height (cm)	146.5 ± 1.8	166.9 ± 1.6*
Body mass (kg)	38.4 ± 2.3	57.4 ± 1.3*
Body mass index (kg m^{-2})	17.8 ± 0.9	20.6 ± 0.4*
MVC torque (Nm)	105.9 ± 7.9	222.1 ± 9.1*
MVC torque: Body mass (Nm kg^{-1})	2.8 ± 0.2	3.9 ± 0.2*

*$p < 0.05$ compared with pre-pubertal girls.

elicited, and 2 min after the last resting twitch was recorded, the subjects were instructed to make a 5 s conditioning MVC and then to relax. Postactivation twitch was elicited within 2 s after the onset of relaxation. The subjects performed three isometric MVCs of the PF, pushing the foot plate as forcefully as possible for 2–3 s. The greatest torque of the three maximal efforts was taken as the isometric MVC torque.

Measurements

The following characteristics of resting isometric twitch were calculated: peak torque (Pt) – the highest value of isometric torque production; contraction time (CT) – the time to twitch maximal torque; half-relaxation time (HRT) – the time of half of the decline in twitch maximal torque, maximal rate of torque development (RD) – the peak value of the first derivate of the development of torque (dF/dt) and maximal rate of relaxation (RR) as the first derivate of the decline of torque (−dF/dt). The percentage increase in post-activation twitch Pt in relation to resting twitch was taken as an indicator of PAP. The resting twitch contraction Pt was expressed in ratio with the MVC torque force (Pt:MVC torque) in per cent. The MVC torque was calculated in relation to body mass of the subjects (MVC torque:BM).

Statistics

Data are expressed as means and standard errors (±SE). One-way analysis of variance (ANOVA) followed by Scheffé post hoc comparisons were used to test for differences between groups. A level of $p < 0.05$ was selected to indicate statistical significance.

Results

Results are presented in Table 54.2. Post-pubertal girls had a greater ($p < 0.05$) MVC torque and MVC torque:BM ratio as compared to pre-pubertal girls. Twitch Pt, RD and RR were also greater ($p < 0.05$) in post-pubertal compared with pre-pubertal girls. No significant differences in Pt:MVC torque ratio, twitch PAP, and CT and HRT were observed between the measured groups.

Discussion

The present results illustrate differences in twitch contractile properties of the PF muscles in pre- and post-pubertal girls, knowing that an evoked twitch provides information of changes in muscle properties independently of volition or central motor control mechanisms. A significantly greater resting twitch Pt, RD and RR was observed in post-pubertal compared with pre-pubertal girls. It can be associated with several morphological, histological and biochemical differences between immature and mature muscles: the diameters of muscle fibres continue to

Table 54.2 Mean (±SE) twitch contractile characteristics of the plantarflexor muscles in pre- and post-pubertal girls

Parameter	Pre-pubertal girls (n = 16)	Post-pubertal girls (n = 15)
Pt (Nm)	17.0 ± 1.1	26.0 ± 1.6*
Pt:MVC torque (%)	16.1 ± 3.6	11.7 ± 3.7
PAP (%)	122.8 ± 5.6	126.1 ± 4.6
RD (Nm·s^{-1})	260.4 ± 18.8	399.2 ± 19.7*
RR (Nm·s^{-1})	160.8 ± 13.7	264.8 ± 16.1*
CT (ms)	97.1 ± 4.0	105.3 ± 3.2
HRT (ms)	75.4 ± 3.6	80.4 ± 3.5

Pt – peak torque; MVC – maximal voluntary contraction; PAP – post-activation potentiation; RD – maximal rate of torque development; RR – maximal rate of relaxation; CT – contraction time; HRT – half-relaxation time. (*$p < 0.05$ compared with pre-pubertal girls.)

increase until growth is complete, the number of sarcomeres increases and muscles become longer with growth, the sarcoplasmic reticulum (SR) protein yield, ATP-dependent Ca^{2+} binding and uptake activity increase due to maturation. One major finding of this study was that there are no significant differences in PAP of the PF muscles between the pre- and post-pubertal girls. The mechanism of PAP is considered to be phosphorylation of myosin regulatory light chains via myosin light chain kinase during the conditioning contraction, which renders actin-myosin more sensitive to Ca^{2+} released from SR in a subsequent twitch and thereby enhances the force of the twitch contraction (Grange *et al.*, 1993), which seems to be highly developed prior to puberty. No significant differences in time-course characteristics of isometric twitch of the PF muscles were observed between the pre- and post-pubertal girls. Similar results have been published previously Gosset *et al.*, (2005). The time-course of isometric twitches is probably highly dependent on the kinetics of excitation-contraction coupling, including intracellular Ca^{2+} movements (Klug *et al.*, 1988).

It was concluded that puberty in girls is characterized by increased voluntary and electrically evoked force-generating capacity of PF muscles with no changes in PAP and time-course characteristics of isometric twitch.

References

Belanger, A.Y. and McComas, A.J., 1989, Contractile properties of human skeletal muscle in childhood and adolescence. *European Journal of Applied Physiology*, **58**, pp. 563–567.

Davies, C.T.M., 1985, Strength and mechanical properties of muscle in children and young adults. *Scandinavian Journal of Sports Sciences*, **7**, pp. 11–15.

Grange, R.W., Vandenboom, R. and Houston, M.E., 1993, Physiological significance of myosin phosphorylation in skeletal muscle. *Canadian Journal of Applied Physiology*, **18**, pp. 229–242.

Grosset, J.-F., Mora, I., Lambertz, D. and Perot, C., 2005, Age-related changes in pre-pubertal children. *Pediatric Research*, **58**, 966–970.

Klug, G.A., Leberer, E., Leisner, E., Simoneau, J.A. and Pette, D., 1988, Relationship between parvalbumin content and the speed of relaxation in chronically stimulated rabbit fast twitch muscle. *Pflügers Archives*, **411**, pp. 126–131.

Pääsuke, M., Ereline, J. and Gapeyeva, H., 2000, Twitch contraction properties of plantar flexor muscles in pre- and post-pubertal boys and men. *European Journal of Applied Physiology*, **82**, pp. 459–464.

55 Muscle force and activation pattern of boys vs men in isometric elbow flexion and extension

C. Usselman, D. Gabriel, R. Dotan, L. Brunton, P. Klentrou, J. Shaw and B. Falk
Brock University, St. Catharines, Ontario, Canada

Introduction

Children's muscle function has been shown to be both quantitatively and qualitatively different from that of young adults (Blimkie, 1989). Maximal muscle force is much lower in children, even when normalized to any measure of body size (Sale and Spriet, 1996).

The gain in muscle strength is partially related to an increase in muscle mass (Sale and Spriet, 1996). However, the rate of strength gain exceeds that expected on the basis of the increase in muscle mass. Therefore, additional maturation-related factors related to neuro-motor control most likely explain the increase in muscle strength (Asmussen, 1973).

The purpose of this study was to compare strength, rate of force development and neuron-motor activation between boys and men in a maximal isometric effort.

Methods and measurements

Subjects

Subjects included 16 men (22.1 ± 2.8 years old) and 15 boys (9.6 ± 1.6 years old). All subjects were healthy, physically active but not athletes, and right-hand dominant. None of the subjects participated in any unilateral sports (Table 55.1). Boys were smaller than men in all physical dimensions, including upper arm cross-sectional area, but were not different in body fat percentage.

Protocol

All subjects participated in one habituation session. Following a warm-up, subjects performed 10–15 maximal elbow flexion and extension contractions (MVC), measured isometrically. The order of flexion and extension was randomized. The mean MVC trace was calculated from 8–10 trials from which peak torque and peak rate of force development were calculated.

Table 55.1 Physical characteristics of boys and men. Data are means ± SD

	Men	Boys
Height (cm)	180.9 ± 2.8	137.5 ± 8.7
Mass (kg)	81.7 ± 7.2	32.8 ± 6.9
Body fat (%)	15.8 ± 4.1	16.4 ± 6.2
Lean body mass (kg)	68.7 ± 5.5	27.1 ± 4.6
Upper-arm CSA (cm^2)	69.4 ± 9.0	3.6 ±1.0

CSA = cross-sectional area. (* = significant difference between groups, $p < 0.05$.)

Anthropometry and body composition

Body height, mass and skinfold thicknesses were measured using standardized methods. Adiposity was estimated from skinfold measurements, using age- and maturity-specific equations (Durnin and Wohmersley, 1974; Slaughter *et al.*, 1988). Circumference of the upper arm, along with the skinfold thicknesses over the biceps and triceps were used to calculate upper arm lean cross-sectional area (Gurney and Jelliffe, 1973).

Muscle force

An isokinetic dynamometer (Biodex II, Biodex, Shirley, NY) was used to evaluate peak torque. The dynamometer was individually adjusted for each subject. The warm-up included six contractions, following which subjects were encouraged to exert maximal muscular force (for both flexion and extension). Verbal encouragement and visual feedback of the torque was provided. For a detailed description of the methodology, see Falk *et al.* (2000, 2005).

Force 'explosiveness'

Force explosiveness (rate of torque production) was evaluated using the above setting (Biodex II). Peak rate of elbow-torque change was calculated by taking the maximum of the first derivative of the torque signal (Gabriel *et al.*, 2001).

Neuro-motor control mechanisms

Surface electromyography (EMG) was used to assess muscle activation. The area under the curve in the first 30 ms of the linear envelope of the detected SEMG signal (Q_{30}) is a measure of the rate of muscle activation and was used to assess changes in neural drive (Gabriel and Boucher, 2000). The onset of SEMG relative to the beginning of force production (electro-mechanical delay, EMD) was used to assess muscle timing of both the flexors and extensors (Gabriel and Boucher, 2000).

The EMG activity was recorded with Delsys 2.1 (Delsys Inc., Boston, MA) bipolar surface electrodes, band-passed filtered (20–450 Hz) using the Bagnoli 4

(Delsys Inc., Boston, MA) bioamplifier. All signals were sent to a 16-bit A/D converter (BNC-2110, National Instruments) and sampled at 2048 Hz using a computer-based oscillograph and data acquisition system (DASYLab, DASYTEC National Instruments, Amherst, NH). Tracings of the 10 highest contractions were used to determine EMG amplitude, EMD, and Q_{30}, as well as EMG during the peak rate of force development (Q_{pk}).

Results and discussion

In absolute terms, men were significantly stronger than boys in both flexion (67.2 ± 11.0 vs 19.5 ± 5.7 Nm, respectively) and extension (54.3 ± 10.2 vs 18.4 ± 5.7 Nm, respectively), as expected. This could theoretically be explained by age-dependent differences in muscle size, muscle activation properties, or muscle composition. To date, muscle composition is believed to be determined sometime after birth and does not appear to differ between boys and men. Therefore, we examined muscle size and activation as possible explanatory factors of differences in muscle strength. When peak torque was normalized to upper-arm CSA, men remained significantly stronger than boys in flexion, with no difference in extension (Figure 55.1). When normalized to agonist EMG activity, peak torque was significantly higher in men during flexion with a trend towards greater strength during extension (Figure 55.2). Therefore, although the differences between groups were minimized when the data were normalized for size or for electrical activity, men were able to produce more force than children. Thus, both muscle size and muscle activation at least partly explained the lower force production in boys.

Men exhibited a more rapid rate of force development compared with boys in both flexion (646 ± 162 vs 132 ± 53 N·m s^{-1}, respectively) and extension (434 ± 123 vs 106 ± 36 N·m s^{-1}, respectively). Figure 55.3 depicts the rate of force development normalized to peak torque, which remained significantly faster in men during flexion, and a similar trend during extension. Men also maintained

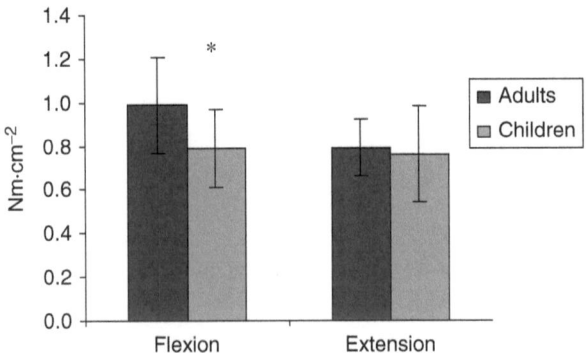

Figure 55.1 Peak torque corrected for upper arm CSA – *p < 0.05.

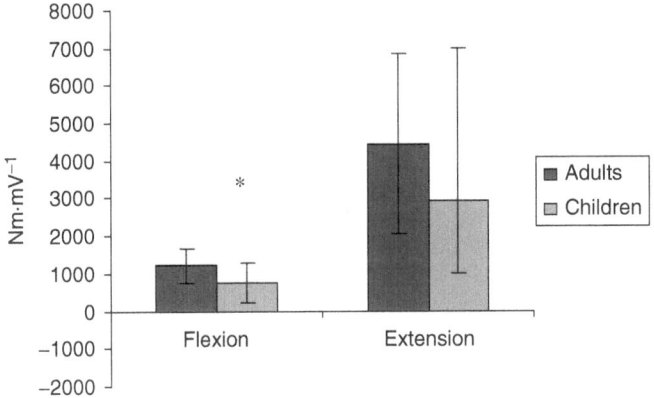

Figure 55.2 Peak torque relative to agonist EMG activity – *p < 0.05.

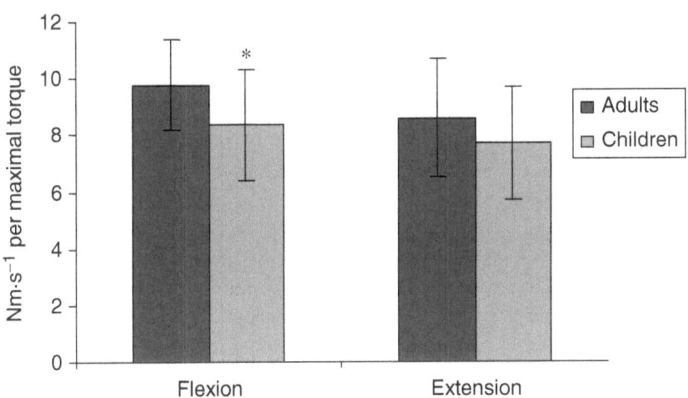

Figure 55.3 Rate of force development per peak torque – *p < 0.05.

a significantly greater rate of force development when data were normalized to agonist muscle activation (Qpk) (Figure 55.4). Therefore, although the differences between groups were minimized when the data were normalized, children had a lower rate of force development compared with men.

During both flexion and extension men exhibited a significantly shorter agonist EMD than boys (flexion: 47.5 ± 17.6 vs 75.5 ± 28.2 ms, respectively; extension: 37.7 ± 13.1 vs 66.3 ± 31.8 ms, respectively). That is, boys needed to activate their agonist groups for a longer period of time before force development occurred. The agonist/antagonist ratio was not significantly different between groups, reflecting no difference in co-contraction between boys and men.

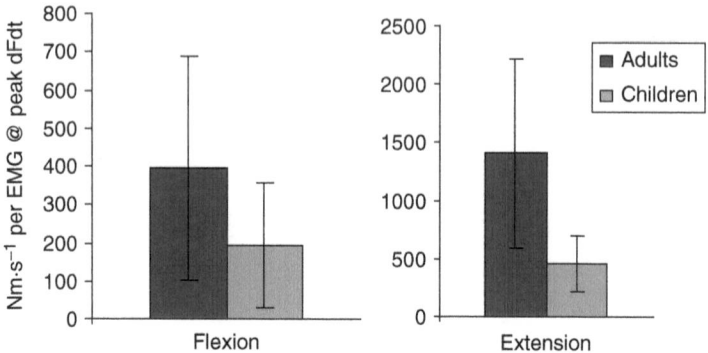

Figure 55.4 Rate of force development relative to agonist EMG activity – *$p < 0.05$.

In summary, children exhibited lower muscle force and rate of force development in absolute terms, relative to muscle size (upper-arm CSA), and relative to EMG activity. In view of the longer EMD in boys, children may be less able to recruit their higher threshold motor units compared with men, resulting in a lower maximal force and lower rate of force development.

References

Asmussen, E., 1973, Growth in muscular strength and power. In: *Physical Activity, Human Growth and Development*, edited by Rarick, G. London: Academic Press, pp. 60–79.

Blimkie, C.J.R., 1989, Age- and sex-associated variation in strength during childhood: Anthropometric, morphologic, neurologic, biomechanical, endocrinologic, genetic, and physical activity correlates. In: *Perspectives in Exercise Science and Sports Medicine, Vol. 2: Youth, Exercise and Sport*, edited by Gisolfi, C.V. Indianapolis, IN: Benchmark Press, pp. 99–163.

Durnin, J.V. and Womersley, J., 1974, Body fat assessed from total body density and its estimation from skinfold thickness: Measurements on 481 men and women aged from 16 to 72 years. *British Journal of Nutrition*, **32**, pp. 77–97.

Falk, B., Portal, S., Tiktinsky, R., Weinstein, Y., Constantini, N. and Martinowitz, U., 2000, Anaerobic power and muscle strength in young hemophilia patients. *Medicine and Science in Sports and Exercise*, **32**, pp. 52–57.

Falk, B., Portal, S., Tiktinsky, R., Zigel, L., Weinstein, Y., Constantini, N., Kenet, G., Eliakim, A. and Martinowitz, U., 2005, Bone properties and muscle strength of young hemophilia patients. *Haemophilia Journal*, **11**, pp. 380–386.

Gabriel, D.A. and Boucher, J.P., 2000, Practicing a maximal performance task: A cooperative strategy for muscle activity. *Research Quarterly in Exercise and Sport*, **71**, pp. 217–228.

Gurney, J.M., Jelliffe, D.B., 1973, Arm anthropometry in nutritional assessment: Nomogram for rapid calculation of muscle circumference and cross-sectional muscle and fat areas. *American Journal of Clinical Nutrition*, **26**, pp. 912–915.

Sale, D.G. and Spriet, L.L., 1996, Skeletal muscle function and energy metabolism. In: *Exercise and the Female – A Life Span Approach. Perspectives in Exercise Science and Sports Medicine*, Vol. 19, edited by Bar-Or, O., Lamb, D.R. and Clarkson, P.M. Carmel, IN: Cooper Publishing Group, pp. 289–359.

Slaughter, M.H., Lohman, T.G., Boileau, R.A., Horswill, C.A., Stillman, R.J., Van Loan, M.D. and Bemben, D.A., 1988, Skinfold equations for estimation of body fatness in children and youth. *Human Biology*, **60**, pp. 709–723.

Index